To True Love

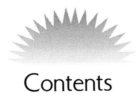

Contents

Healing HIV

HOW TO REBUILD YOUR IMMUNE SYSTEM

Jon D. Kaiser, M.D.

To order additional copies of this publication call:
888-HEAL-HIV
(888-432-5448)
volume discounts available

HEALTHFIRST PRESS
Mill Valley, California

HealthFirst Press
775 East Blithedale, Suite #367
Mill Valley, CA 94941
www.jonkaiser.com

Copyright © 1999 Jon D. Kaiser, M.D.
Cover design by Ray Lobato, RayDesign
Book design by Ray Lobato, RayDesign
Edited by Nancy Grimley Carleton
Additional editing by Jill Jarvie, R.D.

To place your name on Dr. Jon Kaiser's confidential mailing list and receive his free newsletter *Taking Charge,* send your name and address to HealthFirst Press at the address listed above.

The Library of Congress has catalogued the hardcover edition as follows:

Kaiser, Jon D.
    Healing HIV : how to rebuild your immune system / Jon D. Kaiser.
        p.   cm.
    Includes bibliogrphical references and index.
    1. HIV infections – Immunological aspects.   2. AIDS (Disease) –
Immunological aspects.   3. HIV infections – Treatment.   4. AIDS
(Disease) – Treatment.   5. AIDS (Disease) – Alternative treatment.
    6. Immune system.   I. Title.
    RC607.A26K3485   1999
    616.97'9206--dc21   98-35964
                                                                CIP

ISBN 0-9666373-0-5
Printed in the United States of America

Contents

Author's Note

A ll statements contained in this book are based on the experiences and observations of the author. They are meant to provide information to educate patients and their health-care providers on how to integrate alternative and standard medical therapies in the treatment of HIV and other immune system disorders. The natural therapy and emotional healing aspects of this program are designed to be an adjunct to, not a substitute for, conventional medical therapy.

No treatment program, whether alternative, conventional, or a combination of the two, is effective for everyone. Some people may become worse despite any treatment or lifestyle changes. The goal of this book is to provide a program that will help many people improve the status of their health and significantly delay the progression of their HIV infection. It is extremely important that you consult with your doctor before making any changes to your medical program.

Preface

Some 5 years ago, my first book on the treatment of HIV (*Immune Power*, St. Martin's Press, 1993) proposed a highly compelling, commonsense approach to the treatment of HIV disease. The main focus of the book was to teach individuals how to combine natural and standard medical therapies, while maximizing the immune-strengthening benefits of both.

When deciding how to update *Immune Power*, I had 2 choices. I could go through the book page by page and rewrite it entirely. That was clearly unnecessary; much of the information it contained was still valid. Or I could choose to write a sequel to the initial edition, one that contains the newest and most useful advances to my program, plus the essential elements brought forth from my previous book.

One of the main reasons I chose to write this sequel, *Healing HIV: How to Rebuild Your Immune System*, is to serve the thousands of individuals who are in dire need of its message. This book is designed to help HIV(+) individuals *use the least amount of medication possible*, while at the same time helping ensure that the medications that are used work better, last longer, and are better tolerated by the body.

Since the publication of *Immune Power*, the use of natural therapies to support the immune system, as well as standard medical therapies to suppress viral activity, has benefited thousands of HIV(+) individuals. I experience pride and gratitude as many of my patients continue to enjoy good health and stability despite being HIV(+) for upwards of 18 years!

In fact, many of my patients feel that HIV's presence in their lives has produced a healing and joy they never before thought possible. I am humbled whenever a patient shares these feelings because I know how much courage and hard work it takes to reach this point. Learning how to love yourself through good diet, stress reduction, emotional healing, and spiritual growth requires an enormous commitment. These lifestyle adjustments bring forth more than just physical rewards. They tap into a source of love and caring that may have been hidden previously. They can also stimulate tremendous growth in one's life.

During the past several years, I have received many calls and letters testifying to the success of my program. Patients often describe, in great detail, both stabilization and significant improvement in their health and immune system strength. The wife of one HIV(+) prison inmate described how all of his HIV-related symptoms, as well as most of his chronic health problems in general, disappeared at the same time he experienced a tripling of his CD4 count. Instituting the Healing HIV program was the only change he made. Another individual wrote to me stating that his CD4 count, after steadily declining during the past 4 years, went from 234 to over 1000 cells/mm3 without his implementing any changes other than beginning my program.

Of course, the above accounts are anecdotal. My ability to perform clinical trials and collect research data has been somewhat limited during the past few years due to the tremendous growth and change my practice has experienced. However, I have recently conducted a controlled, retrospective analysis of my private practice's patient population. As you will see in Chapter 4, the results of this analysis are extremely positive. They clearly demonstrate that successful outcomes using less antiviral medication are entirely possible. I am also preparing the results of this analysis for submission to a peer-reviewed journal.

Many doctors have also called during this time to express encouragement and thanks for such a reasonable and commonsense approach to HIV patient care. Although physicians who are skilled at both standard and complementary medicine are hard to find, I urge you to keep looking. At the very least, try to find a caring physician who is technically skilled at treating HIV and who also maintains an open mind toward natural therapies. As with everything else, persistence will pay off.

Though the majority of my HIV(+) patients continue to remain healthy and stable, many friends and loved ones have unfortunately passed on. This fact only drives me to work harder, and commit further, to discovering treatments that are safer, more effective, and better able to provide good health and longevity to all HIV(+) individuals throughout the world.

In summary, I intend for this book to make available to the public continued improvements in the Healing HIV program as well as to document its continued record of success. I urge all who would like to share their individual healing stories to write to me at the address listed below. Your examples can serve as guiding lights to the many souls who may also be searching for their path to healing HIV. I also encourage any physicians who are supportive of my work and general philosophy to contact me. I maintain a nationwide referral list of supportive practitioners, and I would be very pleased to see it grow.

Jon D. Kaiser, M.D.
c/o HealthFirst Press
775 East Blithedale, Suite #367
Mill Valley, CA 94941

Acknowledgments

No one publishes a book by themselves. No one is successful in life without the help of countless others. For their assistance in bringing this book to fruition, I would like to thank the following individuals.

My deep gratitude goes to publishers Hal and Linda Kramer for their generous help, without which I could not have identified the resources to publish this book on my own. The entire process continues to be a learning experience, and I can't imagine having done it without their assistance. They are warm, sensitive, and caring people, and the books they publish at HJ Kramer Inc make this planet a better place.

I would also like to thank their daughter, Jan Phillips, who skillfully guided me through the challenging waters of ISBN numbers, Cataloging-in-Publication Data, bar codes, and other technological tidbits that only those in the field of publishing are painfully aware of.

There were 2 editors who worked with me on this book. The first, Nancy Grimley Carleton, is a true professional who, early in the evolution of this project, committed to helping me publish it on an unusually tight time line. She is directly responsible for it being a clear and readable book.

My second editor, Jill Jarvie, supported and nurtured this book and its author every step along the way. She is my friend, colleague, and life partner, and I could not have completed this project without her. She is also the only person who truly knows how hard I worked to get this book into your hands. Thank you, Sweetie!

I would also like to thank my friend and business associate Bill Rosen; my friend and business associate Joe Robinson; Donald Abrams, M.D.; Robert Neger, M.D.; Martin Mass, M.D.; and the members and staff of The Community Consortium of S.F. Bay Area HIV Treatment Providers. They are all hard-working professionals who have dedicated their lives to helping people with HIV live longer, healthier, and more productive life spans.

Next, I would like to thank several additional individuals who have contributed their help along the way: My friend and colleague Peggy Flynn and the members of my HIV support group: You all know how deeply in my heart you reside. Allen Reubin, M.D., an infectious disease specialist in Dallas, Texas, who has been an ardent supporter of my work for over 5 years. He also contributed significantly to Appendix 3 and Appendix 11. I am grateful to him for his continued support. Richard Bowman Pierce, Ph.D., has done extensive work highlighting the ways in which intestinal parasites cause stress to the immune system of chronically ill patients. Corresponding with him helped me immensely as chapters 7 and 8 took form. I am very grateful to Ben Cheng of Project Inform for providing early research for several of the chapters. He is a dedicated individual and excellent medical writer. Gary Wolf, R.N., reminded me that I needed to produce hard data to support my claims, which stimulated me to write Chapter 4. Vincent Fisher, Alison Schwarz, Donna Palmer, Linda Bornholdt, Sandy Rizzari, and Jennifer Clarke provided invaluable support along the way, as well as important bits of information on short notice as my "no longer changeable" deadline rapidly approached. Thanks also to Ray Lobato for his ability to convert ideas in my head into delightful images on the printed page. And finally to Patricia Davis, Greg Monardo, Lee Liskey, M.D., Virginia Cafaro, M.D., Lisa Lewis, M.D., Gordon Sanford, P.A.-C., Ray Mirra, and Marcus Conant, M.D., who all contributed in one way or another to my being where I am today. I thank you all!

The staff of The Jon Kaiser Wellness Center also deserve special mention. In my opinion, they are the most talented and dedicated team of health-care professionals I could possibly be associated with. Pramela Reddi is the clinic's very capable and dedicated administrator who helps me care for its staff and clients; Monica Markiewicz, Lynne Anne Miles, and James Auwae make up our massage and physical therapy department; Sheila Pyatt provides our clients with a rare and gentle type of warm water massage known as Watsu. Buck Ellis, our senior medical assistant, worked especially hard with me to collect and organize the Healing HIV research data; his efforts made a huge difference in helping Chapter 4 to mature. K. C. Esfandiary is the best new patient coordinator I could ever imagine; Gelila Gizaw, is our newest medical assistant; and Jill Jarvie, R.D., our dietitian, provides The Wellness Center's clients with nurturing advice and is an award-winning author in her own right. Martin Kramer, P.A.-C., is the best holistic/integrative medicine P.A. I know; Pat Sanders and Kate Black are our 2 excellent nurse practitioners and licensed acupuncturists who provide our clients with their invaluable talent and expertise. Denis Bouvier, D.O., is our seasoned and experienced hospital specialist; and finally, our staff wouldn't be complete without Jason Tokumoto, M.D., a sensitive, wise, and powerful soul who joined our staff at just the right time to allow me to finish this book. You all have my greatest appreciation, gratitude, and respect.

I would also like to mention a few additional individuals whose talent, bravery, persistence of vision, patience, and ability to get the job done I greatly admire: Albert Einstein, Steven Jobs, Michael Jordan, Dean Ornish, Michelangelo Buonarroti, Mohandas K. Gandhi, the Rev. Martin Luther King, Jr., and his Holiness, The Dali Lama.

And finally to my patients, whose passion for living and dedication to healing provides me with a continual source of inspiration. Their ongoing good health is my greatest reward!

— Jon D. Kaiser, M.D.
Fall 1998

Chapter One

Introduction

The light at the end of the tunnel has finally appeared. After years of wandering in the dark and searching for ways to prevent the progression of HIV to AIDS, we are now able to treat this condition better than ever before. During what felt like an eternity, we fumbled with coarse and imprecise tools such as AZT monotherapy, beta-2 microglobulin tests, and p24 antigen levels. We even entered into a discussions as to whether or not HIV was actually the cause of AIDS. Now, due to aggressive research and new technologies, we are on the verge of being able to strengthen and rebuild our patients' immune systems despite their having declined to previously irretrievable levels. At last, many HIV(+) individuals can now hope to be alive for what amounts to a normal life span.

Though long-term stability in my patients has always been the rule, I can now definitely say that the progression of HIV disease in my practice is an extremely rare event. My experience, which has encompassed the care of over 1000 HIV(+) patients during the past 10 years, allows me to make the following statements:

- Not 1 patient who has come to me during the past 4 years with a CD4 count of greater than 300 cells/mm3 has progressed to below that level.
- Not 1 patient who has come to me during the past 4 years with a CD4 count of greater than 50 cells/mm3 has become seriously ill or died from an HIV-related illness.

This extraordinary level of good health and stability is the result of hard work. My patients follow an aggressive program of natural therapies to support their immune systems. They have also benefited tremendously from new drugs, lab tests, and other recently released treatment options. What a difference a few years has made!

Some 10 years ago, when I opened my private practice, I believed that a comprehensive approach to the treatment of HIV would be more effective at preventing its progression than the limited medical treatment then being prescribed. Some 5 years later, when my book *Immune Power* was released, I revealed how a combination treatment approach helped hundreds of patients achieve a level of good health and stability far exceeding the community standard. Since there weren't many effective antiviral medications available at the time, many looked toward alternative therapies as an important way to help them remain healthy and survive.

Fortunately, we now have protease inhibitors, NNRTIs, and many other highly effective antivirals with which to treat HIV. These therapies have helped thousands of patients outlive earlier predictions. However, these drugs have not worked for everyone. Many HIV(+) individuals are unable to tolerate their side effects or, even worse, have become resistant to all of the currently available medications. Individuals who find themselves in this situation need additional treatment options. The comprehensive treatment program described in this book can help most people living with HIV create a strategy that can enable them to live out normal, healthy lives, far beyond what otherwise might be expected.

I define a comprehensive approach as one which adds a program of *aggressive natural therapies* and *emotional healing techniques* to the standard medical treatment of an illness or condition. An aggressive natural therapies program includes a combination of diet therapy, vitamins, herbs, exercise, and stress reduction. Emotional healing encompasses a proactive program of psychological healing techniques that ideally includes a spiritually oriented practice (prayer, meditation, yoga, etc.), combined with a significant level of social support.

In theory, adding a program of natural therapies to the best that standard medical therapy has to offer invariably improves the results far beyond what would have been achieved utilizing either approach alone. Until modern medicine places greater emphasis on the use of nutrition, vitamins, stress reduction, and other natural healing techniques as part of its recommended treatment, it will always fall short of achieving the best possible results. This book is designed to help both patients and practitioners integrate the 2 approaches.

"Healing" HIV

Some people equate the term *healing* with *cure*. *Cure* is a final achievement which comes from the outside. *Healing* is a dynamic process that occurs within the individual. It is achieved when you go from your present level of health to one that is higher and more stable. It is an ongoing process. With this definition in mind, I can truly say that the vast majority of my patients have healed, and continue to heal, from HIV.

Some of my patients have experienced significant increases in their CD4 counts. Others have achieved undetectable viral loads on fewer than 3 antiviral medications. Still others have completely eliminated chronic symptoms such as fatigue, diarrhea, neuropathy, chronic pain, and lifelong depression. Others possess a state of balance and strength they previously had thought unachievable: Their stories set an example for how to bring forth true healing from HIV.

Healing can also be defined as a growth experience — a process of becoming whole through the integration of body, mind, and spirit. Over the years, many of my HIV(+) patients have grown and blossomed into extremely healthy and happy individuals. As long as their growth continues, I know they will remain healthy.

As I write about healing from HIV, I sometimes wonder whether some of my patients have healed *from* HIV, or were healed *by* HIV. I know this sounds like a radical statement. However, if HIV had never made its way into their lives, many of the changes these patients have made in response to its presence might never have occurred. These changes have included improving their diet, reducing stress, abstaining from drugs, exercising regularly, and embarking upon a path of emotional healing and growth. HIV has stimulated these changes, not only in the patients I directly care for, but in thousands of individuals I have spoken to across the country during the past several years.

I have written this book as a guide for HIV(+) individuals to strengthen and stabilize their health. If you are making progress in this direction that is strong, significant, and sustained, you, too, are healing from HIV. May your journey be filled with growth, joy, and unconditional love.

Chapter Two

What Has Changed?

Before describing the specifics of my program, I believe it is important to review the many changes which have occurred in the HIV treatment landscape over the past several years. I have also included several patient stories, or case histories, in this chapter as well as throughout the book. These stories describe many of the treatment interventions I commonly use.

Viral Dormancy

The belief that HIV lies dormant during an initial latency period has for all practical purposes been debunked. Instead, there appears to be a dynamic equilibrium which occurs between viral replication and the body's immune system. Despite HIV producing up to 10 billion viral particles per day, the body can often maintain stability for long periods of time. Even without antiviral therapy, the majority of HIV-infected individuals do not develop symptoms for upwards of 10 years. Supporting the body with good nutrition and aggressive stress reduction in the midst of this ongoing battle is vitally important.

Since there are now more than a dozen effective drugs to treat HIV, it is easy to become less focused on the importance of diet and natural therapies. One long-term patient of mine, Kenny, began to experience this situation. Kenny was able to remain healthy and stable for several years despite a CD4 count of less than 150 cells/mm3 (normal range:

greater than 400 cells/mm3). With his CD4 count now approaching 400, he finds that he is less motivated to exercise and eat healthfully. Unfortunately, Kenny only has a few antiviral medications left before he runs out of drug treatment options due to resistance. Following an aggressive natural therapies program can help ensure that the efficacy of the medications Kenny is currently taking will last as long as possible. After a thorough discussion regarding the importance of these factors, Kenny once again became committed to following a healthy diet and lifestyle.

I'd like to present to you an important analogy. Envision your body as a race car in the Indy 500. Your vehicle requires high-quality fuel (optimal nutrition), special additives (vitamin supplements), and special care (effective stress management) to last the duration of the race and have a good chance of winning. Optimal nutrition, vitamin supplements, and effective stress management are the keys to living a long and healthy life with HIV.

As we all know, medications are often necessary to treat HIV effectively. But they need to be managed *skillfully* for optimal results. Deciding when to add an antiviral medication to your program, or when to change your combination of drugs, may be one of the most important decisions you make. Mixing and matching the right combination of drugs to provide you with a safe and effective antiviral program has become as much an art as a science. Accomplishing this goal requires knowledge, patience, and creativity. Empowering you, the reader, with this knowledge is the primary goal of this book.

Listed below are several important factors to be taken into account before intervening with drugs to treat HIV:

1) What is your CD4 count?

2) How high is your viral load?

3) Is there a positive or negative trend to your CD4 count during the past 6 to 12 months?

4) Do you have any HIV-related symptoms such as fevers, night sweats, fatigue, or thrush?

5) How sensitive are you in general to medication side effects?

6) Are you interested in being conservative or aggressive with antiviral medications?

These factors need to be taken into account before making medication decisions. Your doctor does not always have the time, or know you well enough, to make the best decisions for you. It is up to you and your doctor to make these decisions *together*. This is why it is important to become fully knowledgeable regarding how to use antiviral medications.

When you finish reading chapters 3, 5, and 6, you will be better equipped to participate in making these decisions. But please remember one thing. Though I initially favor following an aggressive natural therapies program to treat HIV, if complete stability cannot be maintained solely by natural means, it is wise to include antiviral medications as part of your program.

Antiviral Medications

When *Immune Power* was released, there were 3 antiviral medications available. Now there are more than 12. More important, several recently released drugs (saquinavir, ritonavir, indinavir, and nelfinavir) are part of a new class of antiviral compounds called protease inhibitors. Protease inhibitors are among the strongest antiviral treatments yet discovered. They inhibit the ability of HIV to assemble new particles. Protease inhibitors, in combination with reverse transcriptase inhibitors such as AZT, DDI, 3TC, D4T, and DDC, and NNRTIs (non-nucleoside reverse transcriptase inhibitors) including nevirapine, delavirdine, and efavirenz, can completely suppress HIV activity in the majority of cases. Access to these medications has finally given HIV(+) individuals a wide range of effective treatment options.

Another recent change in the way we treat HIV is that the use of a single antiviral medication to treat HIV (monotherapy) has become a thing of the past. Recent studies have conclusively shown that, due to the emergence of resistant viral strains, viral activity is less suppressed, and for shorter periods of time, if only 1 antiviral is used. Utilizing antiviral combination therapy, with 2, 3, and sometimes even 4 antiviral medications, has now become the standard of care.

Protease inhibitors, though highly effective at suppressing HIV activity, often come with significant side effects. Members of this antiviral class can cause liver inflammation, kidney stones, nausea, diarrhea, lipodystrophy, and even diabetes. Furthermore, they can also increase the blood levels of other medications and prohibit the use of some completely. They should not be used cavalierly.

This caveat aside, the emergence of the protease-inhibitor class of drugs now gives us better options for suppressing HIV activity than we have ever had in the past. Accordingly, mild side effects may be a small price to pay for the ability to stabilize and even improve a previously deteriorating situation. The full complement of currently available antiviral medications will be discussed in detail in Chapter 5.

Judy

Judy is a 35-year-old administrative assistant who tested HIV(+) in the mid-1980s. Her initial CD4 count was approximately 700 cells/mm3. At our first meeting in 1995, she told me of her frequent oral and genital herpes outbreaks and loose bowel movements. By that time, her CD4 count had declined to 243 cells/mm3 and her viral load was 22,000 copies/ml.

Judy was very fearful of taking antiviral medications. Instead, she chose to follow an aggressive natural therapies program that included a vegetarian diet, vitamin supplements, and Chinese herbal therapy. By utilizing natural therapies, Judy hoped the need to take antiviral medications could be avoided.

Since Judy's CD4 count had declined significantly during the past several years, I recommended that she not wait any longer to begin antiviral therapy. We chose to start with a combination of D4T/3TC (2 drugs known as reverse transcriptase inhibitors). Judy requested that the D4T be started at the lowest possible dosage, so I prescribed it at 15 mg 2x/day. I also recommended that Judy go on chronic suppressive therapy for her herpes infection with acyclovir 400 mg 2x/day. This would help remove a source of ongoing stress to her immune system. In addition, I started her on 50 mg 1x/day of DHEA (dehydroepiandrosterone, a natural hormone) due to a suboptimal blood level (see Chapter 11 for more information on DHEA supplementation).

I also ordered a comprehensive stool analysis, which showed an excessive growth of 3 yeast species. These were treated with a combination of herbs and a 2-week course of a prescription medication called Nystatin.

During the next several months Judy's viral load progressively declined and her CD4 count began to increase, both good signs. I also convinced her to increase the D4T dosage to 30 mg 2x/day, which was well tolerated. By November 1996, Judy's CD4 count had risen to 332 cells/mm3 and her viral load had become undetectable.

At this time, Judy was still experiencing chronic herpes outbreaks, so I recommended that she switch from acyclovir to valacyclovir 500 mg 2x/day, which is a more potent and effective herpes medication. Some 6 months after the above interventions eradicated the yeast in her intestinal tract and suppressed her herpes outbreaks, Judy's CD4 count climbed again to 518 cells/mm3 with an undetectable viral load while still only taking 2 antivirals.

Judy's story provides an example of how a comprehensive approach to the treatment of HIV can produce highly significant improvement in CD4 counts, viral load values, and quality of life. Judy no longer has any digestive complaints, her energy level is outstanding, and her herpes outbreaks are greatly diminished.

Judy's immune system is clearly stronger now than it has been in a very long time. It is noteworthy to mention that we were able to accomplish all of these results on only 2 antiviral medications due to her aggressive natural therapies program. This has allowed us to save protease inhibitors, as well as NNRTIs (another useful class of antivirals), for use in the future when they may be more beneficial and necessary.

Important Lab Tests

1995 brought the widespread availability of a new, more effective way to track HIV activity known as the viral load assay. This lab test is able to detect, with great accuracy, the number of viral particles present in the bloodstream at any given time. The 2 competing technologies for measuring viral loads, called PCR and branched chain DNA, are similar in cost and accuracy. Also available now are tests to help determine which antiviral drugs your particular strain of HIV has become resistant to. These tests, known as genotypic and phenotypic resistance tests, are available but still considered experimental.

During the past several years, several other lab tests have also become available which are helpful in monitoring the health of HIV(+) individuals. These include tests which measure hormone levels such as testosterone, DHEA, and erythropoietin, as well as the use of comprehensive stool analysis tests which measure the amount of healthful and unhealthful bacteria in the colon. The individual pros and cons associated with each of these tests are discussed in detail in Appendix 2.

Preventing and Treating Kaposi's Sarcoma

Kaposi's sarcoma used to be the second most common AIDS-defining illness. During the late 1980s, thousands of HIV(+) individuals were affected by its potentially life-threatening lesions. Fortunately, the incidence of KS has been declining steadily. This decline is partly attributable to the ability of antiviral treatments to keep HIV activity suppressed to very low levels.

For those patients still dealing with active KS, the availability of liposomal KS chemotherapy (Daunoxome and DOXSL) has greatly improved KS treatment in efficacy and tolerability. These intravenous medications need be delivered only once every 2 to 3 weeks and cause fewer side effects than older regimens. Currently, Daunoxome is approved for the first-line treatment of advanced KS, while DOXSL is approved for use in cases that are unresponsive to other therapies.

Finally, new research into the etiology of KS has revealed the presence of a virus known as KS herpes virus (KSHV). This virus is virtually always present in individuals who have KS. It is also believed to be sexually transmitted. Though additional research is still necessary, this discovery may help further the development of additional KS treatments and make possible effective prophylactic treatments to prevent its occurrence.

Preventing and Treating Fatigue

Your immune system is the most sensitive system of your body to your energy level. When you are tired, your eyes do not shut down, your heart does not stop beating, and your muscles do not stop moving. Your immune system, however, can become depressed.

Evolutionarily speaking, it makes sense that the immune system is the first system of the body to go off-line in times of acute stress. If you were being chased by a saber-toothed tiger or engaged in a fierce battle, your body would appropriately divert all of its energy toward surviving the immediate event. In such situations, the sympathetic nervous system, which controls the heart, lungs, and muscles, predominates. Parasympathetically mediated systems, such as the immune and digestive systems, are therefore temporarily put on hold. If you survived the initial trauma, these systems would come back on-line and help you heal as you rested.

In modern life, chronic stress predominates. Many of us work 12-hour days and are often at the mercy of minds which do not turn off easily. Although at times we may feel fatigued, we still often push ourselves beyond healthful limits. Those of us who do not have HIV in our bodies may eventually catch a cold, get the flu, or possibly even develop high blood pressure. Those living with HIV however, can progressively lose CD4 cells and eventually become seriously ill.

Fatigue is best viewed as your body's first attempt to send you an important message. It may be that your viral load is too high. It may be that your hormones are out of balance. Other causes include an exercise program that is too rigorous, an infection with intestinal parasites, a case of anemia, or the presence of psychological depression. Listening to your body's early warning signs can help you avoid the emergence of stronger messages later on. Discuss the presence of fatigue with your doctor. Let him or her know how much it is bothering you. By intervening early to correct fatigue (being proactive), you can maximize your chances of remaining in balance and staying healthy. A 6-part approach to the prevention and treatment of fatigue is presented in Chapter 12.

Bob

Bob began his initial visit by saying, "I've heard all the good news about protease inhibitors, so I guess it's about time for me to start taking triple-combination therapy." Bob's CD4 count had gradually been declining during the past few years and was now 467 cells/mm3, with a viral load of 25,000 copies/ml. Despite remaining healthy during the past 10 years without using antiviral drugs, Bob had mentally prepared himself to begin taking them starting today.

After a thorough review of Bob's situation, I was not sure I agreed that now was the right time for him to begin taking these medications. Based on his initial lab work, there were several things I suggested he try before resorting to drugs. These included correcting his suboptimal DHEA level by taking DHEA 100 mg 1x/day, adding acyclovir 400 mg 2x/day to suppress any occult herpes activity, and treating the 3 intestinal parasites that we discovered on his comprehensive stool analysis. These treatment interventions were not felt to be "important" by his regular treating physician.

Some 4 months after initiating these changes, Bob returned to my office for his follow-up visit. "I am feeling better now than I ever have," he stated. "I am curious to see what my lab work shows." When I told Bob that his viral load had declined from 28,000 to 7,000 copies/ml and his CD4 count had risen from 467 to 546 cells/mm3, he began to beam with pride and satisfaction. "Well, I guess I didn't need to start taking antiviral medications yet. I'd like to stay off them a while longer if possible." I told Bob that eradicating intestinal parasites, raising his hormone levels into the optimal range, and starting daily acyclovir therapy had given his immune system the boost it needed to decrease his viral load to below 10,000 copies/ml and raise his CD4 count back over 500 cells/mm3.

Some 6 months later, Bob returned for his next follow-up visit to find that his CD4 count had again risen to greater than 600 cells/mm3! His viral load also continued to remain stable at below 10,000 copies/ml. Not surprisingly, he still felt great.

The strategy of eliminating cofactors that can stimulate viral activity (i.e., stress, herpes infections, intestinal parasites) can help the immune system to remain strong and healthy. It can also keep HIV activity suppressed without the need for antiviral drugs for as long as possible.

If at any point Bob experiences a decline in his CD4 count or a rise in his viral load that cannot be corrected by eliminating cofactors, we will add antiviral medications to the program. This stepwise approach is the most intelligent, cost-effective, and healthful way to treat HIV. By supporting Bob's immune system naturally, and only adding antiviral medication if there are signs of instability, important therapies can be saved for later, when their use may be more beneficial and necessary.

Maintaining Optimal Intestinal Health

Our gastrointestinal system is responsible for the digestion of food, absorption of nutrients, and excretion of waste products. To efficiently perform these functions, our body needs help. Most people don't realize that our colons are colonized by 10 billion bacterial organisms that symbiotically assist us in accomplishing these functions. It is imperative that this large number of bacteria be our friends and not our enemies.

There are many factors that can alter the balance of intestinal bacteria from friendly to unfriendly. These include poor eating habits, overconsumption of alcohol, a sedentary lifestyle, and the frequent use of antibiotics, just to name a few.

By implementing proper dietary habits, supplementing your diet with beneficial bacteria, and intervening *early* if any signs of a digestive system imbalance occur, the health of your gastrointestinal tract can remain strong and vital. Specific details on how to achieve these goals, as well as where to obtain testing to measure the levels of healthful and unhealthful intestinal organisms, are covered in detail in chapters 7 and 8.

Body Cell Mass and the Immune System

Wasting syndrome is defined as the loss of at least 10% of normal body weight which cannot be attributed to the presence of a known infection (other than HIV).

In my experience, wasting syndrome is entirely preventable. This statement is based upon the experience I've accumulated treating over 1000 HIV(+) patients during the past decade. During this time, not 1 patient who has come to me with a normal weight has developed wasting syndrome. Furthermore, I have been extremely successful in helping to reverse wasting syndrome in many patients who have come to me with this condition already present.

New technology in the field of body composition testing has greatly improved our ability to identify and prevent wasting syndrome. Muscle tissue, due to its high metabolic rate, produces abundant energy. This energy-producing component of your body is referred to as your *body cell mass.* The use of BIA testing (bioelectric impedance analysis) enables a health-care practitioner to objectively measure and follow the amount of muscle mass present on your body.

Recent studies have also shown that maintaining your body cell mass as close to ideal as possible is as important a predictor of long-term survival as maintaining a high CD4 cell count or a low viral load. Keeping all 3 of these parameters in the most healthful range will ensure that your HIV condition remains stable and does not progress.

If your body cell mass is found to be less than optimal, it can be improved utilizing techniques which enhance appetite, maximize nutrient consumption, raise hormone levels, and maximize the benefits of progressive resistance exercise. A program to teach you how to maximize your body cell mass is presented in chapters 9 and 10. If you institute this program early, you can drastically reduce the possibility of ever developing wasting syndrome.

Casey

Casey first came to my clinic in June 1996 after several months of treating what was thought to be a rectal abscess. Unfortunately, this condition was eventually diagnosed to be rectal cancer.

At that time, Casey had a CD4 count of 0 cells/mm3 and a viral load of 220,000 copies/ml. The presence of cancer along with the absence of CD4 cells gave him a pretty dismal prognosis. Casey's cancer was initially treated locally by removing the 3-inch tumor. Luckily, it did not extend into the surrounding tissue and no further therapy was required at that time.

Casey had been taking the antivirals AZT/3TC/saquinavir with little apparent benefit. He clearly needed to strengthen his immune system quickly before any additional cancers or infections took advantage of his weakened state.

My first conversation with Casey included a pep talk to help keep his hope alive and spirit strong. He needed to have faith that he could improve his situation and regain his health. If he was depressed and despondent, his immune system would not fight as hard as it otherwise could. Fortunately, this was not a problem. Casey displayed a strong spirit and a positive drive to overcome his present set of circumstances.

Since Casey's CD4 count was 0 and his viral load was exceedingly high, I suggested a change in his antiviral program from AZT/3TC/saquinavir to D4T/3TC/indinavir. This is an extremely potent and well-tolerated antiviral combination. Within 1 month of starting this regime, Casey's CD4 count rose from 0 to 65 cells/mm3 and his viral load declined from 220,000 to 1085 copies/ml. His surgical site where the cancer was removed was healing well, and his bowel movements and energy level were returning to normal.

Further lab evaluation revealed suboptimal hormone levels, so I recommended Casey start supplements of DHEA and testosterone (see Chapter 11). He also began meeting with our clinic's dietitian, who advised him to increase his protein intake and begin a program of resistance exercise 3x/week as tolerated.

In December 1996, despite an undetectable viral load and a CD4 count that was continuing to rise, Casey's rectal cancer was found to have metastasized to his colon. He was quickly scheduled to have a large part of his colon removed. In my meeting with Casey prior to his surgery, I suggested that he visualize that his body had placed all of its toxins and negative substances into the tumor. The goal of the surgical procedure was therefore to remove every bit of negative physical and emotional energy from his body so he could become lighter and healthier. This technique is called *visualization* and helps engage the mind to become a partner in your treatment program.

The surgeon predicted that Casey's hospitalization would last 3 weeks and might be complicated by infections and other problems due to his already-weakened state. He was quite amazed when Casey walked out of the hospital 8 days after the surgery was performed. Casey proceeded to receive 20 postsurgical radiation treatments to further diminish any recurrence risk of his cancer. He also tolerated these treatments well.

Despite his amazing recovery, Casey lost 16 pounds during this ordeal. In addition, his CD4 count dropped from a high of 194 back down to 90 cells/mm3. Once again, this did not diminish Casey's resolve to continue healing from his condition. I recommended he start a daily protein drink containing 30 grams of protein and 330 calories per serving. I also increased his testosterone and DHEA dosages to help him regain the muscle mass he had lost.

Some 2 years later, Casey is doing extremely well. His CD4 count has again risen to over 200 cells/mm3 (from 0), and his viral load remains undetectable on D4T/3TC/indinavir. His rectal cancer has been effectively treated and is no longer of concern. He is back to work full-time as the administrator of a local health organization and appears as healthy and vibrant as ever. Casey deserves the success which he has achieved, and I anticipate he will continue healing from HIV as the future unfolds.

Hormonal Therapies

Hormones are extremely potent chemicals that are used by the body to facilitate all of its vital functions. Mood, energy, appetite, sex drive, immune function, heart rate, and body cell mass are all directly affected by your body's hormone levels.

Cortisol, testosterone, and DHEA (dehydroepiandrosterone) are natural hormones which can be accurately measured, and supplemented if necessary, to ensure optimal health and well-being. Identifying and correcting any deficiencies can be one of the most important health-promoting actions an HIV(+) individual can take. Oxandrolone, nandrolone, and recombinant human growth hormone are hormonal supplements that can be used to enhance the effects of your natural hormones if necessary.

Evaluating and correcting suboptimal hormone levels, is an essential part of wise HIV care. Details on how to monitor hormone levels, as well as how to achieve optimal hormone balance through supplementation, are covered in Chapter 11.

Long-Term Survivors

Most HIV(+) individuals in my practice continue to enjoy tremendous good health and stability. This is true despite the fact that many of them have been infected with HIV for upwards of 18 years. Some 10 percent have been able to avoid using antiviral medications and remain healthy during this entire time. All are on the fewest medications and the lowest dosages possible while still remaining stable.

Medications are best viewed as supplemental to a strong natural therapies program, as opposed to being the central pillar of your treatment. If you keep this strategy in mind, you will be able to remain on the middle path of good health and stability — preserving strong immune function, a quiescent viral infection, and the greatest number of future treatment options for a long time to come.

Ben

Ben discovered that he was HIV(+) in 1985. In 1987, he was diagnosed with non-Hodgkin's lymphoma, a cancer manifested by swollen lymph nodes in his neck and chest. He was treated with 3 months of chemotherapy followed by 3 months of radiation therapy and experienced a complete response. Some 3 years later we began working together to combine natural and standard therapies into a comprehensive treatment program for him to follow.

At that time, Ben was taking AZT monotherapy. We initially added vitamins, herbal supplements, and a daily practice of meditation. In addition, I recommended that Ben consider utilizing a mind-body technique which I call "Letters to the Virus." I recommend this technique to many of my patients in an attempt to help them develop a closer understanding of the emotional issues brought about by living with HIV. Here are a few of Ben's letters.

To the Virus:

I didn't choose to enter into this relationship. It's a fact, a reality, so I have to deal with it, and we have to deal with each other. I do everything I can to help keep my body healthy. Also, I do everything I can to keep from getting infections that might stir you up and make you more active. This is not my natural state, being infected, but I can and will live with it. I love and accept who I am, and I will not allow you to work against me on an unconscious level. We will learn to live with each other, if not in harmony, then in a neutral state.

I was weak once, and you manifested yourself by stimulating a tumor called lymphoma in my neck. I learned that I must keep myself strong and respond to you with strength if you don't stay in your place. I must stay strong mentally and physically in order to keep you from overtaking me.

We must learn to peacefully coexist if we are both to live a long life together.

Signed,

Ben

P.S. If I could take a pill tomorrow and sweep you out of my body, thus returning to my natural state, I have to be honest and say that I would. But I am an intelligent being who can adapt to these circumstances and will learn how to live with you!

Dear Ben,

This is my natural state as well. I find a host to live off, and I grow stronger if I can. I don't really want to destroy you, since we would both die in the process. I can exist in a quiet, dormant state if not excited, but if you are weak and my defenses are triggered, I can be deadly. If your immune system grows weak, I will grow stronger. I am held in check by a strong-functioning immune system.

Signed,

Virus

This set of letters highlights a number of things. First, Ben has a significant amount of psychological and emotional strength, which, despite the situation he currently faces, he can use to move positively into the future. Fortunately, there is not an overwhelming level of fear or anger blocking Ben's ability to continue living his life fully. This is very important. Repressed anger and fear can drain your energy. Reducing anger and fear is an important goal for anyone dealing with a life-challenging condition.

Second, it is clear from his letters that Ben does not believe that HIV is "destined to kill him no matter what." This signifies the possibility that Ben can avoid "being at war" with the virus for the rest of his life. Being in a state of war for the rest of your life drains your energy and can prevent you from gaining whatever insights and lessons might come from this difficult, but potentially strengthening, set of circumstances.

Ben continued to take AZT monotherapy and remained healthy and stable until the fall of 1995. At that time, faced with slightly declining lab values, he switched to D4T/3TC dual therapy. In additional, he began DHEA and testosterone supplementation to bring these hormone levels into the optimal range. I also recommended to Ben that he continue taking acyclovir 400 mg 2x/day to completely suppress his chronic herpes. Ben also continued his vitamin supplements, received regular acupuncture, and worked to keep his stress low.

A year after starting D4T/3TC, Ben's CD4 count had risen from 288 to 481 cells/mm3. His viral load, though initially undetectable, unexpectedly increased to 2000 copies/ml after about a year on the above regimen. My suggestion to Ben was that he not rush to change his program since it was helping him maintain a stable CD4 count and feel extremely well.

Ben's next viral load dropped to 846 copies/ml (from 2000). I continued to recommend that Ben stay the course. Ben's other physicians were strongly recommending that he go on triple-combination therapy with either a protease inhibitor or NNRTI (non-nucleoside reverse transcriptase inhibitor) medication. This philosophy, in my opinion, would have caused Ben to go through his future medication options too quickly.

By working to eliminate all of the possible cofactors that might be stimulating Ben's viral infection, we determined that he was not getting enough protein. Inadequate protein intake is clearly a cofactor that can weaken the immune system. After visiting with our clinic's dietitian, and increasing his protein intake to greater than 100 grams/day, Ben found that his CD4 count had risen to 739 cells/mm3 and his viral load had once again became undetectable!

I cannot overemphasize how important it is to make changes to your antiviral medications as infrequently as possible. Following this path requires intelligence, sensitivity, and hard work. For some patients, 3 or 4 antiviral drugs are essential, but for others, 2 antiviral medications can last an exceptionally long time; often more than 3 years when used appropriately. This can allow many additional medication options to be released during the interim.

Ben continues to remain healthy and stable. He has maintained good health for over a decade utilizing a total of only 3 antiviral drugs. I attribute much of his success to his willingness to follow a comprehensive healing program that naturally supports his immune system. This enables his antiviral medications to work better and remain effective longer.

Ben has been taking D4T/3TC for over 3 years now (after 5 years of AZT monotherapy). Hopefully he will not need to change this medication program for several years to come. When he does, there will still be a large number of medication options for him to choose from. Ben's sensitivity, hard work, personal growth, and continued excellent health illustrate that he is indeed healing from HIV.

Keep Hope Alive!

Throughout this book I have included many patient stories like the ones in this chapter; they highlight the tremendous success that has been achieved by patients following the Healing HIV program. Their experiences reinforce my belief that most HIV(+) individuals have the ability to live normal and healthy lives.

I also believe that all individuals, no matter what their CD4 count when they start this program, have the ability to stabilize and improve their condition. By utilizing presently available therapies, they can dramatically suppress viral activity. Soon-to-be-released medications will give us even safer and more beneficial options. Even now, we are able to raise CD4 counts of patients with fewer than 25 CD4 cells to over 300 cells/mm3. This was unheard of just a few years ago. We must keep hope alive!

We must also keep fighting: Fighting to increase research funding. Fighting to increase awareness of the benefits of natural therapies. And fighting to skillfully maintain stability in the present, so that you are here, and in good health, for the next wave of advances and ultimately...the cure! This book can help you achieve these goals.

Chapter Three

The Middle Path
of Good Health and Stability

During the past several years, there has been an explosion of new and effective treatments for HIV. Protease inhibitors, NNRTIs, and viral load tests have moved us into a new era. CD4 cell expansion, chemokine inhibitors, and other potent immune-enhancing therapies will further improve our ability to treat this condition effectively as the future unfolds.

The promise of these new therapies can give all who are HIV(+) good reason to continue fighting as hard as possible to maintain their good health. There is also compelling evidence for those who are not perfectly stable; if you are not already taking antiviral medications, it is time to seriously consider starting them now. With such a large number of effective antiviral options available, patients who have postponed taking these medications due to doubts about their effectiveness would be wise to reconsider this decision.

Conversely, it is important not to succumb to the "take as many drugs as possible" philosophy. When counseling my patients, I frequently refer to a concept that I call walking "The Middle Path." For any individual at any time, there is a middle path of good health and stability which can be found by using just the right combination of natural therapies and medications. If you are currently within the boundaries of this path, you are by definition on a program that is working well for you.

The middle path's goal is the achievement of long-term strength and balance. The ability to stay within its boundaries requires a combination of sensitivity and individual tailoring. By integrating aspects of the following 3 modalities into your treatment program, you can achieve long-term strength and balance:

1) *Aggressive natural therapies:* To support the long-term health of the immune system.

2) *Emotional and spiritually based practices:* To help transform being HIV(+) into a stimulus for positive lifestyle changes and growth.

3) *Antiviral medication:* To help suppress viral activity to safe and manageable levels. It is also wise to employ effective prophylaxis medications to prevent specific opportunistic infections when indicated (see Appendix 4).

The basic premise underlying the Healing HIV program is that HIV is best treated with the *long-term health* of the individual in mind. Taking antiviral medication can help you achieve this goal, but these medications are best used with great care. By adding them to your program only as they become necessary, you ensure that you are staying within the boundaries of the middle path. Taking just the right combination of drugs and natural therapies best suited to your individual needs will allow you to live the longest and healthiest life span possible despite being HIV(+).

You are on middle path of good health and stability if you can give affirmative answers to the following 3 questions:

1) Are you relatively asymptomatic?

2) Is your CD4 count greater than 300 cells/mm3 and stable or improving?

3) Is your viral load low (*at least* under 20,000 copies/ml, and preferably less)?

If you can answer yes to the above 3 questions, you are currently within the boundaries of the middle path. This means that the program you are following is working well for you, and you do not need to make any changes in your medications at this time. If you have determined that you are currently on the middle path, relax and enjoy life for a while. It is important not to worry constantly that you are missing out on a new drug or therapy. You are stable, you feel well, and your lab tests reflect this situation.

If you can only answer yes to 2 of the questions, you may still be on the middle path of good health, but you need to monitor your condition very closely. If you can only answer affirmatively to 1 of the questions, or to none of them, you almost certainly need to make significant changes to your current treatment program. Of course, this is a very general version of my guidelines, and every case needs to be carefully individualized. Please refer to Chapter 6 for specific details on how to treat several commonly encountered clinical situations.

Simply stated, the goal of the Healing HIV program is to ensure that an individual is remaining stable or improving, and is utilizing the minimum amount of medication necessary to continue feeling well.

I'd like to highlight a few individual stories which further describe the benefits that walking "The Middle Path of Good Health and Stability" can bring.

Jason

Jason is a yoga teacher at a nationally recognized healing center. As one might imagine, he is a strong believer in the healing power of natural therapies. After 10 years of excellent stability on a purely natural program, Jason began to experience a slow but steady decline in his CD4 count. He also began to notice fatigue, chronic sinus infections, and a drop in his libido and sex drive.

Initially we began antiviral therapy with D4T/DDI. He quickly experienced a steady increase in his energy, a return to his previous level of well-being, a significant improvement in his CD4 count, and a decline in his viral load to an undetectable level. Now, 4 years later, Jason is still taking the same antiviral medications and remains perfectly stable with a high CD4 count. He is clearly on "The Middle Path of Good Health and Stability."

In addition, Jason has not experienced any side effects from the drugs he is taking. This is partly due to the aggressive natural therapies program he is following. For instance, he effectively prevents peripheral neuropathy by taking oral supplements of calcium, magnesium, and vitamin B$_6$. He maintains a healthy liver through diet, regular exercise, and the avoidance of alcohol and other recreational drugs. The combination of these natural therapies and the antiviral drugs he is currently taking provide his body the balance and strength it needs to remain healthy and stable for a long time.

The next example also describes a patient who is maintaining good health and stability on "The Middle Path."

Scott

Scott is a 42-year-old investment advisor. Based on several negative experiences with antiviral medications in the past, Scott realized he was especially sensitive to these drugs. Despite a decreasing CD4 count and the presence of several KS (Kaposi's sarcoma) lesions, Scott was still reluctant to add antiviral medications to his natural therapies program. I vividly remember the day when Scott lay on my exam table and asked me to try and help him stay alive for just 2 more years. Again, I strongly urged him to try adding antiviral medications to his program. Fortunately, this time he agreed.

To initiate Scott's antiviral program, we first began with 3TC in combination with a very low dose of AZT, 100 mg 2x/day. Slowly, we advanced his AZT dosage to 200 mg 2x/day with no adverse effects. Scott then added ritonavir, the newest protease inhibitor at the time, at a lower than usual dosage, 500 mg 2x/day. Scott tolerated this regimen extremely well for quite some time and has only required a few minor adjustments to his medications since.

It has now been 6 years since the day when Scott begged me to help him stay alive for just 2 more years. Today he is healthy, happy, and has over 500 CD4 cells/mm3. His KS has completely resolved, and his viral load continues to remain undetectable. He is now stronger and healthier than at any point since I have known him. Scott has also not had any serious infections nor been in the hospital for any reason during this entire time.

It is important to work with sensitive patients like Scott in a very gentle fashion. One size does not fit all with these drugs. I tell all of my patients when they first begin antiviral medications that my goal is for them to feel as good or better on these drugs than before they started them. If they do not, I work closely with them until they do. This has to be your goal if you are to achieve long-term good health and stability.

Scott's current good health, sense of well-being, and the complete disappearance of his KS lesions are the result of "The Middle Path" treatment philosophy. If Scott started all 3 antiviral drugs simultaneously, he most assuredly would have experienced significant side effects. He might have had to start and stop medications in a way that would have caused the emergence of resistance. The careful use of these medications, *individualized to each patient's unique sensitivities and needs,* is a key to achieving the most successful outcome. Scott is now pleased to be making new long-term plans for his future.

Long-term stability *is the rule,* not the exception, among my patients. The data I present in the next chapter firmly supports this statement. As more and more treatment options emerge, I hope to continue improving my record of success. The goal of living 20 years or more after exposure to HIV is now a reality. Utilizing potentially toxic medications in as sensitive a manner as possible, and combining them with the aggressive use of natural therapies, is the cornerstone to this success.

Why *not* go on as many beneficial medications as possible? There are several important factors to consider:

1) *Avoiding short-term side effects:* Most antiviral medications have a wide range of side effects which can occur soon after they are begun. These include diarrhea, rash, peripheral neuropathy, liver abnormalities, anemia, and others. Taking antiviral medication only when absolutely necessary helps you avoid these short-term effects.

2) *Avoiding long-term side effects:* In fact, 3 of the 4 currently available classes of antiviral medications have been approved for the treatment of HIV only during the past 2 years. We have no idea what long-term toxicity these medications may possess. Already, there have been over 100 patients who have developed serious diabetes-like elevations in blood sugar that have been linked to the use of protease inhibitors. While this does not discount the enormous benefits these drugs have brought to thousands of HIV(+) individuals, their indiscriminate use should be strongly discouraged.

3) *Avoiding using up your medication options too fast:* This is probably the most important reason to practice the philosophy of minimizing antiviral usage in treating HIV. It is vitally necessary that you keep important medications in reserve so that you can continue to maintain a surplus of powerful and effective antiviral options well into the future. Your goal must be to remain healthy and stable over the long term, always preserving additional treatment options to use if your viral strain develops multidrug resistance. Going through the list of currently available antiviral medications as slowly as possible also allows many newer and potentially more effective therapies to be released during the interim.

4) *Minimizing costs:* If current trends continue, the number and types of HIV medications available to our patients will begin to be rationed. Already, some patients with multidrug-resistant HIV are taking 6 and 7 antivirals in a last-ditch attempt to treat their infection. When the standard treatment of this condition is coupled with a comprehensive program of natural therapies, the need for expensive medications is lessened. This fact is clearly demonstrated by my private practice and research study data.

5) *Long-term health concerns:* There is one final reason to exercise caution. Protease inhibitors frequently cause multiple liver function abnormalities to appear on blood tests. These include rises in the serum levels of cholesterol, triglycerides, liver enzymes, blood sugar, and bilirubin. While these laboratory abnormalities do not cause adverse symptoms for most patients in the short term, they are disturbingly similar to the laboratory abnormalities we see in patients on their way to developing

heart disease, liver failure, and diabetes. What a cruel joke if, in our attempt to aggressively treat HIV, we cause our patients to develop these serious ailments 5 or 10 years down the road. While I certainly hope this is not the case, this consideration again speaks for caution and restraint when taking these medications, especially if you are currently healthy, stable, and within the boundaries of "The Middle Path."

Balance and moderation have always been keys to good health. Endeavor to find your place of balance on the middle path, stay on it as long as possible, and make as few changes to your treatment program as you can. This strategy will allow you to remain healthy and stable for the longest time possible, potentially outliving HIV in the process.

Chapter Four

Private Practice Data

Despite the many outstanding HIV treatments released during the past several years, my philosophy for prescribing antiviral medication has essentially remained the same. I always want to give the body a chance to control HIV first, before adding potentially toxic medications. The only exceptions I have to this rule are if you know you have been exposed to HIV for the first time within the past 6 months or if you are certain you want to be highly aggressive with your antiviral medications. In the first case, please see clinical scenario #3 in the Chapter 6. This outlines my recommendations for treating Acute Retroviral Syndrome. In the second, I always take my patient's general philosophy on medication usage into consideration before deciding exactly how to prescribe these drugs. This is because patients need to be enthusiastic about their treatment program if it is to work as effectively as possible.

If the immune system is well supported with an aggressive program of natural therapies (diet, vitamins, herbs, exercise, stress reduction, etc.), it can often control HIV for many years before needing antivirals to help maintain good health and stability. Even if you are already taking antiviral drugs, an aggressive program of natural therapies will help these drugs work better, *and last longer,* by promoting a strong response by your immune system. However, if you choose to rely *solely* on antiviral medications to treat this condition, you will be employing a Band-Aid approach that may ultimately lead to medication resistance, increased toxicity, and a slowly deteriorating picture of health.

Important: If you do not faithfully follow an aggressive natural therapies program, I strongly recommend that you follow the antiviral treatment guidelines released by the U.S. Department of Health and Human Services Committee on Antiviral Medication (see Fig. 4.1). These guidelines encourage those who are HIV(+) to begin triple-combination therapy as early as possible in the course of their infection. However, if you choose to support your immune system aggressively with a strong natural therapies program similar to the one described in this book, the ability to use less antiviral medication becomes a possibility.

The most important advice I can give you at this juncture is to work very closely with your doctor to choose the treatment options that are best for *you.* If you are not completely satisfied with your health-care provider at this time, start searching for a new one *now.* Do not wait until you are in the midst of a health crisis to begin looking for a new doctor. Your choice of which person helps you care for your health is an extremely important one. Do not settle for anything less than someone who is open-minded and willing to discuss all potential treatment options in a nonjudgmental way. Even if your doctor disagrees with your ideas, he or she needs to be willing to support your decisions. This will ultimately ensure that your treatment program best meets your needs. As always, please do not make any changes to your medical program without first discussing them with your health-care provider.

Private Practice Data

It is not an exaggeration to say that I care for one of the healthiest groups of HIV(+) individuals around. As you will see from the information presented below, they experience a very low rate of progression from this condition. I attribute this success to my "Middle Path" philosophy, which strikes a delicate balance between the *excessive* use of drugs and an *excessive* reliance on natural therapies.

My program also provides the body with the natural support it needs to live healthfully with HIV for an entire life span. I prescribe antiviral medication only when the body's immune system is not sufficiently able

Figure 4.1

Recommended Antiviral Agents
for Treatment of Established HIV Infection
(1998 U.S. Department of Health and Human Services)

Preferred (A1): Strong evidence of clinical benefit and sustained suppression of plasma viral load. 1 highly active protease inhibitor* plus 2 NRTIs (1 from Column A and 2 from Column B. Drugs are listed in random, not priority, order):

Column A	Column B
Indinavir	AZT/DDI
Nelfinavir	D4T/DDI
Ritonavir	AZT/DDC
	AZT/3TC#
	D4T/3TC#

Alternative (B2): Less likely to provide sustained virus suppression; clinical benefit is undetermined.

• 1 NNRTI (Nevirapine)** + 2 NRTIs (from Column B above)
• Saquinavir + 2 NRTIs (from Column B above)
(New soft gel formulation of saquinavir (Fortovase) appears to enhance the efficacy of this combination to the same level as with the other PIs)

Not generally recommended (C1): Clinical benefit demonstrated but initial virus suppression is not sustained in most patients

• 2 NRTIs (from Column B above)

Not recommended (D1)##: Evidence against use, virologically undesirable

• All monotherapies	• DDC/D4T
• D4T/AZT	• DDC/3TC
• DDC/DDI	

---

* The old hard-gel capsule formulation of saquinavir is not recommended due to poor bioavailability.

** The only combinations of 2 NRTIs + 1 NNRTI that have been shown to suppress viremia to undetectable levels in the majority of patients is AZT/DDI/Nevirapine. This combination was studied in antiviral-naive individuals.

\# High level resistance to 3TC develops within 2–4 weeks in partially suppressive regimens; optimal use is in 3-drug antiviral combinations that reduce viral load to < 500 copies/ml.

\#\# AZT monotherapy may be considered for prophylactic use in pregnant women with low viral load and high CD4 cell counts to prevent perinatal transmission.

to stabilize HIV on its own. This approach enables my patients to make as few changes as possible to their antiviral program while continuing to remain healthy and stable. It also allows for the release of many newer, and potentially more effective, medication options during this period.

As a means of highlighting the level of antiviral medication use among my HIV(+) patients, I recently conducted a survey of my private practice. The following sampling of my long-term HIV(+) patients shows an interesting breakdown of medication usage (these are patients who have been followed in my practice for a minimum of 2 years, n=74):

> On 0 antiviral medications. 12%
> On 1 antiviral medications 0%
> On 2 antiviral medications. 31%
> **Less than triple therapy** 43%
>
> On 3 antiviral medications. 37%
> On 4 antiviral medications. 15%
> On 5 antiviral medications 5%
> **Triple therapy or more** 57%

While 57% of my patients are taking at least a standard triple combination of antiviral medications, 43% are taking 2 antivirals or fewer. More important, the patients taking 2 antivirals or fewer are by far the healthier, more stable group. They are, in general, more active and have fewer medication side effects. Also, fewer patients in this group have needed to go on medical disability.

Important point: It is currently not recommended that anyone take 1 antiviral medication for any period of time due to the almost certain emergence of resistance. I also do not recommend that you decrease the number of antiviral medications you are currently taking.

The question that I am usually asked at this point is: "Although they are stable now, how long will patients on 2 antiviral medications or fewer remain stable?"

The answer to this question, based on the past 5 years of my clinical experience using the Healing HIV program, is clear:

••

"As long as these patients utilize their antiviral medication in combination with an aggressive natural therapies program as described in this book, they will remain healthy and stable for a very long time."

••

In our clinic's hands, double-combination antiviral therapy with 2 reverse transcriptase inhibitors (dual RTI therapy), instituted in patients with mild-to-moderate HIV disease (CD4 counts greater then 300 cells/mm3 and viral loads less than 50,000 cells/ml) is effective for at least 2 years, *and oftentimes longer,* in at least 90% of the patients who use it. This allows our patients to go through the present list of antiviral medications more slowly than patients who are following a more aggressive treatment philosophy. This conservative approach allows safer and potentially more potent treatment options to be developed and released during this period of time. Remember, it is the aggressive natural therapies program which I prescribe to my patients that allows this strategy to work. It accomplishes this goal by encouraging the immune system to become a strong partner in the treatment of HIV.

The aggressive natural therapies program I recommend to my HIV(+) patients includes a seamless blend of the following treatment modalities:

1) Nutritional counseling
2) Antioxidant nutrient supplementation
3) Acupuncture and herbs
4) Regular exercise
5) Hormone balancing
6) Stress reduction/psychospiritual interventions
7) Standard medical therapies

Although each therapeutic intervention contained in the above list achieves a positive effect on its own, the Healing HIV program's overall ability to rebuild immune systems is maximized when all of them are combined. Immune reconstitution can then occur even in patients whose health has been declining for years.

While utilizing the Healing HIV program during the past 4 years, not 1 patient starting with a CD4 count greater than 300 cells/mm3 has progressed to below that number. In addition, not 1 patient starting with a CD4 count of greater than 50 cells/mm3 has become seriously ill or died from an HIV-related illness during this same period of time. This experience encompasses the treatment of more than 300 HIV(+) individuals.

Healing HIV Research Study

I know these statistics sound incredible. Many colleagues have told me so. That is why I recently conducted a controlled, retrospective analysis of my HIV patient population (The Healing HIV Research Study). The data for this study was collected by an independent observer who reviewed the charts of all of the HIV(+) patients receiving continuous primary care at my practice for at least the past 2 years. A total of 74 patients met all of the inclusion criteria and were accrued. The majority of these patients live in San Francisco and have been exposed to the HIV virus for more than 10 years.

Each of these patients was given the same aggressive natural therapy and antiviral medication recommendations as per the approach described in this book. Patients accepted or rejected my recommendations based on their personal philosophies and socioeconomic abilities. The extent to which they followed my program was not a criteria for admission to the study.

The control group for this study consisted of 74 HIV(+) individuals cared for by a similar HIV-specialty medical practice located in the same neighborhood in San Francisco. The patients lived in the same geographical area, belonged to the same socioeconomic group, and were similarly aggressive about their care *except* that this group was provided a more standard HIV treatment program. Therefore, the emphasis was mainly on antiviral therapy and little, if any, counseling was provided on the use of diet, vitamins, intestinal health, stress reduction, etc. The control group individuals met the same inclusion criteria, and their charts were randomly selected from this practice's charts by a neutral party without prior knowledge of the study's purposes or goals.

Analysis of the study data revealed that the mean number of *antiviral* medications in use at the end of the 2-year study period was 2.58 per patient in the study group (range: 0–5) and 3.08 per patient in the control group (range: 0–5). In addition, 43% of the patients in the study group were taking *less than triple-combination therapy* compared with only 18% taking less than triple-combination therapy in the control group. This confirms the assumption that there was significantly *less antiviral medication* prescribed to the study group participants.

In addition, the mean number of *total* medications in use at the end of the 2-year study period was 5.96 per patient in the study group (range: 2–12) and 8.46 per patient in the control group (range: 2–22). This confirms that significantly *less total medication* was prescribed to the study group participants.

Healing HIV Study Results

1) The study group participants used less antiviral medication and less total medication than the control group participants.

2) When compared to the control group participants, the study group participants experienced:

- A greater average rise in CD4 cells (45% vs 25%)
- A greater average drop in viral load (-86% vs -72%)
- Fewer opportunistic infections (1 vs 3)
- Fewer hospitalizations (0 vs 1)
- fewer hospital days (0 vs 5)

The results of this study are summarized in Fig. 4.2. The study group achieved results as good as or better than the control group while using fewer antiviral and total medications. I am currently in the process of readying the results of this study for submission to a peer-reviewed journal.

Figure 4.2

HEALING HIV RESEARCH STUDY DATA SUMMARY

	Study Group	Control Group
Total number of patients	74	74
Male:female ratio	69/5	73/1
Mean age	44	41
Baseline mean CD4 cell count	291	361
Ending mean CD4 cell count	423	451
Baseline mean viral load	101,627	31,828
Ending mean viral load	13,840	8894
Avg. CD4 cell change	+45%	+25%
Avg. viral load change	-86%	-72%
Mean # of antiviral medications	2.58	3.08
Mean # of total medications	5.96	8.46
Total # of opportunistic infections	1	3
Total # of HIV-related hospitalizations	0	1
Total # of HIV-related hospital days	0	5

In addition, since a CD4 count of greater than 300 CD4 cells/mm3 usually signifies a normally functioning immune system, I thought it would be interesting to identify how many patients from both groups improved from below 300 CD4 cells to above this level during the 2-year study period. I also looked at how many patients declined from above to below this level. The results of this analysis are represented in Fig. 4.3.

Figure 4.3

HEALING HIV PROGRAM STUDY

	Study Group	*Control Group*
Number of Patients Improving from less than 300 CD4 cells to greater than 300 CD4 cells:	21 of 74	11 of 74
Number of Patients Declining from greater than 300 CD4 cells to less than 300 CD4 cells:	0 of 74	3 of 74

Healing HIV Study Conclusion

This study concludes that:

· ·

"The Healing HIV treatment program can potentially help HIV(+) individuals achieve as good or better outcomes using less antiviral medication than is commonly recommended. Though not specifically measured in this study, it appeared that the study group participants experienced fewer medication side effects and had an overall lower cost of care."

· ·

Despite the fact that there were differences in the outcomes of these 2 groups, a second important conclusion that can be drawn from this study is that HIV(+) patients treated by an HIV specialist can remain extremely healthy over a 2-year period. When data from the 2 groups are viewed together, 148 HIV(+) patients experienced only 4 opportunistic infections and 1 HIV-related hospitalization during a 2-year period. It is also important to note that many of these patients had severe HIV disease

Figure 4.4

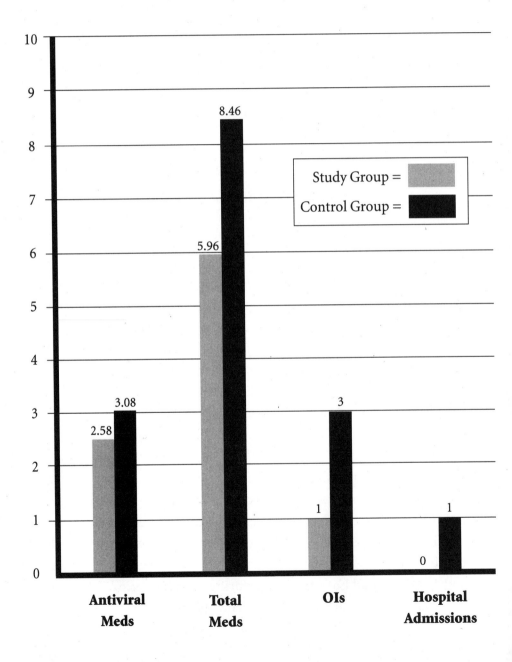

**HEALING HIV RESEARCH STUDY
GRAPHIC ANALYSIS**
(n=148)

(AIDS) at the onset of this study, with 31% having CD4 counts below 200 CD4 cells/mm3. This highlights the high level of care that is often delivered to HIV(+) individuals by physicians who commonly treat this condition. It also provides hope that patients at any stage of HIV disease today can be kept stable and healthy to benefit from newly emerging treatments in the near future.

As a final word with regard to this study, I would like to thank the medical providers who allowed us to use their practice as the control group for this study. I respect the care that they provide very much, and if I were HIV(+), I would not hesitate to be treated at their practice. However, as one might expect, I would add a more aggressive natural therapies program to my treatment.

Chapter Five

Antiviral Medications

"There is no single, absolute answer to the question of when to start antiviral treatment. Some researchers and physicians believe that everyone who is HIV infected, regardless of viral load, symptoms, or CD4 counts, should be on treatment. Some believe that people should begin therapy when their CD4 counts fall below 500 cells/mm3 or their viral load exceeds 10,000–20,000 copies of virus. Others believe that only people experiencing symptoms of HIV disease should consider anti-HIV therapy. One note of agreement is that most researchers and physicians believe that the decision to start anti-HIV therapy should be guided by looking at clinical health and measures of both CD4 cell counts and viral load levels."

— Project Inform Discussion Paper on Antivirals, February 1998

At present, antiviral medications can be thought of as belonging to 1 of the following 4 categories:

1) *Reverse Transcriptase Inhibitors (RTIs):* AZT (Retrovir), 3TC (Epivir), D4T (Zerit), DDI (Videx), DDC (Hivid), abacavir (Ziagen)

2) *Non-nucleoside Reverse Transcriptase Inhibitors (NNRTIs):* Nevirapine (Viramune), delavirdine (Rescriptor), efavirenz (Sustiva)

3) *Protease Inhibitors (PIs):* Saquinavir (Fortovase), ritonavir (Norvir), indinavir (Crixivan), nelfinavir (Viracept)

4) *Miscellaneous Antiviral Medications:* Hydroxyurea (Hydrea), adefovir (Preveon).

The drugs within each of the above categories can generally be thought of as inhibiting HIV replication at a specific point in its life cycle. Fig. 5.1 illustrates the process of HIV replication from the moment it initially fuses onto the cell surface, known as absorption, to the release of mature viral particles, known as budding.

Figure 5.1

Life Cycle of HIV Virus

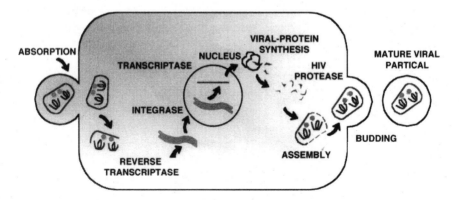

Fusion of HIV onto the cell surface is a very complex process that involves the participation of many proteins, both in the serum and on the cell surface. The serum proteins are known as chemokines. The participating proteins in this part of HIV's life cycle have recently been identified, and the search is currently underway for inhibitory drugs to block this process. The category of drugs that block the fusion and absorption of HIV onto the cell surface are known as fusion and/or chemokine inhibitors. No drugs from this category are presently available.

Once within the confines of the cell, HIV sheds its protein coating to reveal its genetic material in the form of RNA (ribonucleic acid). The virus then attempts to take over the host cell's machinery to reproduce additional copies of itself. Before this can occur, it must first convert its RNA genetic material into DNA (deoxyribonucleic acid). DNA is the form of genetic material compatible with that of the host cell. The process of converting HIV's RNA to host cell–compatible DNA is facilitated by the viral enzyme, reverse transcriptase, which HIV has conveniently brought along. Reverse transcriptase is inhibited (blocked) by the class of antiviral medications known as RTIs or reverse transcriptase inhibitors. This is the class of drugs that includes AZT and was the first class of anti-HIV medications to be released.

These are 3 basic types of reverse transcriptase inhibitors: "nucleoside" RTIs, "non-nucleoside" RTIs (also referred to as NNRTIs), and "nucleotide" RTIs. All of these drugs work at the same stage of HIV's life cycle and accomplish the same result. However, because they have different mechanisms of action, all 3 classes of RTIs can potentiate each other in a beneficial way when taken together.

The next step in HIV's goal of conquering the cell is the incorporation of its new DNA strands into the genetic material of the host cell's nucleus. Once integration of the virus's genetic code into that of the host cell is accomplished, HIV can control the cell's reproductive machinery and make additional copies of itself for export into the bloodstream.

The incorporation process of HIV genetic material into the host cell's nucleus is facilitated by a second enzyme called an integrase. Blocking this step in HIV's reproductive cycle is a current focus of intense research. More information on new antiviral treatments such as integrase, fusion, and cytokine inhibitors can be found in Appendix 3.

The next 2 phases of viral reproduction are known as assembly and budding. These steps are facilitated by the viral protease enzyme. HIV protease cleaves the large protein strands HIV initially manufactures into smaller proteins it needs to produce a mature virus particle. Drugs that block this enzyme are called protease inhibitors (PIs). Protease inhibitors were released in 1995. As you can see in Fig. 5.2, their availability has coincided with a dramatic decline in deaths from HIV.

Figure 5.2

DECLINE IN HIV-RELATED MORTALITY SINCE 1995

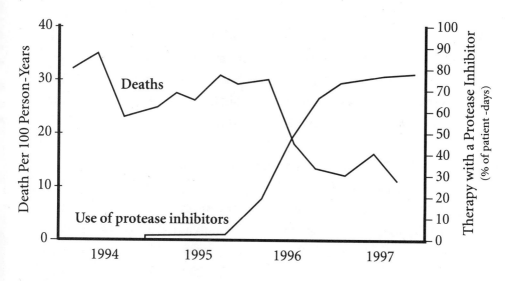

Correlation between mortality and frequency of use of HAART, including a PI, between 1/94 and 1/97 among people w/HIV w/a CD4 cell ct. <100 cells/mm

Palella et al. *N Eng J Med.* 1998; 338:853–860

The last category of antiviral medications, which I call miscellaneous, includes hydroxyurea and adefovir. Hydroxyurea is an antimetabolite. When combined with other antiviral drugs such as DDI, it works to decrease the pool of available raw material HIV needs to replicate itself. Adefovir is a "nucleotide" RTI (see above), which inhibits the reverse transcriptase enzyme of HIV, CMV, and other viruses as well.

The ability to block HIV's replication at multiple sites is a strategy which has produced tremendous benefits during the past several years. As new categories of antiviral drugs become available, they will enable us to block HIV's replication at additional points in its life cycle. This will improve our ability to greatly suppress its replication. Patients with resistance to the older categories of antiviral drugs will benefit tremendously from these new antiviral medications. Many patients in this situation are anxiously awaiting these new categories of antiviral drugs.

The more you know about the drugs you put in your body, the more you can help participate in the decisions surrounding your care. I will now briefly describe each of the currently available antiviral medications, followed by additional comments on how to get the most benefit from their use. Chapter 6 will describe in detail how to use these medications in several commonly encountered treatment situations.

Reverse Transcriptase Inhibitors (RTIs)

AZT (Retrovir)

AZT was the first antiviral medication approved for the treatment of HIV disease. It is a member of the class of antivirals known as nucleoside reverse transcriptase inhibitors. The most common dosing regimen is 300 mg 2x/day, but it has also been dosed at 200 mg 3x/day and 100 mg 5x/day in the past. Many patients still have a great deal of reticence about taking AZT due to the fact that this drug was prescribed at a dosage of 1200 mg/day when it was first released. This dosage was excessive and often produced nausea, anemia, and other serious side effects. The incidence of these side effects has steadily decreased as the dosing recommendations have been revised.

We now know that using a single antiviral agent to treat HIV encourages the quick *emergence of resistant viral strains*. Therefore, it is always best to use AZT in combination with at least 1 other antiviral medication. Common AZT combinations include AZT/3TC, AZT/DDI, and AZT/DDC, with or without additional protease inhibitors and/or NNRTI medications. AZT/3TC is a commonly used combination that has recently been released as a single pill called Combivir. Combivir contains 300 mg of AZT and 150 mg of 3TC. When this formulation is used, both medications are provided as a single pill taken 2x/day.

Side effects: AZT's most common side effect is bone marrow suppression. This can cause low red blood cell counts (anemia), low white blood cell counts (neutropenia), and low platelet counts (thrombocytopenia). AZT can also cause nausea, headaches, and muscle aches that may make you feel as if you had the flu. These symptoms often resolve during the first 2 to 4 weeks of taking this medication.

Comments: Many studies support AZT's effectiveness, especially when taken in combination with 3TC plus a protease inhibitor or NNRTI medication. Unfortunately, AZT's biggest drawback is that it may depress the bone marrow, the very organ that produces all of the body's blood cells. Studies have shown that patients with anemia have more opportunistic infections during the course of their HIV infection than those who don't. Therefore, if you are taking AZT, it is important to monitor your red and white blood cell counts closely.

My goal in treating antiviral-naive patients (patients about to start antiviral therapy for the first time), is to make their medication program as easy to tolerate as possible. Because of AZT's tendency to cause a moderate amount of side effects, I usually choose not to recommend it as part of the initial treatment regimen. However, it can be a valuable medication option when used at a later time. I therefore prefer to keep it in reserve.

DDI (Videx)

DDI is the second RTI to have been released. DDI was originally marketed as a powder, but has since been reformulated into a pleasant, chewable orange-flavored, tablet. The 2 tablets are chewed or dissolved in water, and taken on an empty stomach 1 hour before or 2 hours after a meal.

Several of the original studies of DDI showed that 1x/day dosing of this antiviral demonstrated similar efficacy as 2x/day dosing. Despite these findings, the medication was initially released with the more conservative 2x/day dosing recommendation. Most recently, DDI has been reevaluated as a 1x/day medication. This reevaluation is based on new research data and is part of a trend to make antiviral medication programs as easy to take as possible.

In a recent study of 52 HIV(+) adults who were antiviral naive, patients were administered either DDI 300 mg 1x/day plus D4T 40 mg 2x/day, or DDI 200 mg 1x/d and D4T 30 mg 2x/day. Interim analysis of this study at week 16 showed a greater than 90% drop in HIV viral load from baseline for 91% of the patients, with greater than 75% of the patients achieving undetectable status. CD4 cell counts increased an average of 109 cells/mm3 as well. The interim data analysis concluded that DDI taken once daily in combination with D4T is well tolerated, has potent immunologic effects, and is a highly effective antiviral combination.

A second study looked at 15 HIV(+) patients who took AZT 300 mg 2x/day plus DDI 300 mg 1x/day (if the patient weighed more than 132 lbs) or DDI 200 mg 1x/day (if the patient weighed less than 132 lbs). At 6 months, HIV viral loads had declined greater than 99% and the CD4 counts showed an average increase of 162 cells/mm3 (from a baseline of 278 cells/mm3). These results indicate that, when used in combination with AZT, single-dose administration of DDI has similar efficacy to twice-daily administration of DDI.

Among patients who have enrolled in DDI once-daily dosing studies, no increase in gastrointestinal side effects, peripheral neuropathy, or pancreatitis has been reported. The results of these and other recent studies demonstrate that DDI, administered once daily as part of a combination treatment regimen, is effective and well tolerated.

DDI is also often combined with protease inhibitor and/or NNRTI medications. However, taking DDI and indinavir together is slightly problematic because the administration of these medications must be separated by at least 1 hour despite both of them being recommended to be taken on an empty stomach (indinavir can now be taken with a low-fat, low-protein snack). Does this sound confusing? It is.

To alleviate some of this confusion, Bristol-Myers Squibb, the drug's manufacturer, has funded studies which have proven that DDI is effective and well tolerated when taken 1x/day. This dosing regimen can simplify antiviral drug administration for both the patient and the physician. It is emerging as an attractive option for patients interested in simplifying their HIV treatment program.

Dosage: DDI 400 mg 1x/day, if your weight is greater than 60 kg (132 pounds). This dosage is best achieved by combining 2 150 mg tablets and 1 100 mg tablet taken at the same time. The recommended dosage is 300 mg 1x/day, if your weight is less 60 kg (132 pounds), or if 400 mg 1x/day is tolerated poorly.

Side effects: Peripheral neuropathy is one of DDI's common side effects. It can be prevented to a significant degree by following the nutritional guidelines on preventing peripheral neuropathy presented in Chapter 13 of this book. Indigestion, nausea, and diarrhea also occasionally occur. It is important that your physician evaluate any abdominal pain, nausea, and vomiting immediately, as these can be symptoms of pancreatitis.

Comments: DDI is a very effective antiviral medication which affords the convenience of once-daily dosing. It possesses significant antiviral activity and a reasonably low side-effect profile. It can be combined with almost all of the available antiretroviral agents. Diarrhea may be a problem when DDI is combined with nelfinavir. DDI/DDC combinations may also be problematic since both can cause peripheral neuropathy.

DDI/3TC combinations are not recommended since no additive benefit has been demonstrated. Hydroxyurea, a member of the miscellaneous antiviral category described below, has been shown in several small studies to significantly enhance DDI's antiviral benefit. This combination may prove useful in antiretroviral-experienced patients as a means of potentiating DDI's effect or as initial therapy in protease inhibitor-sparing regimens.

Alan

Alan works as a journalist for a local television station. When he first came to see me in early 1991, he had known about his HIV(+) status for about a year. Alan had always been extremely healthy and had a CD4 count of 756 cells/mm3, well within the normal range.

Alan's preference was to avoid using antiviral medications for as long as possible. Since his antiviral options at the time included only AZT, DDI, and DDC, I supported this desire. We instead chose to support his immune system aggressively with diet, vitamins, herbal therapies, exercise, and stress reduction.

Using natural therapies alone, Alan maintained excellent health and stability for over 5 years. His CD4 count and viral load remained stable, and he experienced no HIV-related symptoms. However, in late 1996 Alan's CD4 count dropped to 425 cells/ mm3. This was confirmed by a repeat lab test and also accompanied by a rise in his viral load to 118,000 copies/ml. Due to the negative trend these numbers were taking, I strongly recommended to Alan that he start dual-RTI (reverse transcriptase inhibitor) therapy with D4T/DDI. These 2 medications have been shown to be a powerful and well-tolerated antiviral combination.

You may wonder why I didn't elect to start Alan on a protease inhibitor. First, because Alan's CD4 count was well above 300 cells/mm3, I felt confident in choosing a conservative treatment program using a protease-sparing, dual-RTI combination. Second, because Alan takes excellent care of himself and follows an aggressive natural therapies program, I have confidence that his immune system has the ability to participate strongly in suppressing his viral infection. Third, Alan was completely asymptomatic. And fourth, because his viral load had only recently gone over 100,000 copies/ml, I believed that his infection was still within the mild-to-moderate range. Though I usually reserve dual-RTI treatment programs for viral loads below 50,000 copies/ml, I felt strongly that it would work in this situation. Sometimes you just have to go with your gut.

In addition, Alan's DHEA-S level had fallen to 144 ug/dl. This was below the optimal range of this important immune-enhancing hormone (the DHEA-S optimal range for men is 300 to 600 ug/dl). I therefore started Alan on an oral supplement of DHEA 100 mg 1x/day. Please see Chapter 11 for additional information on how to evaluate and treat hormone deficiencies in HIV.

During the next 2 years, after beginning dual-RTI therapy with only D4T/DDI, plus starting DHEA supplementation, Alan's CD4 count rose from 425 to over 1000 cells/mm3! His viral load quickly became, and still remains, undetectable.

These are dramatic effects. I see no reason to recommend a protease inhibitor or NNRTI medication to Alan at this time. I fully anticipate, when used in combination with his aggressive natural therapies program, the potent 2-drug combination of D4T/DDI will continue bringing Alan good health and stability for many months and probably years to come. By the time any changes to these medications are necessary, I anticipate that even more antiviral options will be available to choose from. Alan is also currently avoiding the potential side effects recently associated with long-term protease-inhibitor therapy (i.e., high cholesterol, liver abnormalities, elevated blood sugar levels, and lipodystrophy).

Alan is extremely pleased with his current situation. His immune system is as strong as it has ever been and he continues to plan for a long and healthy future. Alan is a clear example of healing HIV in action.

DDC (Hivid)

DDC is the third member of the reverse transcriptase inhibitor class to have been released. In the test tube, DDC exhibits extremely potent anti-HIV effects. Unfortunately, high doses of DDC produced painful peripheral neuropathy in early studies. Later studies utilizing lower dosages, showed a significant reduction in this side effect.

Dosage: DDC is usually prescribed at a dosage of 0.375-0.75 mg 3x/day.

It is important that the dosage chosen balance the need for a strong antiviral effect versus a healthy respect for DDC's ability to cause peripheral neuropathy. Since peripheral neuropathy is common in many HIV(+) individuals, the lower dosage may often need to be used. I once again want to mention that the side effect of peripheral neuropathy can be prevented to a significant degree by following the nutritional guidelines presented in Chapter 13 of this book.

Side effects: Peripheral neuropathy, mouth ulcers, rash, elevated liver enzymes, and low platelet counts.

Comments: DDC is now the least prescribed reverse transcriptase inhibitor partly because there are few studies testing it as part of a triple-combination antiviral regimen. DDC should not be totally ignored though, especially when your antiviral options are limited. If peripheral neuropathy is not a major symptom, and you have never taken DDC in the past, consider it a valuable treatment option.

D4T (Zerit)

D4T also belongs to the reverse transcriptase inhibitor family of antiviral medications. D4T became available in October 1992 as part of an expanded access program through its manufacturer, Bristol-Meyers Squibb. D4T is used as the foundation of many antiviral programs due to its ability to inhibit actively dividing, HIV-infected CD4 cells.

The actions of "nucleoside" reverse transcriptase inhibitors are best understood by dividing them into 2 subcategories. The first of these subcategories are drugs which target *actively dividing* HIV-infected CD4 cells. This subcategory includes AZT and D4T.

The second subcategory of nucleoside RTIs targets *resting* HIV-infected CD4 cells. This subcategory includes 3TC, DDI, DDC, and abacavir. By combining 1 drug from each of these 2 subcategories, both dividing and resting CD4 cells can be targeted. This achieves a more effective antiviral effect.

Protease inhibitors and/or NNRTIs can also be combined with drugs from both of the above-mentioned reverse transcriptor inhibitor subcategories to build highly potent antiviral combinations.

Dosage: 40 mg 2x/day if weight > 60 kg, 30 mg 2x/day if weight < 60 kg, and 20 mg 2x/day if peripheral neuropathy is present or occurs at the higher dosage.

Side effects: Peripheral neuropathy, anxiety, insomnia. Some patients have difficulty sleeping if D4T is taken close to bedtime. If this occurs, it is recommended that your second dose of D4T be taken at 6:00 P.M.

Comments: The combination of D4T and DDI was initially avoided because of concern that their additive toxicities might lead to an increased incidence of peripheral neuropathy. In general, this has not been observed. This is fortunate because the D4T/DDI combination has been shown to possess significant synergy and is associated with excellent viral load suppression and CD4 cell increases.

Multiple trials have studied D4T/DDI, and the results have been very positive. In my opinion, D4T/DDI is one of the strongest and best tolerated dual-RTI combinations currently available. Since dual-RTI therapy is commonly used in our practice to treat mild-to-moderate HIV disease, D4T/DDI is frequently my choice as the initial antiviral combination. When used in this situation, as long as peripheral neuropathy and/or gastrointestinal symptoms do not pose significant problems, the D4T/DDI combination has helped many of my patients maintain undetectable viral loads and clinical stability for extended periods of time. In addition, combining D4T and DDI with hydroxyurea (see miscellaneous category below) provides an extremely potent protease-sparing, triple combination of drugs.

D4T/3TC is another effective dual-RTI combination. These 2 medications afford a level of convenience and tolerability that is extremely favorable. The ability to take 1 pill of each 2x/day, with or without food, is very attractive. A large study recently showed that this combination affords a level of viral suppression equal to the more commonly prescribed combination of AZT/3TC (Combivir). Based on my clinical experience with dual-RTI regimens and these study results, I continue to view D4T/3TC as an extremely useful 2-drug antiviral combination. Finally, D4T can be combined with virtually all of the PI and/or NNRTI medications to build potent 3- and 4-drug antiviral programs.

Elliot

When Elliot and his wife Susan came into my office in 1995 for their initial consultation, they were extremely concerned. Elliot had probably been exposed to HIV from a blood transfusion in 1984 and had found out about his infection less than a month ago. Thankfully, Susan had tested HIV negative.

Elliot stated that his CD4 count was 465 cells/mm3 though his viral load had not yet been tested. He still felt well and had no symptoms. His examination was normal, and his demeanor belied nothing out of the ordinary.

1 week later, Elliot and Susan returned to review his labs. While his CD4 count remained stable in the 400s, his baseline viral load came back at 221,000 copies/ml. A repeat of this test yielded a similar result.

Despite a relatively normal CD4 count and the lack of any significant symptoms, it has been my experience that extremely high viral loads usually lead to the uncontrolled spread of HIV throughout the body. Therefore, I recommended to Elliot that he begin combination antiviral therapy with D4T/DDI immediately. In addition, due to a suboptimal DHEA-S level of 207 ug/dl, I started Elliot on a supplement of this naturally-produced hormone at a dosage of 200 mg 1x/day. The optimal DHEA-S level for an HIV(+) man is 300-600 ug/dl.

Last but not least, 2 intestinal parasites were identified with a comprehensive stool analysis and these were appropriately treated utilizing the parasite elimination protocol described in Chapter 8.

Utilizing the combination of D4T/DDI, it was my belief that Elliot could bring his viral load down to a more healthful level and more potent medications such as protease inhibitors could be saved for the future, if and when they might be more necessary.

After 6 months on the Healing HIV program, including D4T/DDI dual-RTI therapy, Elliot's CD4 count rose from 482 to 811 cells/mm3 and his viral load declined from 221,000 copies/ml to undetectable. Now, 3 years after beginning this program, his CD4 cell count has risen to over 1000 cells/mm3 with a continued undetectable viral load.

The comprehensive treatment of HIV includes much more than just prescribing antiviral medication. Optimizing intestinal health, supplementing immune-enhancing hormones, and the installation of hope and confidence (working with a patient's mental attitude) are integral components of a comprehensive approach to HIV care. As you can see from the results described above, this multidimensional treatment of HIV works extremely well.

Important point: The notable success of this 2-drug combination (D4T/DDI) is due to the comprehensive nature of Elliot's program. It includes a healthy diet, vitamin supplements, and efforts toward the reduction of stress in his life. When complementary therapies are combined with an effective antiviral strategy, a 2-drug regimen can sufficiently maintain a patient's good health and stability much longer than if no effort was put in this direction. I fully anticipate that Elliot's good health and stability are going to last a very long time.

3TC (Epivir)

3TC was approved for use in 1994. It is made by Glaxo Wellcome, the same pharmaceutical company which makes AZT. In fact, before protease inhibitors became available, AZT/3TC was the leading antiviral combination in use.

Multiple studies of this 2-drug combination have been performed which show that AZT/3TC works extremely well together. Though it was initially believed that adding 3TC to AZT monotherapy helped reverse AZT resistance, the long-term validity of this hypothesis has never been clinically proven.

Dosage: 150 mg 2x/day.

Side effects: Side effects to 3TC are rare but may include anemia, liver inflammation, and gastrointestinal upset.

Comments: Many studies of protease inhibitors have used AZT/3TC as the 2 RTI antivirals of the triple-drug combination. Most recently, a randomized, comparative study of AZT/3TC/indinavir (a protease inhibitor) versus D4T/DDI/indinavir showed both triple-combination regimens to have similar effects on viral load levels and CD4 counts over the first 6 months of available data. A second study which compared AZT/3TC/indinavir to D4T/3TC/indinavir also showed comparable viral suppression and CD4 count increases. The point here is that all of the 3TC-containing regimens mentioned above are highly potent and effective at suppressing viral replication.

3TC is well tolerated and easy to take, and combines well with most of the other antiviral medications. The only significant drawback to 3TC is the fact that resistance to this medication requires very few changes to the viral genome (genetic map). It can therefore develop quickly. It is important to understand that as soon as the viral load begins to rise significantly, resistance to 3TC has probably occurred.

In summary, 3TC is an excellent, easy-to-take, and well-tolerated antiviral medication.

Alex

Alex is a 42-year-old gay man who tested HIV(+) 8 years ago. He works as a hairdresser and lives a quiet, simple life. Although his initial CD4 count was 585 cells/mm3, his numbers steadily dropped to 255 cells/mm3 by the time he arrived at my office for his initial consultation. At the time, Alex complained of depression, severe fatigue, blurry vision, and some numbness and tingling in both of his feet. His viral load was 97,000 copies/ml. Since he felt his health beginning to spiral downward, Alex decided he needed to take a more active role in improving his health.

At our first visit, Alex voiced concern about his declining CD4 count. I recommended a full laboratory evaluation including hormone levels and a comprehensive stool analysis. Alex's blood tests showed a DHEA-S level of 163 ug/dl. This is below the optimal range for men (300-600 ug/dl). I therefore recommended he begin supplementation with DHEA at a dosage of 100 mg 1x/day. The rationale for using this hormone to stabilize and enhance immune functioning is presented in Chapter 11.

I was also not surprised that Alex's comprehensive stool analysis showed the presence of 2 intestinal parasites, Endolimax nana and Entamoeba coli. These organisms weaken the intestinal tract and are a source of chronic stress to the immune system. After Alex took my parasite elimination program for 10 days (see Chapter 8), they were completely eliminated. Alex's experience provides an example of how a chronic intestinal infection can be present for a long time without investigation or treatment by most other physicians.

Alex next met with our dietitian for a BIA analysis (body composition test) which showed that his body cell mass was only 91% of ideal. We recommended increasing his protein intake and starting a program of resistance exercise. Finally, in response to his persistently high viral load, Alex started on a dual-RTI antiviral combination with D4T/3TC.

Since our first visit, Alex's life has transformed dramatically. His fatigue, neuropathy, and blurred vision have completely resolved. His mood, appetite, and body cell mass are now normal. Most important, his CD4 count is once again over 500 cells/mm3 accompanied by a completely undetectable viral load. This stability has now been present for 3 years. Alex's viral load continues to remain undetectable and he has not needed to change his medications during this entire time.

Alex's story represents a simple but dramatic example of how significant improvement can occur within a relatively short period of time when using the Healing HIV program. Alex has achieved significant improvement using a minimum of medications because aggressive natural therapies enable his immune system to participate fully in healing HIV.

Abacavir (Ziagen)

Abacavir, formally known as GW1592, is currently in clinical trials. It is a reverse transcriptase inhibitor with potent activity against HIV. In antiviral-naive patients, the maximum median reduction in plasma viral activity during monotherapy studies with abacavir (300 mg 2x/day) was 1.7 logs (about 96%) at 4 weeks. Abacavir in combination with each of the 4 available protease inhibitors has been shown to reduce plasma HIV viral activity by approximately 2.0 logs (99%) at 4 weeks. Studies with abacavir in antiviral-experienced patients are presently ongoing.

In vitro studies have demonstrated synergy between abacavir, AZT, nevirapine, and amprenavir (an investigational PI). Additive effects were observed with 3TC, DDI, D4T, and DDC. Abacavir does not compete with DDI, 3TC, D4T, DDC, or AZT for intracellular activation.

In vitro resistance studies using abacavir alone have demonstrated that abacavir may not develop rapid high-level resistance. This may be due to the fact that abacavir requires multiple stepwise mutations before it develops high-level resistance. Cross-resistance studies have also demonstrated little cross-resistance between AZT, DDI, 3TC, DDC, and abacavir individually. HIV strains with resistance to multiple reverse transcriptase inhibitors do show increased resistance to abacavir.

Dosage: 300 mg 2x/day. Abacavir can be taken with or without food.

Side effects: Fatigue, abdominal pain, liver inflammation, nausea, fever, dizziness, and rash.

Important note: If a flu-like illness characterized by fatigue, malaise, low-grade fever, and/or rash occurs while taking abacavir, see your doctor immediately. This syndrome has been described in a small percentage of patients after beginning abacavir and can signify a hypersensitivity reaction to the drug. **If you stop abacavir due to these side effects, do not restart this medication. Serious, life-threatening reactions have occurred upon rechallenge.**

Non-nucleoside Reverse Transcriptase Inhibitors (NNRTIs)

In June 1996 the Antiviral Drugs Advisory Committee of the FDA recommended accelerated approval for nevirapine, the first non-nucleoside reverse transcriptase inhibitor (NNRTI) to receive such approval. NNRTIs attack the same enzyme targeted by the original class of antiviral drugs, nucleoside reverse transcriptase inhibitors, but interfere with it in a different way. While it is not entirely known how NNRTI medications work, it is known that they attack the structure of the reverse transcriptase enzyme.

More than 2500 NNRTI drugs have been screened and their resistance patterns mapped. While any antiretroviral drug used as monotherapy will cause some level of resistance within a short period of time, initial studies of monotherapy with NNRTI drugs indicated that viral resistance to them emerged quickly. This finding dampened early enthusiasm for the class of drugs as a whole.

Now that antiviral therapy using combinations of drugs is common practice, the development of resistance to NNRTIs can be delayed. While the amount of research data is somewhat limited, it is thought that resistance to 1 NNRTI drug usually results in some measure of cross-resistance to the entire class. However, despite the occurrence of in vitro resistance, clinical benefits are often seen to continue beyond the point when laboratory resistance is detected. The key to using NNRTIs is to combine them with at least 2 other potent antiviral medications.

Nevirapine (Viramune)

Nevirapine was the first NNRTI to be approved for the treatment of HIV disease. Recent studies demonstrate significant increases in CD4 counts as well as decreases in viral load when nevirapine is used as initial therapy in combination with 2 RTIs.

There are 3 advantages to using nevirapine in initial triple-therapy combinations such as D4T/3TC/nevirapine, D4T/DDI/nevirapine, AZT/3TC/nevirapine, AZT/DDI/nevirapine, or AZT/DDC/nevirapine. First, this medication is conveniently dosed at 1 pill 2x/day. Second, when given as part of a triple combination to a patient who has never taken antiviral medications before (antiviral naive), it is potent and usually well tolerated. Third, if used as initial therapy, it can preserve the protease-inhibitor category for future use.

The first clinical trial to report on NNRTI medications was presented at the 11th International Conference on AIDS in Vancouver (1996). Julio Montaner, an organizer of the meeting, presented publicly for the first time 12-month data on a trial of AZT/DDI/nevirapine vs. AZT/DDI vs. AZT/nevirapine. All 151 patients were treatment naive prior to study entry. The CD4 count at entry was 200–600 cells/mm3, the patients were all asymptomatic, and the mean viral load was 30,000 copies/ml.

Over 60% of the patients in the triple-combination arm (AZT/DDI/nevirapine) had undetectable viral loads (less than 500 copies/ml) at 12 months, findings similar to that seen at the time with protease inhibitor–containing combinations. In contrast, no patient in the AZT/nevirapine arm, and only 25% in the AZT/DDI arm, had undetectable viral loads at 12 months. The percentages of patients with viral loads below the ultrasensitive level (less than 20 copies/ml) at week 52 were 51% (AZT/DDI/nevirapine), 12% (AZT/DDI), and 0% (AZT/nevirapine) CD4 counts in the triple-therapy arm increased by 100 cells, which was sustained. Side effects were common but mild, usually a rash. Only 7 of the 102 patients taking nevirapine needed to discontinue therapy due to rash.

Dosage: 200 mg (1 tab) 1x/day for 14 days, then 200 mg (1 tab) 2x/day thereafter. This medication is begun at a dosage of 1x/day for the first 2 weeks to help prevent the occurrence of rash.

Side effects: Rash is, at present, a side effect common to the entire NNRTI class. It is often mild and fades over time. Sometimes the rash will need to be treated by your practitioner with allergy-suppressing medications. It is important for you to have any rash that develops after starting a new medication inspected visually by your health-care practitioner.

Comments: Nevirapine can be an effective contributor to a triple-combination regimen in patients who are beginning antiviral therapy. There are 3 important points to remember about nevirapine:

1) Although nevirapine is a potent antiviral medication, resistance can develop quickly and preclude later utilization of other medications within the NNRTI class.

2) Nevirapine increases the activity of the liver enzyme system responsible for clearing most protease inhibitors from the bloodstream. This means that *protease-inhibitor blood levels may become decreased when*

using this drug. At this point, the only protease inhibitor that requires a dosage change when taken in combination with nevirapine is indinavir (increased to 1000 mg 3x/day).

3) If your viral load does not become completely undetectable within the first 6 months of using an NNRTI for the first time, it is important to consider adjusting your medication program to prevent high-level resistance to the entire class from developing.

Jeffrey

Jeffrey knew of his HIV(+) status for 1 year when he first arrived at my office in 1996. During that year, he had experienced severe HIV-related symptoms. These included night sweats, fever, diarrhea, chronic fatigue, weight loss, sinus infections, and depression. He also described having several months of memory loss, confusion, and decreased libido. I remember Jeffrey stating that the past year had been one of the worst of his life. He was losing his way and really needed to get back on track. Recently, he had started meditating 1 or 2 times a day, and had even begun to "accept and embrace HIV as his spiritual challenge."

Jeffrey's initial lab testing revealed a CD4 count of 324 cells/mm3 and a viral load of 79,000 copies/ml. His comprehensive stool analysis showed the presence of 2 intestinal parasites, Endolimax nana and Blastocystis hominis. His hormone tests showed suboptimal levels of testosterone and DHEA. His body composition test revealed a borderline phase angle of 5.9 and a body cell mass that was only 88% of ideal (please see Chapter 9 for a complete description of body composition testing).

My initial recommendations to Jeffrey included starting vitamins and taking a DHEA supplement. I also asked him to eat more protein and progressively increase his resistance exercising to 3x/week. His intestinal parasites were treated with my parasite elimination program, and his diarrhea promptly resolved. Last but not least, I recommended that Jeffrey start taking an antiviral combination consisting of

D4T/DDI/nevirapine. I made this recommendation because of his declining CD4 count, high viral load, and HIV-related symptoms. This is a very potent 3-drug combination that is easy to take and tolerated well.

Some 2 months after beginning this program, Jeffrey returned for his follow-up visit. He could not believe how much better he was feeling in so short a time. His energy level, mental clarity, and sense of well-being had all improved dramatically, and he was no longer feeling depressed. In fact, Jeffrey told me that he never felt better in his life!

A repeat CD4 count and viral load test 6 months after starting the above program showed that Jeffrey's CD4 count had now risen to 510 cells/mm3 (up from 324), and his viral load had dropped from 79,000 copies/ml to undetectable. Over 2 years later, his CD4 count continues to remain above 500 cells/mm3 with an undetectable viral load.

By using a combination of RTI and NNRTI medications, the protease-inhibitor class of antivirals was preserved as a valuable future option. By integrating an aggressive program of natural therapies in combination with his drugs, Jeffrey is clearly on the path of healing HIV.

Delavirdine (Rescriptor)

Delavirdine was approved for the treatment of HIV in April 1997. Though similar in many ways to nevirapine, delavirdine is different in others. Delavirdine requires 3x/day dosing and does not penetrate the central nervous system as well. However, delavirdine *raises the levels of most protease inhibitors in the blood.*

Taking a drug that increases the blood level of protease inhibitors is more often associated with benefit than with harm. The drug can potentiate the protease inhibitor's antiviral effect without having to use more of it. In so doing, GI side effects such as nausea and diarrhea can be minimized.

Some patients with multidrug resistance have significantly benefited from this effect. Small studies have demonstrated that the use of a PI plus delavirdine as part of a "salvage regimen" (or "salvation regimen" as one of my patients prefers to call it), is associated with significant clinical benefit and CD4 cell increases.

Dosage: 400 mg (4 tablets) 3x/day. Delavirdine tablets can be mixed in 3 ounces of water and consumed as a slurry. Delavirdine may soon be able to be taken 2x/day in combination with some protease inhibitors. A study is currently underway looking at administering delavirdine and nelfinavir together in this fashion.

Side effects: Rash.

Comments: Given the large number of pills and the current 3x/day dosing schedule, I usually reserve delavirdine for second-line therapy. This is not to say that it isn't effective. When taken in combination with 1 or 2 protease inhibitors plus at least 2 RTIs, delavirdine significantly adds effectiveness to the regimen. Whether this is due to its increasing the blood level of the protease inhibitor, decreasing the virus's ability to kill CD4 cells, or a combination of the 2 is unknown. However, sometimes patients on 3 or more antiviral medications who were previously deteriorating often begin to stabilize upon adding delavirdine to their regimen.

Efavirenz (Sustiva)

Efavirenz (formerly known as DMP-266) is a new NNRTI medication that is currently only available through an expanded-access program. Individuals with less than 400 CD4 cells who have exhausted all other antiviral options can qualify for this program. Efavirenz is scheduled to be released in late 1998. This medication is highly attractive due to its high potency, once-daily dosing, and penetration into the central nervous system.

At the 12th World AIDS Conference in Geneva (1998), Staszewski and colleagues presented 24-week data from a Phase lll multicenter, open-label study looking at the antiviral effect and tolerability of 3 antiviral combinations: AZT/3TC/indinavir vs. AZT/3TC/efavirenz vs. the 2-drug combination, indinavir/efavirenz. This 3-arm study randomized 450 asymptomatic or mildly symptomatic HIV(+) patients, of which 85% were completely antiviral naive, to the above 3 arms. The mean CD4 count of the 3 groups was 345 cells/mm3 and the viral load at baseline was greater than 10,000 copies/ml.

At the 24-week analysis, all 3 groups demonstrated viral load decreases of at least 99% (2 logs) accompanied by CD4 cell increases of at least 150 cells/mm3. These numbers demonstrated an excellent response to all 3 combinations. However, the AZT/3TC/efavirenz group had a significantly higher percentage of patients with plasma viral loads suppressed below a detectable level (<400 copies/ml) when compared to the AZT/3TC/indinavir group (94.5% vs. 88.6%, respectively). When the AZT/3TC/indinavir and indinavir/efavirenz arms were compared, there was no statistically different effect on viral load suppression.

Discontinuation of efavirenz in this study due to side effects was relatively rare. All 3 groups tolerated their medications well; however, patients on the indinavir-containing combinations did report a higher incidence of gastrointestinal side effects, including gas, bloating, abdominal pain, and diarrhea.

The authors of this study concluded that AZT/3TC/efavirenz may offer antiviral-naive patients a potent alternative that can allow protease inhibitors to be saved for use as second line therapy. This strategy may help prevent or delay some of the side effect that have recently been associated with long-term PI therapy (see section below on Protease Inhibitors). The authors also mentioned that efavirenz, dosed once daily in combination with indinavir, may be an attractive initial 2-drug regimen for asymptomatic HIV(+) individuals to consider. Based on these study results, indinavir/efavirenz offers similar potency and durability as that seen with more commonly accepted 3-drug regimens (2 RTIs + 1 PI). The dosages used in this study were: AZT (300 mg 2x/day)/3TC (150 mg 2x/day)/indinavir (800 mg 3x/day); AZT (300 mg 2x/day)/3TC (150 mg 2x/day)/efavirenz (600 mg 1x/day); and indinavir (1000 mg 3x/day)/efavirenz (600 mg 1x/day).

A second study of 137 asymptomatic, antiviral-naive HIV(+) patients (DuPont Merck Protocol 005) tested the combination of AZT/3TC/efavirenz when compared to AZT/3TC/placebo. The 24 week data revealed that 100% of the 21 patients randomized to the triple combination with efavirenz showed undetectable viral loads compared to fewer than 50% of those randomized to the AZT/3TC plus placebo arm.

A subset of patients taking efavirenz in the above-described studies are participating in another study to test efavirenz's penetration into the cerebrospinal fluid (CSF). Maintaining adequate drug levels in this compartment of the body may help prevent HIV from seriously impacting the central nervous system. In this study, both plasma and CSF HIV viral loads were measured in patients taking efavirenz in combination with other antiviral agents. The mean plasma viral load at baseline was 52,963 copies/ml. After an average of 24 weeks of therapy, plasma and CSF viral loads were below the level of detection (< 400 copies/ml) in all 8 patients studied. This data suggests that efavirenz, in combination with indinavir or AZT/3TC, effectively suppresses HIV replication in both plasma and CSF.

Dosage: 600 mg (3 tablets) 1x/d. Take before bedtime to avoid lightheadedness or dizziness. The total dosage can be split into 2 tablets in the evening and 1 tablet in the morning if there is a problem with tolerability.

Side effects: Side effects of efavirenz include lightheadedness, dizziness, and dysphoria. These symptoms are less likely to happen if this medication is taken before bedtime and may resolve after a few weeks. Other side effects can include headache, nausea, diarrhea, and, similar to all the members of the NNRTI class, a rash. Due to its inhibition of the P450 liver enzyme system, efavirenz should not be taken concurrently with the following medications: Seldane, Hismanal, Propulsid, Halcion, or Versed. It has also been recently shown to lower saquinavir blood levels by 60% (see below). Efavirenz has also been found to cause birth defects in monkeys and should never be taken during pregnancy.

Comments: Efavirenz appears to be highly effective at suppressing HIV viral activity when administered as either a 2- or 3-drug combination. At present, it appears to be the most potent drug of the NNRTI class. It can be combined with indinavir and is probably also effective when combined with other protease inhibitors as well. Recent data has shown that efavirenz, when taken concurrently with saquinavir (Fortovase), lowers saquinavir blood levels by 60%. This combination of protease inhibitors is therefore not recommended.

Efavirenz penetrates the cerebral spinal fluid (CSF) and currently does not appear to require any dosage adjustment when used with most other medications. Due to the ease at which resistance can develop to any of the NNRTI medications, the only 2-drug efavirenz-containing combination that has been proven effective at this time is efavirenz 600 mg 1x/day plus indinavir 1000 mg 3x/day. More data is necessary before combinations with efavirenz other than those described above can be recommended.

Protease Inhibitors

The HIV protease enzyme cleaves long intracellular polypeptide strands into viral proteins. This process occurs during the final stage of viral assembly and is a critical step in the completion of HIV's life cycle.

Protease inhibitors as a class have demonstrated potent antiviral and clinical benefits when administered at all stages of HIV infection. Their effects have been most dramatic and sustained when they have been used in combination with at least 2 reverse transcriptase inhibitors. Their major limitations are intolerance, questionable penetration into the central nervous system, and the development of cross-resistance within the class.

Protease Paunch

Crix belly was the original term used to describe the phenomenon of increased abdominal girth often seen in patients taking protease inhibitors. It is now more appropriately referred to as *protease paunch,* since the phenomenon has been observed to occur in a proportion of patients taking all of the currently approved protease-inhibitor medications.

This syndrome is characterized by a redistribution of peripheral fat from the limbs and face to the organs and surrounding tissue of the abdomen. Less commonly, a fatty mass develops at the back of the neck between the shoulder blades. When this occurs, it is often termed a *buffalo hump*. Women may also experience a narrowing of the hips and enlargement of the breasts. Studies have estimated that, on average, 25% of patients taking PIs develop some degree of these changes.

The specific medical term for this syndrome is *protease inhibitor-induced peripheral lipodystrophy syndrome*. The mechanism for its occurrence is possibly linked to the metabolic effects that occur when these drugs are administered to HIV(+) individuals. These may include elevations of serum triglycerides, cholesterol, and glucose, as well as resistance to insulin and low testosterone levels. It is unclear at this point whether 1 or a combination of these factors causes this syndrome to occur.

The same morphologic changes associated with peripheral lipodystrophy are also common to a condition known as Cushing's syndrome. This syndrome is caused by an increased production of the adrenal hormone cortisol, usually as a result of an adrenal gland tumor. Extensive investigation has failed to find any evidence that the hormonal imbalances observed in Cushing's syndrome are present in PI-associated peripheral lipodystrophy.

At present, the prevailing hypothesis attributes the changes of PI-induced peripheral lipodystrophy to be related to insulin resistance and high levels of serum triglycerides. Researchers have also reported evidence that the PIs may interfere with a protein produced by the liver that clears lipids (fats) from the blood. This protein's molecular structure strongly resembles the active site of the HIV protease molecule. Protease inhibitor drugs may block the ability of this liver protein to clear fats from the blood with concomitant accumulation in the abdomen and other regions.

A similar syndrome of increased abdominal girth and metabolic changes has also been described in HIV negative subjects and has been termed syndrome X. Symptoms of syndrome X include obesity, glucose intolerance, hyperlipidemia, and below normal testosterone levels. It has also been reported in both men and women. Similar findings between HIV(+) individuals and those with syndrome X is cause for concern, since individuals with syndrome X experience an increased incidence of heart disease.

Many physicians are closely monitoring the elevations in serum triglycerides and cholesterol associated with PI-induced peripheral lipodystrophy and treating them when they are high. A healthy diet, avoidance of alcohol, and the use of medications such as gemfibrozil (Lopid) and clofibrate have been successfully used to lower blood lipids in many cases. It is also extremely important to exercise regularly and monitor your testosterone and DHEA levels (see Chapter 11). A small study looking at the use of recombinant human growth hormone (Serostim) to treat the morphologic effects of peripheral lipodystrophy (truncal obesity and buffalo hump) showed preliminary positive effects in all 4 study subjects. These data were presented by Torres and colleagues at the 12th World AIDS Conference in Geneva (1998).

The decision on how to best treat the metabolic and morphologic changes associated with PI therapy need to be individualized. When the changes are mild, little needs to be done in the short term. In more severe cases, frequent monitoring, nutritional counseling, and the lipid-lowering medications described above may be indicated. These decisions need to be made on an individualized basis after a thorough discussion with your physician.

Finally, cosmetic surgery such as liposuction and/or facial implants have in some cases achieved positive results. Other patients have been happy to trade a little bit of protease paunch, for the good health and stability that this class of medications can bring.

The following medications make up the currently available protease-inhibitor class of antiviral medications.

Saquinavir (Fortovase)

Saquinavir was the first protease inhibitor to become available toward the end of 1995. Although it is a well-tolerated medication with good potency in the test tube, the oral bioavailability of the old hard-gel formulation known as Invirase was extremely low. Only 4% of the orally administered drug ultimately made its way into the bloodstream.

The new soft-gel formulation, called Fortovase, has much improved bioavailability. Efficacy studies presented at the 12th World AIDS

Conference showed that when Fortovase is taken by protease inhibitor–naive patients as part of a triple-combination regimen, its effect is similar to that of other protease inhibitors. Because of its enhanced absorption and higher dosage, saquinavir blood levels are now 4 times what they used to be. Saquinavir is commonly taken in combination with other protease inhibitors, such as ritonavir, to further increase its level in the bloodstream.

Dosage: 1200 mg (6 caps) 3x/day. Saquinavir needs to be taken with a high-fat meal for optimal absorption.

Side effects: Nausea, diarrhea, headache, lipodystrophy, and liver inflammation.

Comments: Currently, very few individuals are taking the old, hard-gel formulation of saquinavir (Invirase). The new soft-gel formulation (Fortovase) is often combined with other protease inhibitors, most commonly ritonavir, to improve the overall efficacy of the treatment program. Common protease inhibitor combinations that include saquinavir are ritonavir 400 mg/saquinavir 400 mg both taken 2x/day, and nelfinavir 750 mg/saquinavir 600–1200 mg both taken 3x/day.

Ritonavir (Norvir)

Ritonavir is extremely potent, highly bioavailable, and has been shown to raise the blood level of many other medications, including other antiviral drugs. This effect occurs due to ritonavir's ability to inhibit the hepatic P450 CYP-3A enzyme system. This enzyme system clears many medications from the bloodstream.

When given as the sole protease inhibitor in a triple-combination regimen, ritonavir has been shown to cause significant side effects during the first few weeks of treatment. These may include nausea, vomiting, diarrhea, malaise, fatigue, and numbness around the mouth. The dosage of ritonavir may be adjusted over a 2-week period to lessen these side effects (see below). Ritonavir is also commonly prescribed in combination with saquinavir to increase saquinavir blood levels. When this combination is used, the ritonavir dosage is decreased to 400 mg 2x/day. This lesser dosage can help reduce some of ritonavir's side effects.

Dosage: 600 mg (6 capsules) 2x/day when taken as the sole protease inhibitor of a PI-containing regimen. 400 mg (4 capsules) 2x/day when taken in combination with saquinavir. Ritonavir must be kept refrigerated for long-term storage although a single dose can be kept without refrigeration for up to 12 hours.

Side effects: As mentioned above, adverse effects of ritonavir may include nausea, vomiting, diarrhea, flatulence, malaise, fatigue, and numbness around the mouth. These effects are usually worse during the first few weeks of ritonavir therapy and can be ameliorated by gradually increasing the dosage from 3 caps 2x/day to 6 caps 2x/day during the initial 2-week period. Additional side effects may include elevations in liver enzymes, cholesterol, and triglycerides; sometimes to extremely dangerous levels. Finally, there is a long list of medications which cannot be taken with ritonavir. Potentially life-threatening drug interactions may occur if ritonavir is taken with Seldane, Hismanal, Propulsid, Halcion, or Versed. If you are on ritonavir, never start a new medication, either over-the-counter or prescription, without first consulting your physician.

Comments: Many patients taking the recommended dosage of ritonavir (6 caps 2x/day) can tolerate this medication only for a limited period of time before experiencing some toxicity. These effects include elevated levels of blood lipids or liver enzymes that may be unhealthy if sustained over a long period of time. In addition, ritonavir can cause the blood levels of many other medications to become very high. Ultimately, some patients just begin to feel toxic when taking this medication.

Fortunately, these problems seem much less pronounced when ritonavir is prescribed at a lower dosage (4 caps 2x/day) in combination with saquinavir. When used in this fashion, the ritonavir/saquinavir combination represents a highly potent, usually well-tolerated antiviral combination.

Ritonavir is also being studied in combination with indinavir (see below). When this combination is used in my practice, I prescribe the following dosages of these medications: indinavir 800 mg (2 pills) 2x/day and ritonavir 200 mg (2 pills) 2x/day.

Indinavir (Crixivan)

Indinavir is a highly potent protease inhibitor with good oral bioavailability. When indinavir entered clinical trials, the antiviral effect of indinavir plus 2 RTIs was so dramatic that the criteria for evaluating antiviral regimens began to change. From this point on, researchers looking at the effect of antiviral combinations on HIV activity began to report the percentage of patients who achieved viral suppression to below detectable levels. The excellent results achieved by several large studies using indinavir as part of a triple-combination antiviral regimen set a new standard for antiviral therapy and are summarized below.

1) The Merck 020 study compared indinavir monotherapy with AZT/DDI and AZT/DDI/indinavir. After 24 weeks, patients in the triple-therapy arm had a viral load decrease of 3.1 logs (99.9%) and a CD4 cell increase of approximately 100 cells/mm3. Overall, 60% of the patients in the triple-therapy arm had undetectable amounts of plasma HIV RNA (undetectable viral loads), compared to an average of 15% for the other groups.

2) The Merck 035 study compared individuals taking indinavir monotherapy to AZT/3TC and AZT/3TC/indinavir. All patients had received prior treatment with AZT, but not with 3TC or a protease inhibitor. At 44 weeks, 83% of the patients taking the triple combination with indinavir had undetectable viral loads versus 0% in the AZT/3TC arm. At 120 weeks, over 80% of patients taking the indinavir triple combination still have undetectable viral loads.

3) The AIDS Clinical Trials Group 320 study looked at 1156 HIV(+) individuals with less than 200 CD4 cells and randomized them to receive AZT/3TC or AZT/3TC/indinavir. The results of the triple-combination arm were so successful that the study was prematurely stopped because of a 50% reduction in mortality in the indinavir-containing triple-combination arm.

These results helped establish protease-inhibitor, triple-combination therapy as the community standard for treating individuals with advanced HIV disease. Triple-combination antiviral therapy with protease inhibitors often brings viral activity to below detectable levels for a sustained period of time. This effect is probably responsible for the large decrease in opportunistic infections and mortality described in recent epidemiological studies.

Dosage: 800 mg (2 tablets) every 8 hours taken on an empty stomach or with a low-protein, low-fat meal (less than 300 calories, less than 6 grams protein, and less than 2 grams fat). If you are also taking the NNRTI nevirapine (Viramune), the indinavir dosage should be increased to 1000 mg every 8 hours. This dosage can be achieved using 2 400 mg tablets plus 1 200 mg tablet and is designed to counterbalance nevirapine's indinavir-lowering effect.

Though indinavir was originally recommended to be taken on a completely empty stomach, further studies have found that a low-protein (less than 2 gms), low-fat (less than 6 gms) low-calorie (less than 300 calories) snack does not significantly interfere with its absorption. Examples of these include a toasted bagel with jam, cornflakes with skim milk, apple sauce, crackers, a piece of fruit, and so forth. A complete listing of suggested light meal options has been compiled by the American Dietetic Association and can be obtained by calling Merck at 1-888-CRIXIVAN. Taking indinavir with a light snack may also diminish any nausea that may be associated with its intake.

Michael

Michael is a 38-year-old person with AIDS who complained of a long list of symptoms at his initial visit. The worst of these was constant pain in both of his legs. This symptom began 2 months before as a side effect to 1 of his antiviral medications. The pain was currently so severe that he could hardly walk. Not surprisingly, Michael was becoming more and more depressed. In his new patient questionnaire he wrote, "I feel that I am losing both of my legs and feet."

Michael next explained that his previous doctor wanted to "drill a hole in his chest." This was the way he interpreted his doctor's request to perform a lung biopsy stemming from Michael's 3-month history of cough and shortness of breath. A CAT scan had revealed a nonspecific abnormality that his physician wanted to biopsy with a large needle.

At that time, Michael had a CD4 count of 37 cells/mm3 and a viral load of 513,000 copies/ml. He also smoked 2 packs of cigarettes a day, drank extensively, and periodically used IV drugs, usually amphetamines.

Clearly, Michael presented a challenge. My initial suggestion was for him to begin my nutritional program for peripheral neuropathy, which includes high doses of vitamin B6, calcium, and magnesium (see Chapter 13). I also recommended that he begin a program of regular massage and meet with our dietitian to learn how to improve his eating and drinking habits. Furthermore, I recommended that Michael begin taking DHEA to correct a suboptimal level of this important immune-supporting hormone.

Our dietitian found Michael's body cell mass (lean muscle tissue) to be only 78% of ideal. She therefore recommended that he start consuming a high-protein diet with small, frequent meals and begin a gradually progressive resistance exercise program. Every practitioner at our clinic also continued to reinforce to Michael the importance of eliminating his alcohol consumption, decreasing his cigarette smoking, and discountinuing his use of HIV drugs.

Because of Michael's extremely high viral load, I strongly recommended that he begin adding back the antiviral medications which he had discontinued. I reassured him that I would use the lowest possible dosages of the safest drugs to achieve the goal of suppressing his viral load without producing side effects. Once again, I reiterated my philosophy that being on the right medication regime would enable him to feel better, not worse.

With this reassurance Michael restarted 3TC and indinavir (a protease inhibitor). After a 2-week period, he felt significantly better. The symptoms of his peripheral neuropathy continued to diminish as well, and he started to walk again without pain. I then recommended that Michael restart D4T, at a dosage of 30 mg 2x/day, since he was now taking the vitamins and minerals that could help protect his nerves from its potential toxicity.

Some 3 weeks later (6 weeks after our initial visit), Michael arrived in my office looking terrific. His energy had improved, he no longer had any cough or digestive complaints, and the pain in his legs had disappeared. I kept reinforcing to Michael that continued improvement in his health depended on his following a healthy diet and lifestyle, as well as continuing to abstain from alcohol, cigarettes, and IV drugs. By implementing these changes, he had already sent a positive, life-affirming message to his body, and it was responding in kind with more energy and a renewed sense of well-being.

When it comes to following this new diet and lifestyle program, Michael's behavior is definitely not perfect. Figuratively speaking, he sometimes slips and needs a helpful, supportive hand to regain his balance. However, he represents a perfect example of how a wellness-oriented treatment program can bring about tremendous improvement in an individual's health in a very short time. Because of the right mix of caring, reassurance, and aggressive natural therapies, Michael was able to safely add back all 3 of his antiviral medications, and achieve a level of health and well-being far superior to what he otherwise would have experienced had he continued to use antiviral drugs *alone*.

Michael's program will require continued hard work and fine-tuning. Giving up alcohol, IV drugs, and cigarettes has not been easy. But the work he is doing is paying off in better health, and has provided him, to use a common cliche, "a new lease on life."

Several recent studies presented at the 12th World AIDS conference in Geneva (1998) showed preliminary positive results using indinavir in combination with ritonavir + 2 RTIs. By adding ritonavir to an indinavir-containing regimen, indinavir levels are substantially elevated allowing indinavir to be taken 2x/day without regard to food. The most common dosages of these 2 PIs being studied is indinavir 800 mg (2 pills) and ritonavir 200 mg (2 pills) both taken 2x/day.

Merck originally requested that patients taking indinavir rigidly adhere to an every 8-hour dosing schedule or risk diminished antiviral effects. These criteria have been gradually relaxed as additional data describing indinavir's pharmacokinetics have become available. However, several small studies recently showed that taking indinavir 2x/day does not adequately suppress HIV replication. Taking indinavir 2x/day as the sole protease inhibitor in your program is therefore *not* currently recommended.

I have always told my patients taking indinavir that the most important priorities were: 1) Take the medication at least 3x/day, 2) Have as close to an empty stomach as possible, and 3) Strive to take the medication as close to every 8 hours as possible. By following these guidelines, the balance between adequate viral suppression and the ability to comply with complex dosing schedules can best be achieved.

Side effects: Indinavir's most significant side effect is kidney stones, which occur in approximately 4% of patients per year. The risk of kidney stones can be reduced if patients drink a large amount of fluid every day. The official recommendation is to drink 1.5 liters of fluid per day (6 glasses), but I have always instructed my patients to drink closer to 3 liters (12 glasses) of fluid per day (not coffee or alcohol which can be dehydrating). Very few of my patients who follow this recommendation develop kidney stones. Other side effects of indinavir may include elevated bilirubin levels, nausea, abdominal distention, lipodystrophy, and dry skin.

Comments: When indinavir was first released, the treatment of HIV infection took a quantum leap forward. Within 1 year of its availability, over 75,000 HIV(+) individuals were taking this medication. Indinavir remains a potent therapeutic option for HIV(+) individuals needing to begin protease-inhibitor therapy.

Howard

Howard knew he was HIV(+) for only 3 months before first arriving at my office. As a 40 year old detective on the police force of a large city, he was admittedly uncomfortable about disclosing his status to anyone without a need to know. Howard was also reluctant to take antiviral medication because of the possible side effects they might cause.

Unfortunately, Howard very much needed to consider taking these medications. His CD4 count had dropped to 34 cells/mm3, and his viral load was very high at 170,000 copies/ml. These numbers indicated a severely weakened immune system that was progressively being broken down by his HIV infection.

Howard also complained of gastrointestinal discomfort that had bothered him for several years. His symptoms included chronic bloating, cramping, and urgent bowel movements. He was also routinely having night sweats.

Howard otherwise took very good care of himself. He had been clean and sober for 21 years, quit smoking 10 years ago, exercised regularly, meditated, and took a multitude of vitamins and other nutritional supplements. Despite an aggressive natural therapies program, his immune system was continuing to lose ground.

Shortly after Howard began receiving care at our clinic, he met with our dietitian and had his body composition tested. This test showed that he was dehydrated. Fortunately, his body cell mass and phase angle (see Chapter 9) were still close to ideal levels. After 6 weeks on an enhanced nutritional program, these numbers improved further.

Next, a comprehensive stool analysis was obtained which showed that Howard an infection with a parasite called Giardia lamblia. There is no way of knowing how long this organism was present, but it may explain most (or all) of Howard's chronic GI symptoms during the past several years. Howard followed my parasite elimination protocol, and his chronic intestinal symptoms quickly resolved.

Another part of Howard's evaluation included testing his anabolic hormone levels. These tests revealed suboptimal levels of both testosterone and DHEA. He was prescribed topical testosterone cream and an oral DHEA supplement and his energy level and state of well-being greatly improved.

Finally, I recommended triple-combination antiviral therapy with

D4T/3TC/indinavir. My goal was to bring Howard's viral load down to an undetectable level and allow his immune system to rebuild. Despite his initial fear and hesitation, Howard has tolerated these medications extremely well. Interestingly, if we had not improved Howard's diet and treated his intestinal parasites, he may not have tolerated these medications as well. A worsening of his GI symptoms due to a combination of intestinal parasites and a protease inhibitor might have required us to make a change in his medications. This might have caused him to go through the list of available antiviral medications too quickly. Fortunately, this scenario did not occur.

A month after beginning the Healing HIV program, Howard's CD4 count rose from 26 to 113 cells/mm3; 3 months after his initial visit, his CD4 count was 285 cells/mm3 with an undetectable viral load. Just as important, Howard felt much better now than he had in several years.

Part of the reason for Howard's improved sense of well-being, despite being on multiple medications, is the significant nutritional and hormonal support he is receiving. He is also very pleased to be working with practitioners who strongly support his belief that natural therapies are a vitally important part of his treatment program.

Nelfinavir (Viracept)

Nelfinavir was the fourth protease inhibitor to be approved by the Food and Drug Administration. Its initial dosing recommendations were fortunate in that it could be taken 3x/day with food. This dosing schedule was invariably easier than that initially recommended for indinavir, which was 3x/day on an empty stomach. Furthermore, the pattern of mutations associated with nelfinavir resistance was initially reported to be different from that seen with the other PIs. It was therefore proposed that patients who developed resistance to nelfinavir could subsequently be treated successfully with other protease inhibitors. Clinical studies are presently ongoing to fully evaluate this claim. At the present time, triple-combination therapy with nelfinavir appears to be as potent and beneficial as triple-combination therapy with either indinavir or a ritonavir/saquinavir combination.

A randomized, double-blind, placebo-controlled study of nelfinavir was begun in February 1996 (ACTG 511). This study enrolled 297 antiviral-naive HIV(+) patients who had viral loads of greater than 15,000 copies/ml. The mean CD4 count of the participants at baseline was 288 cells/mm3. The mean baseline viral load was 153,044 copies/ml. All patients received triple-combination therapy with AZT/3TC/placebo, AZT/3TC/nelfinavir 500 mg 3x/day, or AZT/3TC/nelfinavir 750 mg 3x/day.

Results out to 52 weeks show that HIV viral loads remain below 500 copies/ml in 81% of the patients treated. This data also suggests that patients who begin nelfinavir with a low baseline HIV viral load have a better and more durable response. At 1 year, 90% of the patients who began the study with a viral load of less than 50,000 copies/ml were still doing well. Data from this study out to 21 months shows that approximately 70% of patients on nelfinavir continue to have viral load levels below the limit of detection (400 copies/ml).

Dosage: The recommended dosage of nelfinavir is 750 mg (3 capsules) 3x/day, to be taken with a high-fat meal. Ongoing studies are currently investigating the efficacy of taking nelfinavir on a 2x/day dosing schedule. The amount currently being studied is 1250 mg (5 capsules) 2x/day taken with food. The preliminary results of these studies look extremely promising. Based on preliminary data, recent clinical observations, and the long half-life of the drug, I am currently recommending 1250 mg (5 capsules) 2x/day to the majority of my patients.

Side effects: Nelfinavir is generally well tolerated. Its major side effect is diarrhea or loose stools, which are experienced by 10 to 30% of the patients taking this medication. This side effect often occurs within 1 to 2 hours of taking the drug and can be ameliorated with antidiarrheal agents such as loperamide (Immodium) or diphenoxylate hydrochloride (Lomotil). Recently, a small study showed that coadministration of nelfinavir with 1 to 2 capsules of a high potency digestive enzyme (containing amylase, protease, and lipase, e.g., Ultrase) may significantly lessen the diarrheal symptoms associated with this drug. The results of this study are also supported by numerous anecdotal reports. Other side effects which may occur while taking nelfinavir include abdominal distention, elevated liver enzymes, and flatulence. However, in controlled clinical trials, only 1.6% of patients taking nelfinavir needed to discontinue it due to diarrhea and only 4% needed to stop it due to any adverse effect.

Comments: Nelfinavir-containing triple-combination regimens are highly effective. Given the probability that nelfinavir can be prescribed 2x/day with meals, this medication also affords a high level of convenience. The complexity of HIV antiviral dosing regimens has reached such an unpleasant level that it is doubtful pharmaceutical companies will release any antiviral medications which need to be taken more than 2x/day in the future. This is a welcome occurrence!

While the gastrointestinal side effects of nelfinavir therapy can be somewhat ameliorated by taking symptom-reducing medication, it is also important to make sure that there are no intestinal parasites present in the gut (please see chapters 7 and 8). It is also very important that there is nothing in your diet contributing to the occurrence of diarrhea. Foods which can contribute to diarrhea include fats, oils, fried foods, and to some degree, dairy products. It may also be helpful to increase your intake of cooked whole grains and other sources of soluble fiber, such as oat bran. These help to absorb excess water in the colon and lessen diarrhea symptoms.

Finally, recent data from an ongoing clinical trial suggests that salvage therapy using other protease inhibitors may in fact be effective after virologic failure occurs while on nelfinavir therapy. These data seem to support some of the manufacturer's initial claims that starting protease-inhibitor therapy with nelfinavir might allow subsequent and relatively effective treatment with other protease inhibitors. In this study, 26 patients who had 2 consecutive viral loads of greater than 5000 copies/ml while taking nelfinavir, were switched to a regimen consisting of ritonavir 400 mg 2x/day and saquinavir 400 mg 2x/day, plus D4T and 3TC. These patients had taken nelfinavir for an average of 56 weeks. They had a mean viral load of 46,000 copies/ml and a mean CD4 count of 200 cells/mm3 prior to switching therapy. Some 24 weeks after switching from nelfinavir-containing regimens to the D4T/3TC/ritonavir/saquinavir combination, 68% of the patients (13/19) had viral loads below 500 copies/ml. This data suggests that some patients who take nelfinavir and develop subsequent resistance to it may benefit from treatment with other PIs.

Miscellaneous Antiviral Medications

Hydroxyurea (Hydrea)

Hydroxyurea is a medication that has previously been used for the treatment of cancer. It also decreases the intracellular pool of raw materials used by the HIV virus as building blocks for viral replication. When the supply of these building blocks is diminished, the potency of DDI, and possibly of the other RTIs as well, is enhanced.

Dr. Franco Lori, who performed early in vitro work on hydroxyurea in Robert Gallo's laboratory, has also conducted a few small clinical trials. His data demonstrates that the combination of hydroxyurea and DDI exhibit antiviral activity often greater than that seen with DDI alone. Lori has also reported on 1 patient who, after receiving DDI, hydroxyurea, and indinavir for 6 months, had a viral load that continued to remain below the limit of detection several months after all antiviral therapy was discontinued. In the largest study to date involving hydroxyurea, 144 patients are participating in a trial comparing D4T/DDI/hydroxyurea to D4T/DDI/placebo. The 12-week data suggest a superior antiviral response in the hydroxyurea group that approaches a 99% decline in viral load when compared to baseline. In addition, the percentage of patients with viremia suppressed below the limits of detection was greater in the hydroxyurea-treated group (54%) when compared to the placebo-treated group (28%).

Trials to date with hydroxyurea have only included patients who are either naive or limited in their treatment experience to DDI. Despite fairly significant drops in viral load, increases in CD4 counts have been modest. This phenomenon is probably due to hydroxyurea's tendency to suppress bone marrow function. Its effect on CD4 counts should therefore not be considered as important as its effect on diminishing viral loads.

Dosage: 500 mg (1 tab) 2x/day.

Side effects: Nausea, fatigue, low red blood cell count (anemia), low white blood cell count (neutropenia), low platelet count (thrombocytopenia). May interact negatively with AZT due to additive toxicities.

Comments: Hydroxyurea may be effective in a variety of situations. One of these is when DDI has been used in the past, developed some measure of resistance, and is used again in combination with hydroxyurea. In this situation, low-level resistance that has developed to DDI may be able to be overcome.

A second situation in which hydroxyurea can also be effective is as part of an initial triple combination also containing D4T/DDI. Based on preliminary results mentioned above, the combination of D4T/DDI/hydroxyurea may allow HIV(+) individuals to begin highly effective antiviral therapy without needing to use either a PI and NNRTI medication. This strategy can preserve these classes of medications for future use when they may be more necessary.

Individuals with significant anemia or low white blood cell counts are wise to avoid hydroxyurea due to its negative effects on bone marrow health. In addition, due to this effect, CD4 cell increases may not be as robust as would otherwise be seen with a triple-combination regimen not containing this medication.

Finally, more data is expected shortly to determine whether hydroxyurea's effect on lowering viral load is as potent when it is combined with other RTIs such as D4T, 3TC, DDC, and abacavir, as it is with DDI.

Adefovir (Preveon)

Adefovir is the first member of a new class of antiviral medications called "nucelotide" reverse transcriptase inhibitors. Given that this class of antiviral agents inhibits reverse transcriptase in a somewhat different fashion than AZT and its relatives, it may be effective in patients who have developed resistance to these other drugs. Also, this medication is active against other viral infections, including CMV, hepatitis B, and Epstein-Barr virus.

At the 12th World AIDS Conference in Geneva (1998), Kahn and colleagues at the University of California, San Francisco, presented 48-week data from a multicenter, randomized, double-blind, placebo-controlled study of adefovir vs. placebo in addition to a stable combination of other antiviral medications. The study participants had a median HIV viral load of 9800 copies/ml and a mean CD4 count of 326 cells/mm3. Some 39% were receiving a protease inhibitor as part of their baseline antiviral program. Treatment with adefovir was associated with a steady decline in mean viral load by week 24, compared with no change in the placebo group. This difference was statistically significant. The decline in viral load was maintained during the following 24 weeks of open-label use. There was no statistically significant increase in CD4 counts when compared to the placebo group. These data demonstrate that adding adefovir to the treatment of HIV(+) patients on otherwise stable combination-drug regimens results in a statistically significant decline in HIV viral load that persists for at least up to 48 weeks.

At the present time adefovir is only available through a research study or as part of an expanded access program provided by its manufacturer, Gilead Sciences. As of June 1998, more than 5,000 HIV(+) individuals have taken this medication in clinical trials. Approval for its wide use is anticipated sometime in mid-1999.

Dosage: 60 mg 1x/day. Adefovir is taken in combination with L-carnitine, a nutritional supplement, at a dosage of 500 mg 1x/day because of its tendency to lower carnitine blood levels.

Side effects: Serious adverse events have affected 4% of patients taking adefovir in clinical trials. Gastointestinal events (1%) and kidney events (1%) have been the most common. Other side effects have included liver inflammation, electrolyte abnormalities, nausea, and diarrhea. The most common renal side effect has been leakage of protein into the urine. It is important to analyze a urine sample every several months to monitor your kidney function while on adefovir therapy.

Comments: Adefovir represents the first of a new class of medications for the treatment of HIV infection. Its positive aspects include once-daily dosing, an unusual mechanism of action, and the ability to simultaneously inhibit multiple viral infections. It may also take a long time for HIV to develop resistance to adefovir. The most common situation in which I use adefovir in my practice is as part of a newly initiated combination of antiviral medications in patients who have developed resistance to other antiviral agents.

Antiviral Drug Combinations Not Recommended

RTIs

AZT and D4T	*Reason:* Competitive inhibition; decreases effectiveness of each.
3TC and DDI	*Reason:* Similar resistance pattern; recent study showed no increase in effect for the combination.
D4T and DDC	*Reason:* Additive toxicities may cause peripheral neuropathy.
DDI and DDC	*Reason:* Additive toxicities may cause peripheral neuropathy.
3TC and DDC	*Reason:* Competitive inhibition; decreases effectiveness of each.

PIs

saquinavir/indinavir	*Reason:* Competitive inhibition; decreases effectiveness of each.
saquinavir/efavirenz	*Reason:* Efavirenz causes a 60% decrease in saquinavir levels.

Chapter Six

Clinical Treatment Scenarios

I offer the following treatment scenarios as thought-provoking examples of commonly encountered clinical situations. The choice of which antiviral medications to use in each of these situations is not always clear. There are often several options which may all work well. The best choice takes into account the patient's previous experience with each antiviral medication, their personal philosophy on medication use, and their sensitivity to medications in general.

Scenario #1

The antiviral-naive patient

John has never taken antiviral medications in the past. However, he has been experiencing a progressive decline in his CD4 count from 550 to 350 cells/mm3 during the past 12 months, and currently has a viral load of 12,000 copies/ml. Otherwise, he takes very good care of himself and is already following an aggressive natural therapies program.

Though John's viral load is relatively low at 12,000 copies, the fact that his CD4 count has progressively declined indicates that his immune system is losing ground. Since his natural therapies program is maximized, I would strongly recommend that he add antiviral medication to his present program.

In this situation, I do not see the addition of antiviral medications as a sign of failure. They have clearly become necessary at this point and will serve to strengthen John's overall treatment program. When used in this fashion, antiviral medications can help suppress HIV activity to a level which allows his immune system to rebuild.

My initial goal is to raise John's CD4 count back to at least 500 cells/mm3. I also want to suppress his viral activity to an undetectable level (< 500 copies). Furthermore, I would hope that whatever medication program we choose, we would not need to make any changes for at least 2 to 3 years. These are all realistic goals that are commonly achieved in my practice when antiviral medication is added to an existing program of aggressive natural therapies.

After thoroughly discussing with John his philosophy on the use of antiviral medication in general, and also discussing any physical conditions he has which might be exacerbated by their side effects, I would suggest 1 of the following treatment options:

Potential Antiviral Combinations*

2 Drugs	3 Drugs	4 Drugs
D4T/3TC	D4T/3TC/nevirapine	D4T/3TC/ritonavir/saquinavir
D4T/DDI	D4T/3TC/nelfinavir	AZT/3TC/ritonavir/saquinavir
AZT/3TC	D4T/3TC/indinavir	
AZT/DDI	D4T/3TC/efavirenz	
AZT/DDC	D4T/DDI/nevirapine	
	D4T/DDI/efavirenz	
	D4T/DDI/hydroxyurea	
	AZT/3TC/nevirapine	
	AZT/DDI/nevirapine	
	AZT/3TC/nelfinavir	
	AZT/3TC/indinavir	
	AZT/3TC/efavirenz	

* I have chosen to exclude abacavir as an initial choice in this situation due to a lack of extensive treatment experience with this newly available RTI antiviral medication.

Comments

As you can see from the above list, there are many possible options to consider for antiviral therapy in this situation. All of the above combinations can be taken 2x/day with the exception of those which contain indinavir which is a 3x/day medication. Though 2x/day dosing of nelfinavir is currently in clinical trials and showing positive preliminary results, taking this medication 2x/day has not been formally approved by the FDA.

Since this patient is deciding to commit to taking antiviral medication potentially for the rest of his life, convenience and ease of use are important factors. Compliance studies have shown that 2x/day dosing achieves greater than 90% compliance, while 3x/day dosing diminishes compliance to around 65%. Convenient regimens are therefore greatly preferred because they mean fewer missed doses.

Before deciding on which treatment program to recommend, I want to take into consideration John's general philosophy with regard to medication use. If he would like to be conservative when taking these medications, a 2-drug regimen combined with an aggressive natural therapies program can usually bring the viral loads of patients with mild-to-moderate HIV infection down to undetectable levels for periods greater than 2 years. *I define mild-to-moderate HIV infection as a CD4 count greater than 300 cells/mm3 in addition to a viral load less than 50,000 copies/ml.*

Utilizing this philosophy, 1 of the 2-drug, dual-RTI combinations listed above can enable 2 entire classes of antiviral medications to be saved for future use when they may be more necessary (protease inhibitors and NNRTIs). It also allows the initial medication regimen to be as simple and well tolerated as possible. Finally, it affords the opportunity for more effective, and potentially safer medications, to be studied and released while the initial 2 drugs are being used.

I often sit with my HIV(+) patients who are currently on dual-RTI therapy and discuss how well they have done during the past several years. Virtually all are stable, free of medication side effects, and very pleased at how many medication options they still have at their disposal. Their list of available treatment options remains long.

Conversely, many patients in the community who have been highly aggressive with antiviral treatments from the start of this epidemic have not had stellar results. Many have exhausted their list of treatment options too quickly, or are currently dealing with serious side effects caused by an overuse of these medications (e.g., diabetes, hyperlipidemia, peripheral neuropathy, liver abnormalities, and lipodystrophy syndrome). A conservative treatment approach clearly offers many long-term advantages when used to treat mild-to-moderate HIV disease.

When using dual-RTI therapy, I try to squeeze as much time as possible out of the initial combination of drugs (potentially 2 to 3 years) before making a change. If and when the initial 2 medications need to be discarded, the patient can switch to a new 2- or 3-drug regimen for another long run of potent viral suppression. This philosophy allows the patient with mild-to-moderate HIV infection to go through the list of available antiviral medications *as slowly as possible,* while continuing to maintain excellent health and stability. Remember, this philosophy *only* works when an aggressive natural therapies program is used in conjunction with these medications.

In most standard physician practices, 2-drug antiviral combinations have not been found to provide long periods of potent viral suppression. There have also been several published studies that have looked at comparisons between dual versus triple antiviral drug regimens. They all show that 2-drug regimens provide relatively short periods of viral suppression. *Our experience is completely different!* I attribute this difference to the fact that we combine aggressive natural therapies programs with standard medications, *and* with our zealous commitment to eliminating all cofactors that can potentially stimulate HIV activity (please see clinical scenarios #5 and #6 described below). These interventions support the immune system's role as a partner in suppressing HIV activity. We need to attend not only to the virus *but to the immune system within each individual* as well. A strong immune system can then participate fully in enhancing the effects of whichever antiviral medication program a patient is taking.

Most standard physicians have a difficult time believing the success we have had utilizing this approach. This stems in part from their lack of experience with what natural therapies can do. They are skeptical because they have never seen them work. They are also skeptical because there is a shortage of published research data on the benefits of combination programs such as ours. Hopefully, this situation will change.

Joe

Joe can trace his HIV exposure to 1981. Since that time, he has remained healthy except for a brief hospitalization for bacterial pneumonia in 1990. Joe has always taken very good care of himself and is a sensitive and successful middle-aged architect.

In 1992, Joe tested HIV(+). Not long after, he came to my office for his initial consultation. At that time, Joe's CD4 count was 363 cells/mm3. Unfortunately, viral load testing was not available at the time.

Joe had never been tested for intestinal parasites. It is standard procedure in my practice to screen every new patient for intestinal parasites with a comprehensive stool analysis. Despite being asymptomatic, Joe's test identified the presence of 3 intestinal parasites, including Entamoeba coli, Blastocystis hominus, and Endolimax nana. Joe was treated with the Parasite Elimination Program (see Chapter 8), and a repeat stool test came back completely normal.

Joe began the Healing HIV program, including vitamin supplements, herbs, acupuncture, exercise, and aggressive stress management in 1992. His CD4 count steadily climbed to 460 cells/mm3 within 1 year without taking any antiviral medication. Joe and I also continued discussing measures that would further reduce his stress at work, and by mid-1994 his CD4 count had risen to above 500 cells/mm3.

In mid-1995, Joe's CD4 count gradually began to decline. Despite an aggressive natural therapies program, his CD4 count dropped to 326 cells/mm3 by the fall. At this point, Joe could no longer answer yes to the 3 questions which I believe signify clinical stability. These are:

1) Are you relatively asymptomatic? (This was still true for Joe.)

2) Is your CD4 count greater than 300 cells/mm3 and stable or improving ? (Joe's CD4 count was 326 cells/mm but was steadily declining.)

3) Is your viral load low (at least under 20,000 copies/ml and preferably less)? (Joe's viral load was now significantly elevated at 167,000 copies/ml.)

Due to the gradually progressive decline in his laboratory parameters, I recommended that Joe begin dual-RTI therapy with D4T/3TC toward the end of 1995. Joe agreed to start these medications without hesitation. At the same time, Joe's testosterone and DHEA levels were found to be low and we therefore supplemented these hormones appropriately (see Chapter 11). Since that time, Joe has tolerated his medications extremely well, he has had no side effects, and he feels better now than before he began them.

Since starting D4T/3TC 3 years ago, Joe's viral load has been undetectable on only 2 occasions. Usually it ranges between 500 and 2000 copies/ml. Most physicians who specialize in treating HIV feel *very* strongly that achieving an undetectable viral load is essential if you are to prevent the quick emergence of resistant virus to the medications you are taking. Most physicians would also have *strongly* recommended that Joe add a protease inhibitor or switch to a triple combination when this first occurred.

I sympathize with this view. Several recent studies on 2-drug versus 3-drug antiviral combinations have shown that 3-drug combinations are superior at achieving an undetectable viral load and maintaining a long duration of response. However, the fact that I, and my colleagues at The Wellness Center in San Francisco, continue to see tremendous benefit with dual-RTI therapy in mild-to-moderate HIV infection suggests that the Healing HIV program is able to enhance our patient's immune response to a level which allows dual-RTI therapy to work effectively.

It has been *more than 3 years* since Joe began D4T/3TC dual-RTI therapy. His most recent follow-up visit showed that he his CD4 count was now up to 1159 cells/mm3 (from a starting value of 326), with his viral load holding steady at 1925 copies/ml (down from an initial value of 167,000). Joe remains stable due to his strong, well-supported immune system.

Joe is very pleased that he only needs to take 2 pills, 2x/day (aside from his vitamin supplements) to manage his HIV infection. He has also experienced no side effects and continues to feel healthier now than ever in the past. Joe is looking forward to a long, happy, and productive life as he continues to heal from HIV.

When used in mild-to-moderate HIV disease, our patients are currently achieving durable viral suppression with dual-RTI therapy for at least 2 to 3 years, Again, I define mild-to-moderate HIV disease when a patient has a CD4 count greater than 300 cells/mm3 *plus* a viral load less than 50,000 copies/ml. In Joe's case, I took the liberty of implementing dual-RTI therapy despite the fact that his viral load was greater than 50,000 copies/ml for 2 reasons. First, I knew how compliant he was with his natural therapies and stress-reduction programs. Second, he strongly desired to take as few antiviral medications as possible. Our decision to use only 2 drugs to treat HIV at this time has clearly produced satisfactory results.

Individuals who want to be more aggressive with medications, or who are unwilling to make the prescribed changes in diet, lifestyle, and stress necessary to follow the Healing HIV program, should strongly consider taking triple-combination therapy based on the current Department of Health and Human Services, Committee on Antiviral Guidelines (see Fig. 4.1 on page 31).

Triple-combination antiviral therapy will ensure that you are suppressing HIV viral activity as much as possible. The risk of breakthrough is therefore low. Predictably, this aggressive philosophy may allow the greatest time before needing to change your antiviral regimen. However, if your HIV disease is mild-to-moderate, the main reason to consider postponing triple-combination therapy in favor of dual-RTI therapy is to avoid side effects which could lessen your quality of life. These can include diarrhea, liver inflammation, kidney stones, diabetes, lipodystrophy syndrome, GI discomfort, plus others.

As you can probably gather, there is not a single path for every patient to follow. These decisions need to be made with the counsel of an open-minded, nonjudgmental physician. Once you are well informed, it is best to choose your course from a place of inner peacefulness, clarity, and calm. Do not feel pressured or forced. Once you have decided on the path you want to follow, it is important to believe that you have made the right decision, and to embrace it with spirit and grace.

<u>Scenario #2</u>

A patient on dual-RTI therapy whose viral load has begun to rise from a previously undetectable level

James has been on D4T/3TC dual-RTI therapy for 2 1/2 years and has tolerated this regimen extremely well. His CD4 count is 450 cells/mm3 and though his viral load had been completely undetectable, his most recent test came back at 2500 copies/ml.

This situation presents no cause for alarm. The first point I need to make is that "a single test does not a trend make." What a shame it would be if due to a lab error, James were to discard his antiviral program and switch to a new combination of drugs. This would cause him to begin going through the list of available antiviral options too fast.

Instead of rushing to switch medications, James and his doctor need to begin searching for the possible reason (or reasons) why his viral load increased. In addition to such factors as a recent immunization or ongoing infection, there may be 1 or more cofactors suppressing his immune system which, *if corrected,* could decrease his viral load to undetectable once again.

<u>Elimination of Cofactors Checklist</u>
1) Herpes infections
2) Intestinal parasites
3) Unhealthy intestinal environment
4) Low protein intake

5) Inadequate antioxidant vitamins

6) Hormonal imbalances

7) Substance abuse

8) Emotional distress

These 8 cofactors constitute a checklist to help review the completeness of your comprehensive treatment program. If they are not *all* adequately addressed, the potential for increased viral activity exists. *This statement is true whether you are taking antiviral medication or not.*

I always review this checklist with my patients at their quarterly follow-up visits to make sure they are addressing all of the above-stated factors. As you will see, doing this helps us avoid totally relying on antiviral drugs to control the virus's activity. Most important, eliminating these cofactors can ensure that your medications work as well, *and for as long,* as possible.

Since immune system cells that are infected with HIV produce large amounts of viral particles when stimulated, completely eliminating the activity of other infections can minimize HIV replication. At the 5th Conference on Retroviruses and Opportunistic Infections (Chicago, 1998), a study was presented which showed herpes viral activity occurs even in the absence of visible herpes lesions. This study also demonstrated that, in patients with a history of herpes infection, the group taking daily suppressive acyclovir therapy (800 mg 3x/day) had HIV RNA viral loads less than one-third that of the control group subjects not taking daily suppressive acyclovir therapy. The authors of this study stated that they believed a lower dosage of acyclovir would produce similar results.

This study supports my recommendation that anyone who is HIV(+) with prior exposure to genital herpes or herpes zoster infection (shingles) take daily suppressive therapy with either acyclovir (Zovirax) 400 mg 2x/day or valacyclovir (Valtrex) 500 mg 1x/day. These are exceptionally safe, well-tolerated medications that can be taken for long periods of time by generally healthy HIV(+) patients.

Another easy way to eliminate a potential cofactor is to increase the amount of protein you consume each day. This single intervention can correct a hidden deficiency and often reverse a potent cause of immune suppression. The average recommendation for protein consumption for an HIV(+) individual is obtained by multiplying your body weight in pounds by 0.6. This gives you the minimum number of grams per day required to keep your immune system strong. After making this calculation, many people realize that they are not getting the necessary amount of protein to remain healthy and stable with HIV. Increasing your protein intake may also directly boost your CD4 count. (Please see Chapter 10 for additional information on this important subject.)

Any of these 8 individual cofactors, and often several of them combined, may be the reason a patient's viral load begins to rise. Eliminating as many of them as possible will help your viral load remain completely suppressed on as few drugs as possible. Furthermore, eliminating these cofactors can return a slightly increased viral load back to undetectable once again. *I have seen this happen many times.* It is essential to review the "Elimination of Cofactors Checklist" frequently, especially if your antiviral medications are not suppressing your HIV viral load to as low a level as you would like.

What Should James Do Now?

After instituting measures to eliminate all of the above-listed cofactors, there are 3 possible scenarios James may experience: 1) His viral load may return to undetectable when checked 1 or 2 months later. 2) His viral load may continue to stay in the range of 500 to 10,000 copies/ml. 3) His viral load may progressively rise to greater than 10,000 copies/ml. I will address each of these scenarios below.

1) *The patient's viral load returns to an undetectable level when checked 1 or 2 months later.* This is the simplest scenario to address. James makes a few, fine-tuning adjustments to his program which are effective, and can now continue taking the same medications for an additional period of time. In this scenario, I would advise James to continue taking his current dual-RTI combination, and try to squeeze as much time as possible out of it. This will allow newer and more effective medication options to continue becoming available.

2) *His viral load continues to remain in the 500 to 10,000 copies/ml range.*

In this scenario, as long as James's CD4 count remained relatively stable at above 300 cells/mm3, I would not change his medications at this point. Instead, I would continue to closely monitor his lab values and request that his viral load and CD4 cell count be checked every 2 months instead of every 3.

Furthermore, I would continue to review the "Elimination of Cofactors Checklist" with James at future visits. Hopefully, we can find additional ways to strengthen his immune system and return his HIV infection to an undetectable level once again. I have seen this happen many times, either by reducing stress, adding protein, starting antioxidant vitamins, or eliminating a hidden infection with intestinal parasites.

As long as James's CD4 count remained greater than 300 cells/mm3 with a stable, fairly low viral load, there is no reason to switch his drugs. This would only hasten the speed at which he exhausted his currently available treatment options. At this point, I am trying to squeeze as much time as possible out of his current regimen before I discard it in favor of the next. This approach gives us the most time for additional treatment options to be released. Since I have never had an HIV(+) patient become ill with a CD4 count above 300 cells/mm3 and a viral load less than 10,000 copies/ml, I am very confident that James's good health will continue despite the persistence of low-level viral activity.

I know this is a controversial position. Most physicians and patients feel uncomfortable tolerating any level of detectable viral activity, especially if there are good medication options to switch to. However, you need to have *faith* in your immune system's ability to keep you healthy and stable as long as your CD4 count exceeds 300 cells/mm3, even if you have a small amount of persistent viral activity. If James can squeeze another year of good health and stability out of the 2 drugs he is currently taking, he will use up his drug options much more slowly and tremendously benefit down the road.

The only exception to this rule would be if James's viral load had risen to a detectable level while taking his first protease inhibitor or NNRTI medication. In this situation, switching early to a new antiviral combination might prevent high-level resistance from developing to either of these general classes of medications. Hopefully, by switching quickly (within 3 to 6 months), undetectable status can be regained and viral sensitivity to 1 or both of these classes can be retained. I would *first* make sure that any possible cofactors had been eliminated *before* switching the drugs. Please see scenario #4 for more information on how to address this specific situation.

3) *His viral load continues to rise and becomes greater than 10,000 copies/ml.* If this situation were accompanied by a decline in James's CD4 count to below 300 cells/mm3, I would strongly recommend taking action. This situation clearly indicates that the current 2-drug antiviral regimen has lost its effectiveness. It is best discarded and replaced with a new antiviral combination.

The way to decide whether the new intervention should be with 2 or 3 drugs is similar to the initial decision-making process. It is based upon the individual's belief system, his sensitivity to medications in general, his ability to follow a complex medication regimen, the aggressiveness of his natural therapies program, and the number of his remaining antiviral options.

During the past 2 years, while James was taking dual-RTI therapy, 5 new medications became available. It is now a more appropriate time for him to "hit the virus hard." At this point, and in this situation, I would therefore recommend he begin a triple-combination regimen with 3 completely new drugs. We will hopefully not need to make a change in his new antiviral program for at least several more years. Additional treatment options will invariably become available during this time as well, *keeping him ahead of the virus.*

Keith

Keith is the 48-year-old CEO of a San Francisco clothing manufacturing company. He tested HIV(+) in the late 1980s and has remained healthy and stable during the past 10 years without needing to take any antiviral drugs. Although his stress level is too high, Keith eats a healthy diet, takes nutritional supplements, exercises regularly, and otherwise follows a healthy lifestyle.

In November 1995, Keith came to see me for his initial visit. Upon reviewing his most recent lab tests, Keith was surprised to learn that during the past 6 months his viral load had increased from undetectable to over 200,000 copies/ml! His CD4 count, however, remained stable at 750 cells/mm3.

Before impulsively starting Keith on triple-combination antiviral therapy, as most other physicians might have, I asked him a few important questions. These included his state of health when he had his blood drawn, whether the tests were from the same lab, and whether he had received any recent immunizations.

These questions are important for several reasons. First, concurrent infections such as intestinal parasites, herpes outbreaks, influenza, and others can affect these tests. Second, results from different laboratories can cause CD4 counts and viral load values to vary tremendously. Third, immunizations (flu, tetanus, and possibly others) can often increase your viral load for up to 12 weeks. Changes in your medication program, when based upon these errant values, may be unnecessary and counterproductive.

In response to my questions, Keith revealed that he had received a flu shot approximately 3 weeks prior to having his most recent blood test. We therefore decided to postpone starting any antiviral medications at that time, since his viral load was possibly elevated from the flu shot. I asked Keith to return for a repeat blood test in a month.

Keith's viral load dropped from 215,000 to 50,000 copies 1 month later without the use of antiviral medication. Unfortunately, his CD4 count also dropped from 750 to 574 cells/mm3. This probably occurred as a result of his viral load being so high during the previous month. Since Keith's CD4 count was still in a healthful range, and we had recently begun an aggressive program of natural therapies, I decided to wait 2 additional months before recommending that Keith go on combination antiviral therapy for the rest of his life.

We met 2 months later, with Keith still not on antiviral medication, to review his new lab values. His tests now showed a viral load which had declined to 12,000 copies/ml and a CD4 count that had climbed back to 621 cells/mm3 (from 574)!

Some 3 months after that and a full year after the initial extremely high value of >200,000 copies/ml, Keith's viral load was once again undetectable and his CD4 count had risen back to 735 cells/mm3. This level of success was achieved without the use of any antiviral medication. Keith's lab results have continued to remain stable for an additional 18 months.

Keith's health has also greatly improved during this time. After 15 years of chronic diarrhea, this symptom has completely resolved. He has also experienced tremendous improvement in his asthma. His program of aggressive natural therapies has clearly contributed to this success.

What did we accomplish by not beginning triple-combination antiviral therapy based on 1 aberrantly high viral load? We saved the usefulness of these medications for an indefinite period of time. We avoided the occurrence of potential side effects, and we saved Keith and his insurance company $25,000/year in drug costs, lab tests, and doctor visits for as many years as Keith continues to remain stable without them.

Of course, Keith's case is just one example of how an aggressive program of natural therapies, combined with a little patience, can produce a successful outcome without needing to use antiviral medication. Accordingly, patients who have a stable CD4 count, a low viral load, and are currently asymptomatic may want to examine whether they really need to start or change antiviral medication at this time. It may be far wiser to ride your current wave of stability as long as possible and save these tremendously valuable medications for later, when their use may become more necessary.

Scenario #3

A case of acute HIV infection (acute retroviral syndrome)

Renee just found out that she is HIV(+). She knows her exposure most likely occurred 2 months ago during an episode of unprotected sex with someone she met at a party. Within 3 weeks of that night, she felt fatigued and began to have fevers and night sweats that lasted for a month. Her last HIV test was negative a year ago. Based on her history, it is almost certain that this recent sexual encounter exposed her to HIV. A blood test confirmed this suspicion.

Comment: This patient is currently experiencing what is known as acute retroviral syndrome. She had a flu-like illness which occurred approximately 1 to 4 weeks after exposure to HIV. The next statement is very important: **if you are relatively sure you have been exposed to HIV within the past 6 months, it is important to be very aggressive with your treatment and quickly begin a triple-combination antiviral drug regimen.**

The reason for this departure from my usual conservative treatment guidelines is that HIV infection behaves very differently during the first few months when compared to after the infection has matured.

During the first few months of acute HIV infection, the virus is rapidly extending itself throughout the immune system. It is infecting CD4 cells at a very fast rate. These are the cells the immune system needs to remain healthy in order to control the infection later on. If a large percentage of them become infected with HIV, as occurs within the first few months after initial exposure, the immune system's ability to manage the infection over the long term will become significantly compromised. That is why HIV is such a challenging virus for the immune system to control. The cells it needs to control it progressively become infected and destroyed.

However, if you begin triple-combination antiviral therapy *at a point before HIV fully extends itself throughout the CD4 cell line,* the immune system gains a great advantage. It can retain its ability to effectively fight the infection and, *in combination with antiviral drugs,* possibly eradicate it completely from the body.

This is an exciting possibility. And given what we currently know about how HIV behaves, it would be a shame not to act aggressively in this situation. An acutely suppressed HIV infection behaves much differently than one which has extended itself throughout the body.

Scenario #4

A case of early resistance to a protease inhibitor or NNRTI medication

Trevor began a triple-combination antiviral regimen approximately 5 months ago. It was his first use of antiviral medications. The reason he began taking these drugs was because his CD4 count had progressively declined over the past year from 425 to 275 cells/mm3. His viral load had also risen to 150,000 copies/ml. I believe his intervention was appropriate.

After beginning AZT/3TC/indinavir 5 months ago, his CD4 count again rose to 450 cells/mm3 (from 275) accompanied by a decline in his viral load to 15,000 copies/ml (from 150,000). Otherwise he is asymptomatic, but decided to see me for a second opinion.

Comment: With lab values that have improved so quickly, it would be easy to have a false sense of security in this situation. Personally, I would have expected his viral load to become completely undetectable soon after beginning this potent 3-drug cocktail.

My thinking in this situation is very straightforward. The first protease inhibitor you take (or the first NNRTI medication) is going to provide you the greatest amount of suppression because your viral strain has never been exposed to this drug class before. If you do not achieve undetectable status quickly, at least within the first 3 to 6 months, the emergence of a resistant strain of HIV will probably occur. This will lessen the antiviral effect of any drugs chosen from this class in the future.

Before changing Trevor's medications, I would ask the following important question: "Why did a proven triple-combination regimen such as AZT/3TC/indinavir not work perfectly well in a previously antiviral-naive patient?" For the answer to this question, I would refer you to the "Elimination of Cofactors Checklist" repeated below.

<u>Elimination of Cofactors Checklist</u>

1) Herpes infections
2) Intestinal parasites
3) Unhealthy intestinal environment
4) Low protein intake
5) Inadequate antioxidant vitamins
6) Hormonal imbalances
7) Substance abuse
8) Emotional distress

In scenario #2, I discussed how eliminating cofactors can improve your immune system's ability to suppress HIV. Suffice it to say that each of these cofactors can put stress on your immune system, thereby stimulating HIV activity. If a state of incomplete viral suppression is present, *whether you are on antiviral medication or not,* you may need to address and correct 1 or more of these factors. I cannot overemphasize the importance of eliminating these stimulants to HIV activity. The majority of the remaining chapters in this book are devoted to helping you understand how each of these factors weaken the immune system, as well as showing you how to eliminate them.

If all efforts have been made to identify and eliminate the above factors, and despite these efforts Trevor's viral load continues to remain at or above 15,000 copies/ml, switching to a different regimen, or adding additional medications, will raise the chances of achieving complete and long-term viral suppression. The key here is not to wait any longer than 6 months. Otherwise, cross-resistance will develop, and the next combination of antiviral medications will not work as well.

My Recommendations
If Trevor's viral load continues to remain high despite eliminating all of the above cofactors, my recommendation would be that he switch to 1 of the following new antiviral combinations:

- D4T/3TC/ritonavir/saquinavir
- D4T/3TC/nelfinavir/saquinavir

- D4T/DDI/nelfinavir/saquinavir
- D4T/DDI/hydroxyurea/nelfinavir
- D4T/DDI/nelfinavir
- D4T/abacavir/nelfinavir

If we implement this change of medications in a quick and decisive manner, it will most likely suppress Trevor's viral infection to an undetectable level. If this occurs, it will preserve the effectiveness of the PI class of antiviral medications into the foreseeable future. I would not switch Trevor to an NNRTI-containing regimen at this time *because I would like to preserve at least 1 entire class of potent antiviral medications for future use.*

In summary, Trevor needs to make several adjustments to help him avoid losing the entire protease-inhibitor class of medications to resistance. These include rapidly ensuring that his infection is not being stimulated by any of the above cofactors and changing his current medication program if his elevated viral load persists beyond 6 months.

Scenario #5

A case of multidrug resistance

Rob has been HIV(+) for the past 16 years and taken virtually all of the currently available antiviral drugs. Though he appears well and has a CD4 count of 240 cells/mm3, his viral load is 108,000 copies/ml on a 5-drug antiviral regimen. His current antiviral medications include AZT/3TC/delavirdine/nelfinavir/saquinavir. This combination includes 2 RTIs, 1 NNRTI, and 2 PIs.

Though he appears well, Rob has anemia (a low red blood cell count) neutropenia (a low white blood cell count), and frequent diarrhea. Otherwise, he has no complaints. Rob is interested in what his best option is for his next antiviral medication program, and when to begin it.

The Next Antiviral Program

Clearly, the process of choosing Rob's next antiviral program is complex.

Because he is clinically stable, the ability to squeeze a few additional months from his current antiviral program exists. This extra time may prove valuable later on.

The first step in choosing a new antiviral program is to collect a thorough antiviral drug history. A sample antiviral drug history form for this patient is included in Fig. 6.1. This form enables the patient and practitioner to identify which drugs still retain potency against HIV and therefore still remain on Rob's list of current antiviral options.

Figure 6.1

ANTIVIRAL DRUG HISTORY FORM
(Clinical Scenario #5)

Drug Combination	Dates	Side Effects	Level of Resistance *
AZT monotherapy	many yrs	neutropenia	high
3TC combinations	many yrs	none	high
DDI combinations	1–2 yrs only	mild GI symptoms	moderate
DDC combinations	6 mos only	neuropathy	high
D4T combinations	2 yrs only	minimal	moderate
Saquinavir	presently on it	none	high
Ritonovir	6 mos	severe diarrhea	moderate
Indinavir	6 mos	mild diarrhea	low (VL 2500)
Nelfinavir	presently on it	mild diarrhea	moderate
Nevirapine	never taken	—	—
Delavirdine	1 yr	none	high
AZT/3TC/Delavirdine Nelfinavir/Saquinavir	6 mos	mild diarrhea and neutropenia	moderate

* None, Low, Moderate, or High

When making up a list of current antiviral drug options, one begins by assigning a priority level to each potential drug based on the following guidelines:

1) *Priority level 1: A drug from a previously unused class of antiviral medications.* Each class of antiviral medications inhibits HIV activity in its own way. A drug from a class which has never been used has the least chance of encountering viral resistance. Drugs with this priority level will have the most potency when included in a new antiviral program. They are given the highest priority (priority level 1). Examples include 1) using a PI when one has never been used before; 2) using an NNRTI when one has never been used before; or 3) using a "nucleotide" RTI such as adefovir, a completely new class of antiviral agent, since it has never been used before.

2) *Priority level 2: An individual drug that you have never taken before.* Even though the possibility of cross-resistance exists throughout any given class of antiviral agents, the greatest chance of efficacy exists with a drug that your HIV viral strain has never encountered before. Examples of this situation include 1) taking indinavir (Crixivan) though you have previously tried and failed other PIs (saquinavir, ritonavir, or nelfinavir); 2) taking efavirenz (Sustiva) though you have previously failed 1 of the other NNRTI drugs (nevirapine or delavirdine); 3) taking DDI (possibly in combination with hydroxyurea); or 4) taking abacavir (Ziagen) though AZT, 3TC, and D4T have all developed resistance. The priority score for this category of medications is priority level 2.

3) *Priority level 3: Antiviral drugs that may have worked moderately well in the past but were discarded prematurely due to other reasons.* In our desire to achieve undetectable viral loads, many patients and physicians discard drugs which, though working fairly well at the time, have not achieved what is considered the virologic holy grail, "an undetectable viral load." Although it may have seemed like the right thing to do at the time, a review of why you discarded each of your previous antiviral medications may disclose a drug that still holds some benefit. These drugs can be added to your list of antiviral options as priority level 3. Examples include 1) using indinavir if an indinavir-containing 3-drug combination was changed due to a viral load that only decreased to 2500 copies/ml; 2) taking half-dose D4T if full-dose D4T initially worked but was discarded because of peripheral neuropathy (numbness or pain in the extremities)

that has subsequently resolved; 3) reintroducing DDI in combination with hydroxyurea, which has been shown to enhance its antiviral effects.

4) *Priority level 4: Antiviral drugs you have taken and failed in the past but have not been on for a long time.* Although it is known that HIV can quickly regain resistance to a drug you have taken in the past, the ability for this to occur with a drug you took over 5 years ago may not be as great as with a drug you have taken in the more recent past.

There have not been any research studies that address this particular question. However, clinical experience reveals this to be a reasonable assumption. I would still like to see a study designed to determine whether drugs discarded 5 years ago, when used as part of a salvage regimen, have a better chance of working than drugs discarded only a year ago.

An example of this particular strategy would be to reuse D4T/DDI, which was discontinued more than 3 years ago, because it has not been used for the greatest period of time when compared to the other RTI options. This combination should not be used alone but combined with other drugs on your currently available options list. Drugs in this category should be added to your antiviral options list as priority level 4.

5) *Priority level 5: Antiviral drugs which you have failed in the past due to resistance but which may still possess some clinical utility due to their ability to decrease viral fitness.* The discussion of "viral fitness," contained in scenario #6 describes how HIV needs to progressively contort its structure to develop resistance to a multitude of antiviral medications. Although still able to replicate, it often loses its ability to effectively kill CD4 cells. This situation may explain why a person with a high viral load (greater than 20,000 copies/ml) can often maintain a stable CD4 count. The viral particles being produced, though detectable, may be defective in their ability to kill CD4 cells. This fact supports my recommendation that you continue to take your antiviral medications even if your viral load is high, but only if you are tolerating them well.

Examples of this strategy include 1) restarting delavirdine after failing efavirenz (due to side effects) though you have taken delavirdine in the past; or 2) adding 1 or 2 RTIs that you are able to tolerate to a new regimen to force the virus to remain in a mutated state. This may keep it "less fit."

I would admit this strategy of choosing antivirals is more hopeful than scientific, but there is anecdotal experience to support its rationale. We need to see additional research studies on this subject to test this strategy or a lab test which can accurately measure viral fitness. Please see the next clinical scenario for a more thorough description of this topic. Drugs in this category possess the least proven benefit and can be listed as priority level 5.

Antiviral Drug History Form

An example of the antiviral drug history form for this patient was provided in Fig. 6.1. In many instances, it may be impossible to recall all of your dates and antiviral combinations. An example of a more complete antiviral history is shown in Fig. 6.2. A blank antiviral drug history form is provided for your personal use in Appendix 7.

Figure 6.2

ANTIVIRAL DRUG HISTORY FORM
(General Example)

Drug Combination	Dates	Side Effects	Level of Resistance *
AZT monotherapy	4/89 – 6/91	fatigue	high
AZT/DDI	6/91 – 6/92	fatigue, gas	high
AZT/DDC	7/92 –12/92	neuropathy	moderate
D4T monotherapy	1/93 – 2/95	neuropathy	moderate
D4T/3TC	3/95 – 3/96	neuropathy	moderate
AZT/3TC/saquinavir	3/96 – 9/96	fatigue	high
D4T/nevirapine/indinavir	10/96 – present	neuropathy	none

* None, Low, Moderate, or High

Though not entirely complete, the information recorded in Rob's antiviral history form is adequate and allows us to compile the following list of antiviral options from which to choose his next program:

Antiviral Options	Priority Status
Efavirenz (Sustiva)	1
Adefovir (Preveon)	1
Hydroxyurea (Hydrea)	1
Abacavir (Ziagen)	2
DDI (Videx)	3
D4T (Zerit)	3
Indinavir (Crixivan)	3
Ritonavir (Norvir)	3

Rob's best "next program" will best include at least 1 drug from each of the 4 different antiviral classes. These classes include RTIs, NNRTIs, PIs, and the class I refer to as miscellaneous. The miscellaneous class currently includes adefovir, a "nucleotide" RTI (as opposed to "nucleoside" RTIs like AZT, DDI, 3TC, etc.) and hydroxyurea, which is an antimetabolite that has been shown to enhance the antiviral effect of DDI (and possibly other RTIs). I would also order a genotype resistance lab test to gather as much information as possible before coming up with my final recommendation. See Appendix 2 for a review of this testing method.

Antiviral Recommendations for Rob

	Drug Name	Class	Dosage
Core program	Efavirenz (Sustiva)	RTI	3 pills 1x/day
	Adefovir (Preveon)	Misc.	1 pills 1x/day
	Indinavir (Crixivan)	PI	2 pills 2x/day*
	Ritonavir (Norvir)	PI	2 pills 2x/day*
plus either:	Hydroxyurea (Hydrea)	Misc.	1 pill 2x/day
	DDI (Videx)	RTI	2 tabs 2x/day
or:	Abacavir (Ziagen)	RTI	2 pills 2x/day
	D4T (Zerit)	RTI	1 pill 2x/day

* Dosage adjusted because of 2-PI combination.

One reason I would favor the D4T/abacavir option over DDI/hydroxyurea for this patient's new program is that he is currently experiencing anemia and neutropenia. Hydroxyurea can potentially cause bone marrow suppression, thereby exacerbating these conditions.

This regimen, though complex, achieves several important goals. First, it gives us medications from each of the 4 different antiviral categories. This strategy suppresses viral activity from several different angles, thereby increasing our chances of effective inhibition. Second, it does not include any medications with toxicities that might exacerbate Rob's current symptoms. Third, no medication needs to be taken more than 2x/day. This improves both his compliance and quality of life.

When he is ready to start this program, I would ask Rob to start 1 of these 2 regimens and then check a viral load in 2 to 4 weeks. If this test comes back less than 5000 copies/ml, I would continue the regimen he started and recheck the viral load 2 weeks later. If the initial viral load came back significantly greater than 5000 copies/ml, I would continue adding additional medications to his program in an attempt to achieve undetectable viral activity. The reason I would be very aggressive in this situation is because Rob is virtually out of medication options at this point. I want his program to succeed so other effective medications may have a chance to be released while he is taking these.

The reason I would not ask Rob to start this new regimen *immediately* is because I want to exhaust the utility of his current medication program *completely* before starting his new one. Because he is clinically stable and feels well, and recently had one of his highest CD4 cell counts in years (395 cells/mm3), I hesitate to discard his current program just yet. If his most recent lower CD4 count was either a lab error or a "temporary dip" in his numbers, we would be discarding his current program prematurely, before it had completely exhausted its usefulness.

I would therefore ask Rob to return for a repeat CD4 count in 1 month. If his numbers improved, I would keep him on his current regimen as long as possible. In this fashion, we can squeeze as much additional time as possible out of his current medication program, as newer drugs come closer to availability. If a declining trend in his numbers becomes clear, our next program has already been chosen and is ready to go.

Note: Anemia and neutropenia can be compensated for by using injectable red and white blood cell growth factors (Procrit and Neupogen). By giving an injection of 1 or both of these substances 3x/week, low red and white blood cell counts can often be raised back to normal levels. Hydroxyurea might then become a more attractive treatment option.

Scenario #6

Another case of multidrug resistance

Laurie has also taken most of the currently available antiviral medications (see Fig. 6.3). In 1989 she started AZT monotherapy with a CD4 count of 685 cells/mm3. This treatment lasted for 3 years as her CD4 count continued to decline.

When DDI was released, her physician switched her to DDI monotherapy, but Laurie developed neuropathy to this medication after 6 months. Because of her neuropathy, she could not take DDC, so she went off all antiviral medication for a year. Her CD4 count progressively fell during this time and, after developing an infection with Pneumocystis pneumonia in 1994, her physician placed her back on AZT in combination with 3TC (Epivir), the newest available antiviral. On AZT/3TC, her viral load stayed at about 30,000 copies/ml for the next 6 months. When protease inhibitors were released in 1995, Laurie tried saquinavir, ritonavir, indinavir and nelfinavir in succession, all with limited success. Despite aggressive pharmaceutical intervention, Laurie has never has attained complete suppression of her viral infection.

Presently, Laurie is taking the following 5 antivirals: AZT/3TC/ nevirapine/ritonavir/saquinavir. Her CD4 count is 85 cells/mm3, her viral load is 120,000 copies/ml, and she does not feel well. This combination includes 2 RTIs, an NNRTI, and 2 PIs. On this regimen, she is experiencing fatigue, anemia, neutropenia (low white blood cells), frequent sinus infections, and has diarrhea that is barely controlled by the medication diphenoxylate hydrochloride (Lomotil). Fortunately, her antivirals can all be taken 2x/day with meals, though she is always nauseated after taking them.

Figure 6.3

ANTIVIRAL DRUG HISTORY FORM
(Clinical Senario #6)

Drug Combination	Dates	Side Effects	Level of Resistance *
AZT monotherapy	4/89 – 6/92	fatigue	high
DDI monotherapy	7/92 – 1/93	neuropathy	moderate
Off all drugs	2/93 – 2/94	—	—
AZT/3TC	3/94 – 3/95	fatigue	high
AZT/3TC/saquinavir	3/95 – 3/96	fatigue	high
AZT/3TC/ritonavir	3/96 – 9/96	nausea	high
D4T/3TC/indinavir	10/96 – 4/97	neuropathy	moderate
D4T/3TC/nelfinavir	4/97 – 8/97	diarrhea	moderate
AZT/3TC/nevirapine ritonovir/saquinavir	9/97 – present	fatigue diarrhea nausea	high

* None, Low, Moderate, or High

Comments: Although this patient's situation is extremely complex, it is not uncommon. Many patients took sequential monotherapy starting with AZT in the late 1980s, then moved to dual-RTI (reverse transcriptase inhibitor) therapy in the early 1990s, only to try 1 protease inhibitor after another adding them to an already-failing regimen. When the NNRTI class of medications became available, they became quickly resistant to them as well.

Because Laurie does not currently have any opportunistic infections, my first priority is to keep her from getting sick. We can accomplish this by ensuring that she is on adequate OI (opportunistic infection) prophylaxis.

Prophylaxis Medications

Trimethoprim-sulfamethoxazole (a.k.a. Bactrim or Septra) is a medication that helps prevent Pneumocystis pneumonia in immuno-compromised individuals. If your CD4 count is *less than* 200 cells/mm3,

I recommend taking this medication 1 double-strength tablet 3x/week or, if sulfa allergy was a problem and you have been desensitized, 1 single-strength tablet a day. I make this dosing recommendation instead of the more commonly recommended 1 double-strength tablet every day for an important reason. Taking an antibiotic *every day* kills most of the healthful bacteria (friendly flora) which normally inhabit the body. This creates an environment in which pathogenic bacteria can overgrow and cause bloating, gas, diarrhea and, in women, chronic vaginitis. Overgrowth of unhealthful bacteria and/or yeast places a significant stress on the immune system.

In patients following the Healing HIV program, trimethoprim-sulfamethoxazole, taken at the above-recommended dosage, will usually provide complete protection from infection with Pneumocystis carinii pneumonia, as long as your CD4 count is above 50 cells/mm3.

If an individual's CD4 count drops below 50 cells/mm3, I would increase the dosage of trimethoprim-sulfamethoxazole to 1 double-strength tablet every day. At that CD4 count, I could not rely on the immune system to be adequately protective even if it is supported by a strong natural therapies program. Also, recent studies have shown that 3x/week dosing of trimethoprim-sulfamethoxazole becomes less effective the lower the CD4 count drops.

If Laurie's CD4 count were to fall below 50 cells/mm3, I would also suggest that she take the following additional prophylactic medications:

Prophylactic Medications

1) *To prevent MAC (Mycobacterium avium complex)*
   - Azithromycin (Zithromax) 1200 mg 1x/week or
   - Clarithromycin (Biaxin) 500 mg 3x/week
2) *To prevent fungal overgrowth*
   - Fluconazole (Diflucan) 100 mg 3x/week
3) *To prevent herpes virus activity (if a patient has had genital herpes or herpes zoster)*
   - Acyclovir (Zovirax) 400 mg 2x/day or
   - Valacyclovir (Valtrex) 500 mg 1x/day

The next step in stabilizing Laurie's condition is to *establish a sound foundation of natural therapies.* This will strengthen her immune system so it may better participate in suppressing her HIV infection. The most straightforward way to initiate an aggressive natural therapies program is to review the "Elimination of Cofactors Checklist" presented earlier and reviewed here. Each of the following items can be thought of as directly or indirectly stimulating HIV activity.

Elimination of Cofactors Checklist

1) Herpes infections
2) Intestinal parasites
3) Unhealthy intestinal environment
4) Low protein intake
5) Inadequate antioxidant vitamins
6) Hormonal imbalances
7) Substance abuse
8) Emotional distress

Please refer to the clinical scenarios presented earlier, as well as the remaining chapters in this book, for a thorough description of how to eliminate these cofactors.

Choosing Laurie's New Antiviral Program

After a strong natural therapies and effective prophylaxis program are implemented, it is time to begin adjusting Laurie's antiviral medications.

Despite being on 5 antiviral medications, Laurie's viral load continues to be very high (120,000 copies/ml). It is therefore obvious that significant resistance to all of the commonly used classes of antiviral medications (RTIs, NNRTIs, and PIs) has occurred. Because of this, we need to be creative in choosing a new antiviral regimen for the present, while also looking to develop "a new crop" of antivirals for the future.

We also need to keep in mind that the surest way to waste any newly available antiviral drug is to add it to a program that is currently failing. It would be much smarter to maintain Laurie's good health and stability with aggressive natural therapies, OI prophylaxis, and previously used antiviral medications, while planning to add at least 2 or 3 new drugs as soon as we can accumulate them. This strategy may well enable Laurie to maintain her present stability without wasting any of the new drugs.

At this juncture, the key laboratory value to watch becomes the CD4 count, not the viral load. As long as the CD4 count remains stable, or even increases, her immune system is remaining stable and not losing ground.

Some patients are amazed to discover that, despite viral loads which may run in the thousands, their CD4 count can remain stable or even rise. This unusual situation often occurs in patients who continue to take their multidrug combinations despite a persistently high viral load. A viral load in the hundreds of thousands in a patient who is not on any antiviral protection will almost always cause the CD4 count to drop. Continuing your antiviral medications, despite the presence of multidrug resistance, appears to contribute some measure of protection. This may be due to the virus becoming "less fit."

Viral Fitness

HIV is best able to kill CD4 cells in what is called its "wild-type" state. Wild-type HIV is defined by the genetic makeup and physical form that HIV takes when it is not being inhibited by an antiviral medication. If 1 or more antiviral medications are present, they will inhibit HIV's ability to replicate itself until the virus figures out how to genetically mutate, thereby developing resistance to that particular drug or combination. When only a few mutations are present, HIV may still be able to replicate itself, and effectively kill CD4 cells, to the extent it could before the drugs were taken.

However, if HIV needs to develop 10 or 15 mutations to escape the replication-inhibiting effect of 4, 5, or 6 antiviral drugs taken simultaneously, its ability to kill CD4 cells may become compromised. The reason for this is that each mutation changes HIV's shape away from its most desired wild-type state. Eventually the laws of physics intervene and, though the virus can still replicate itself, its progeny are malformed and significantly compromised in their ability to infect and kill CD4 cells.

The viral strain is therefore termed "less fit." Consequently, your CD4 count can remain stable or even rise despite the presence of a high viral load.

Important point: Good health and stability can be maintained while future medication options are being explored and acquired. For this to occur, it is essential to also maintain an aggressive natural therapies program and effective OI prophylaxis. Most important, as long as your antiviral program is well tolerated, I recommend continuing to take these medications even if your viral load is high.

What Medications Does Laurie Need to Change?

Laurie is currently taking AZT/3TC/nevirapine/ritonavir/saquinavir with a persistently high viral load of 120,000 copies/ml. Her CD4 count is also declining and she doesn't feel well.

In deciding which antivirals to change, I would first take a thorough antiviral history. I would review each antiviral medication she has taken and the order in which she took them. Laurie's antiviral drug history form was shown in Fig. 6.3 on page 107. This record can be extremely useful when trying to decide upon your next antiviral combination.

I would also want to know how each of Laurie's previous medications were tolerated and how well, and for how long, they worked. This gives me a sense of which medications might still possess utility, which ones she has been off of the longest, and which, if any, she cannot tolerate due to previous side effects. I would then formulate a list of "potential antiviral options" and assign a priority level to each of them. Please see the previous clinical scenario for a thorough discussion on how to assign priority levels to your current list of antiviral options. Finally, I would consider ordering a genotype or phenotype resistance test (please refer to Appendix 2). Although these tests can be expensive, somewhat difficult to obtain, and not always accurate, they may still provide some guidance in a situation as complex as this.

Based on Laurie's antiviral history and current circumstances, the following assumptions can be made:

1) There is high-level resistance to all of the antiviral medications she

is currently taking (AZT/3TC/nevirapine/ritonavir/saquinavir).

2) The fitness of her viral strain is high because her CD4 count is continuing to decline.

3) Many of her symptoms (i.e., fatigue, nausea, anemia, neutropenia, and diarrhea) may be related to 1 or more of the antiviral medications she is taking.

4) Her present situation is unacceptable. A creative and aggressive change to her antiviral program needs to occur immediately.

Based on her previous history, Laurie's present treatment options would consist of 1 of the following:

1) D4T/DDI/ hydroxyurea/efavirenz/indinavir *or*

2) D4T/abacavir/efavirenz/indinavir *or*

3) DDI/hydroxyurea/efavirenz/indinavir/adefovir *or*

4) D4T/DDI/hydroxyurea/indinavir/ritonavir/adefovir.

My goal is to diminish the fitness of her viral strain, stabilize or improve her CD4 count, and subsequently begin to collect "a new crop" of previously unused medications for her to switch to next. Depending on which of the above treatment programs we choose, I would place the following antivirals on her list of medication options for the future:

1) Adefovir (Preveon)

2) Efavirenz (Sustiva)

3) Abacavir (Ziagen)

I would also begin looking for research studies that were testing new therapies. I know that as long as I can keep Laurie healthy and stable, the chance for newer and more effective antiviral medications becoming available exists. It is also possible for a surprising novel therapy to be released during this time as well. This is similar to what happened when protease inhibitors were discovered and quickly brought to market in 1995. They saved the lives of thousands of patients who previously thought they were completely out of antiviral options. This is why it is so important to always keep your hope alive!

In this complicated and difficult-to-manage situation, I would make sure to use aggressive natural therapies to support Laurie's overall health. Diet, vitamin supplementation, meditation, massage, and acupuncture go a long way to help maximize the strength of the immune system. In addition to encouraging Laurie to remain hopeful, I would also recommend that she take time every day to relax and focus on her healing. The mind-body connection can also be a powerful force, especially when your medication options are exhausted. These are simple, but often not appreciated, recommendations. Our goal is still to rebuild Laurie's immune system and raise her CD4 cell count until it rises above 300 cells/mm3. I will not give up until this is achieved and neither should she!

SUMMARY OF CLINICAL TREATMENT SCENARIOS

1) Your immune system needs to be supported with an aggressive program of natural therapies to ensure that any antiviral medication you take will work as well as possible.

2) The "Elimination of Cofactors Checklist" can help you eliminate as many stimulants to HIV activity as possible.

3) Initiating antiviral medication may be postponed as long as your immune system is continuing to remain healthy and strong without them. This situation can be defined as a stable or improving CD4 count greater than 300 cells/mm3 and a viral load that is less than 50,000 copies/ml.

3) Dual-RTI therapy is a viable option for individuals with *mild-to-moderate HIV infection* (defined as a declining CD4 count that is still greater than 300 cells/mm3 plus a viral load less than 50,000 copies/ml) who prefer to be conservative with antiviral drugs. This strategy is only recommended when an aggressive natural therapies program is used as well.

4) If you have recently started your first PI of NNRTI, strive to achieve a completely undetectable viral load within 3 to 6 months.

5) Acute exposure to HIV that is identified *within the first 6 months of infection* should always be treated with triple-combination antiviral therapy. This strategy will help prevent HIV's aggressive colonization of the immune system.

6) I am often asked by patients currently on triple-combination therapy if they can decrease the number of antiviral drugs they are taking. This course of action carries significant risks, and I almost always recommend against it.

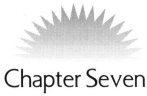

Chapter Seven

Optimizing Intestinal Health

Inarguably, a healthy GI (gastrointestinal) system plays a major role in helping to maintain a person's health. Unfortunately, the large number of drugs HIV(+) individuals need to take can cause significant adverse effects on the GI tract. Protease inhibitors, antibiotics, and other strong medications can cause nausea, diarrhea, malabsorption, heartburn, bloating, and abdominal pain, as well as unwanted changes to the bacteria that inhabit the gut.

Your GI tract gets a great deal of help when it comes to breaking down and absorbing nutrients. In addition to the processes of physical churning (peristalsis) and chemical digestion (hydrochloric acid and digestive enzymes), the GI system is inhabited by healthful bacteria whose presence is essential for good digestion to occur. In fact, the number of bacterial organisms within the intestines exceeds 10 billion; collectively, these tiny organisms would weigh over 3.5 pounds.

These bacteria live in a symbiotic relationship with their human hosts. In return for a warm, dark, and nutrient-rich environment, they help us digest our food, absorb nutrients, and eliminate harmful toxins. They also protect us from becoming infected with other organisms that may not be so kind. They have evolved along with us for millions of years and fill an important, beneficial niche.

The "Inner Garden" Analogy

It is helpful to think of the GI tract as your own private inner garden. This analogy is accurate since bacteria are actually plants. Your private inner garden can be beautiful and healthy, or overgrown with weeds, pests, and mold. It can also be of intermediate health, with many strong, beautiful plants accompanied by a few unwanted weeds. When your inner garden is healthy and vital, it helps your body remain balanced and strong. When it is weak and overrun with pathogenic organisms, the immune system becomes stressed and your health can decline. An imbalanced population of gastrointestinal organisms can disrupt your body, your immune system, and your life in the following ways:

Overstimulation of the immune system: Macrophages are a type of immune system cell that scavenge for invaders throughout the body. Many of these cells are based in the lymph nodes surrounding the GI tract. When your inner garden becomes overgrown with parasites, mold, or unhealthful bacteria, macrophages must work overtime to deal with the waste products and toxins that are produced. This process stimulates these important cells to become activated.

Macrophages are also often infected with HIV. When these immune system cells become activated, they produce large numbers of infectious HIV particles. This event can precipitate an increase in your viral load. If it continues, the probability of developing resistance to your antiviral medications greatly increases. In general, if you are infected with HIV, it is best to keep your gastrointestinal system as healthy and calm as possible.

A hidden cause of fatigue: The presence of intestinal parasites living in the GI tract is always detrimental to your health. Parasites, by definition, drain nutrients and vital energy from their hosts. This vital energy could otherwise be utilized for healing, tissue regeneration, and other immune-restorative activities.

Diminished appetite: Low appetite can lead to decreased food intake, malnutrition, and weight loss. Research has shown that one of the greatest contributors to wasting syndrome in HIV(+) individuals is the inadequate intake of calories and protein. An unhealthful intestinal environment can lead to a decreased intake of these vital nutrients.

Chronic gas and bloating: How many people are bothered by intermittent bouts of bloating and malodorous gas? Many more than I'm sure would like to admit. In fact, I know most patients rarely discuss this symptom with their doctor. Gas and bloating is often just accepted as a part of normal GI functioning. However, these symptoms indicate that an unhealthful intestinal environment is present and should always be investigated with appropriate laboratory testing, which I'll discuss later in the chapter.

Diarrhea and malabsorption: Chronic diarrhea and malabsorption can be caused by infection, medication side effects, and a poor diet. These symptoms can often be prevented if a program to strengthen the GI tract is put in place at an early stage. Unfortunately, the longer diarrhea continues, the more difficult it is to treat. Diarrhea is very irritating to the gastrointestinal tract and progressively destroys its normal architecture. This doesn't mean that long-standing diarrhea is impossible to reverse. In fact, I've had tremendous success helping patients eliminate chronic diarrhea that had persisted for years. The process begins with taking a little test that can help you evaluate your current level of gastrointestinal health.

Evaluating Your Gastrointestinal Health

The key to maintaining a healthy GI tract is to be *proactive.* Mild symptoms should always be listened to, evaluated, and corrected. Preventing GI imbalances starts with healthful eating, supplementing your diet with fermented foods, such as yogurt, miso, and kefir, taking probiotic bacterial supplements (acidophilus, bifidus, etc.), and obtaining a yearly screening for intestinal parasites.

The evaluation of your gastrointestinal health is based on 2 sources of information:

1) Any symptoms you may have.

2) A comprehensive stool analysis.

Your level of symptoms can be quantitatively determined by answering the following questions and determining your "Intestinal Health Score." A copy of this evaluation tool is also printed in Appendix 8.

Intestinal Health Score

1) How's my appetite?
   - ☐ good [1]
   - ☐ medium [2]
   - ☐ poor [3]

2) What is my weight compared to a year ago?
   - ☐ higher [1]
   - ☐ same [1]
   - ☐ lower [3]

3) How many bowel movements do I have per day (on average)
   - ☐ greater than 5 [3]
   - ☐ 3–5 [2]
   - ☐ 1–3 [1]
   - ☐ less than 1 [2]

4) What is their most common appearance?
   - ☐ watery diarrhea [4]
   - ☐ loose and unformed [3]
   - ☐ soft and pasty [2]
   - ☐ well formed [1]
   - ☐ hard [2]

5) Are any of the following symptoms present most of the time?
   - ☐ heartburn [2]
   - ☐ gas/gurgling [2]
   - ☐ nausea [2]
   - ☐ bloating [2]
   - ☐ smelly gas [3]
   - ☐ none [0]

6) What is my "TP" index (how many pieces of toilet paper do I usually have to tear off before I am completely clean)?
   - ☐ greater than 5 [3]
   - ☐ 3–5 [2]
   - ☐ less than 3 [1]

To find out the general health of your intestinal environment, add up the small numbers next to your answers and refer to the scoring key below:

5–10 = Excellent health
10–15 = Intermediate health
greater than 15 = Unhealthy

The next step in determining the health of your intestinal system is to obtain a comprehensive stool analysis. This should be done at least once a year as a screening test and more often if you are experiencing unpleasant GI symptoms or a precipitous drop in your CD4 cells.

There are good reasons to get a yearly screening for intestinal parasites even if you are asymptomatic. At least 50% of patients with intestinal parasites or other significant intestinal imbalances report themselves to be completely asymptomatic. Since our goal is to optimize intestinal health, not just treat acute symptoms, a yearly screening will identify hidden infections that can then be easily corrected. If not addressed early, these minor imbalances can progress to more extensive problems such as diminished appetite, malabsorption, and increased HIV activity.

Comprehensive Stool Analysis Testing

Comprehensive stool analysis testing is available from several reputable laboratories that are listed in the Resources section in the back of this book. Most of them will send a test kit by mail if requested by the patient's health-care professional.

There are several reasons why a comprehensive stool analysis from these labs offers significant advantages over local hospital laboratories. First, these labs usually concentrate much of their time and resources performing stool analyses. Their equipment is also superior and more expensive. Their technicians are specially trained in the evaluation of intestinal health. While a technician working at a large city hospital may process only 8 to 12 stool samples per day, technicians at specialized stool analysis labs routinely process upwards of 50 samples a day.

A comprehensive stool analysis also includes tests which are not routinely performed by local hospital laboratories. One of these is the beneficial bacteria culture. This test quantitates the amount of Lactobacillus acidophilus and Bifidobacter bacteria living in the gut. These organisms must be present in significant quantities for healthful GI functioning to occur.

These labs also perform sensitivity testing to help practitioners use herbs and other natural substances to treat many intestinal infections. They test the sensitivity of these infections to various antibiotics as well, so the physician can have a choice. Finally, these tests measure the ability of the digestive system to break down and absorb specific, hard to digest foods such as fats and meats. Furthermore, all the information described above can be gleaned from a single stool sample.

Extensive research literature supports the accuracy and health-promoting nature of these tests. This kind of testing has helped hundreds of patients at my clinic eliminate chronic GI symptoms, previously unknown parasitic infections, and other GI disturbances. The health of our patients' GI systems is maintained at very high standards. By minimizing excessive activation of the immune system, these interventions have a very calming effect on my patients' HIV infection.

HMOs

One problem that has arisen with the pervasive presence of managed care in medical practice is that most HMOs (health maintenance organizations, or *health minimizing organizations* as I prefer to call them) do not cover the costs of comprehensive stool analysis testing. HMOs are designed to pay the absolute least money for your health care. This makes the most money for their CEO, board of directors, and stockholders. By giving you nothing more than the minimum medical care allowable by law, they often prevent doctors from obtaining lab tests which might sometimes help their patients obtain the best possible care. Because you may switch your insurance in a year or two, the prevention of long-term health problems is often not their highest priority.

I was recently asked by a patient's insurance company (an HMO) to acquire the approval of the head of the hospital laboratory before the company would pay for a comprehensive stool analysis in a patient who had HIV infection and symptoms of chronic gas, bloating, and diarrhea. All the previous stool tests from this hospital had come back negative, *though the patient continued to lose weight and suffer.*

The lab director, a prominent pathologist, flatly refused. He stated that the tests were unnecessary and that their results could not possibly be useful. When I offered to send him research studies to support their use in this specific situation, he bluntly stated that the laboratories performing these tests had accumulated invalid research studies to support their case.

I then told him of my years of experience in utilizing this information to help cure dozens of patients with chronic diarrhea who had previously had negative test results from standard laboratories. I told him that my experience in this area should support his approval of a limited number of these tests on a trial basis. He rebutted that he had never heard that this kind of testing could be worthwhile (although as a pathologist he doesn't see any patients). The only option I could propose at this point was to send the patient to a gastroenterologist for an expensive and invasive procedure that would cost 4 times the price of a comprehensive stool analysis. This is what he then suggested I do.

Albert Einstein once said, "The mind is like a parachute; it works best when open." I believe that this particular pathologist would hit the ground pretty hard if his mind needed to operate as his parachute.

Tony

Tony is a 49-year-old landscape architect who initially tested HIV(+) in 1986. At that time, he had 400 CD4 cells and was completely asymptomatic. At our first visit in early 1995, he stated that his CD4 count had dropped to 11 cells/mm3. He had also recently been hospitalized with PCP (Pneumocystis carinii pneumonia) and been diagnosed with a chronic infection called MAC (Mycobacterium avium complex). This had caused him to lose 40 pounds from his baseline weight. Though he was now on triple-combination therapy with AZT/DDC/saquinavir, his viral load was persistently high at 45,000 copies/ml.

Tony explained that one of the reasons he had done so poorly a few months ago was that he chose to completely stop all of his antiviral medications and instead try to treat his condition solely with herbs. It had now become clear to him that a skillful integration of natural and standard medical therapies was the best path to follow.

Presently, Tony's problems included a CD4 count of 11 cells/mm3, a viral load of 45,000 copies/ml, oral candida, constant watery diarrhea, gas, bloating, fatigue, and a 40-pound weight loss during the past 4 months.

The foundation of Tony's treatment program, given his acute gastrointestinal symptoms, needed to include an extremely rigorous nutritional program. We thoroughly reviewed Tony's diet, and I advised him to increase his protein intake to 100 grams per day. He also started taking vitamin supplements, and we sent off a comprehensive stool analysis.

In addition, I performed a thorough review of Tony's hormone levels. His DHEA-S level was found to be significantly low, and he started taking a DHEA supplement at 250 mg 1x/day in addition to testosterone and nandrolone (muscle building hormone) injections every 2 weeks. Tony also began monthly massage therapy and acupuncture to reduce his stress and encourage his body to heal.

Tony's comprehensive stool analysis revealed a severe intolerance to fatty foods, the complete absence of beneficial bacteria, such as Escheria coli and Lactobacillus acidophilus, and an overgrowth of a probable pathogenic bacteria, Klebsiella pneumoniae. Thankfully, there were no intestinal parasites.

To help strengthen his digestive functioning, I recommended that Tony begin taking digestive enzyme supplements with all meals that had a high-fat content. After we treated the unhealthful Klebsiella pneumoniae bacteria with a week's course of antibiotics, Tony started taking high-dose acidophilus supplementation

Tony responded immediately. His energy quickly began to improve, and within a couple of months his diarrhea was reduced by 50%. Over the next few weeks, Tony's improvement continued. His weight increased from 110 to 130 pounds during his first 3 months on the program, and his diarrhea continued to decline from constant to once every 7 to 10 days.

As far as his antiviral medications were concerned, Tony began taking a new triple combination consisting of D4T/3TC/indinavir. His viral load quickly dropped to an undetectable level and, 6 months after beginning this program, his CD4 count had climbed back up to 116 cells/mm3 (from 11).

A year after beginning the Healing HIV program, Tony's weight had increased by 40 pounds, his fatigue had completely resolved, his CD4 count was greater than 200 cells/mm3, and he felt like a new man.

It has now been over 3 years since our initial visit. Tony's CD4 count is now 345 cells/mm3 and his viral load continues to be undetectable. He has also successfully gone off his MAC treatment, his weight is totally normal at 155 pounds, and he exercises every day. All of this has occurred while continuing to take the same antivirals he began more than 3 years ago. Tony is a perfect example of healing HIV in action.

Where to Obtain Comprehensive Stool Analysis Testing

Several labs that perform this type of stool testing are listed in the Resources section in the back of this book. Comprehensive stool analysis testing is usually covered by Medicare, Medicaid, and many insurance plans which allow you to see the doctor of your choice. If you do not have an insurance plan that covers this kind of testing, I recommend 3 specific ways to keep its cost to a minimum.

First, order this test only once a year for screening purposes or when more standard tests have not proved useful. Second, if cost is a significant factor, do not order the most comprehensive test available. An analysis specifically targeted to your needs may be more cost-effective. You should find out what each test provides, and its cost, before you decide. Third, pay up front. If you enclose a check or credit card number, the laboratory will charge you the minimum price. If they bill you, you will incur additional charges for this service.

What You Need to Know

A comprehensive stool analysis should provide you and your doctor with the following information:

A beneficial bacteria culture: To measure the level of Lactobacillus acidophilus and Bifidobacter bacteria growing in your colon.

A pathogenic bacteria culture: To detect mildly pathogenic bacteria which can grow in the colon and cause chronic symptoms. These unfriendly organisms include Citrobacter freundii, Klebsiella pneumoniae, and Staphylococcus aureus. Most hospital labs do not test for these organisms because the level of symptoms they cause is not felt to be severe. These culture results should be accompanied by specific pharmaceutical *and* herbal treatment recommendations.

A fungal culture: To test specifically for Candida albicans, a common mold. This should also include pharmaceutical and herbal treatment recommendations.

Direct microscopy: To detect yeast and intestinal parasites.

Immunofluorescence testing: To detect Giardia lamblia, Entamoeba histolytica, and Cryptosporidium parasites. If cost is an issue and you are currently asymptomatic, this particular component of the testing may be eliminated.

The first 2 tests mentioned above are almost always *not* available from standard hospital laboratories. This is unfortunate since knowledge of the amount of healthful *and* unhealthful bacteria growing in the gut can greatly aid in balancing your intestinal health. In addition, sensitivity testing for herbal treatments that can be used to eliminate unhealthful bacteria or fungi can enable the health practitioner to treat these infections naturally *first*, moving to stronger antibiotics only if necessary.

Specific Scenarios and Their Treatment

I will now provide a more in-depth discussion of the causes of an unhealthful intestinal environment and specific measures to address them. Always discuss treatment recommendations with your physician before implementing them.

Inadequate beneficial intestinal bacteria

Lactobacillus acidophilus, Escheria coli, and Bifidobacter infantis are the 3 major species of friendly bacteria that reside in the adult colon. In fact, Bifidobacter infantis comprises up to one-quarter of the normal colonic bacteria. High levels of these bacteria indicate a healthy colonic environment. They produce vitamin K, vitamin B complex, intraintestinal nutrients, and other factors to aid in normal digestion. Furthermore, these healthful bacteria produce substances which also inhibit the growth of pathogenic bacteria, yeast, and parasites. In the pursuit of optimal health, they are our true allies.

Friendly bacteria are extremely vulnerable to the toxicity of antibiotics. Many HIV(+) patients are commonly prescribed broad-spectrum antibiotics for the treatment of sinusitis, bronchitis, prostatitis, and other infections. By destroying a significant number of the healthful bacteria living in the gut, taking antibiotics creates a conducive environment for unhealthful organisms to gain a foothold. When this happens, gas, bloating, diarrhea, decreased appetite, fatigue, and increased HIV activity can occur. This is just one reason why minimizing the use of antibiotics and supplementing your diet with healthful organisms is so important!

By culturing healthy bacteria from the gut, a comprehensive stool analysis provides a more comprehensive picture of gastrointestinal health. If healthy bacteria levels are found to be low (0, +1, or +2 out of a maximum of +4), they can be supplemented in liquid or capsule form to raise their numbers, thereby strengthening your GI health.

If these bacteria are already present in healthful amounts (+3 or +4), you might look elsewhere for the cause of any symptoms you might be experiencing. Other causes of chronic gastrointestinal symptoms include intestinal parasites, an overgrowth of mold (Candida albicans), food allergies, medication side effects, or the need to take digestive enzymes to help aid in digesting your food.

Restoring the normal balance of healthful intestinal organisms can be accomplished in 2 steps:

1) *Dietary and lifestyle adjustments:* Eat at least 1 cup of cooked whole grains every day (brown rice, barley, oatmeal, quinoa, amaranth, 9-grain hot cereal, etc.). Do not add large amounts of butter, margarine, oil, or milk. Adding grease to your food can exacerbate the symptoms of gas, bloating, and diarrhea. Keep the amount of sugar, alcohol, and dairy products you eat to a minimum. Avoid iced drinks, drink plenty of filtered water, and exercise regularly. Rest for 15 minutes after every meal.

2) *Supplementation:* Your diet can be supplemented with acidophilus/bifidus bacteria and FOS (fructooligosaccharides) (see Intestinal Rejuvenation Program, Fig. 7.1). This accomplishes what I call "reseeding and fertilizing your inner garden." This program provides plentiful amounts of healthful bacteria as well as nutrients to stimulate their growth. It is an effective way to "grow" a more healthful population of bacterial organisms. I have had outstanding results with this protocol.

Figure 7.1

Intestinal Rejuvenation Protocol

1) **High-potency acidophilus/bifidus supplement**
   This supplement populates the colon with 2 healthful strains of bacteria.
   Directions: Take the recommended dosage 2 times a day

2) **Fructooligosaccharide (FOS) supplement**
   FOS provides nutrients so healthful intestinal bacteria can grow quickly.
   Directions: Take the recommended dosage 2 times a day

3) **Daily Fiber Supplement (oat bran, rice bran, psyllium seed husks)**
   Fiber supplementation provides a matrix to support healthy bacterial growth.
   Directions: 1 tablespoon 2 times a day

Instructions: Mix the above powders in 6 oz of water or dilute fruit juice and take 2x/day (with or without meals) for 1 month, then 1x/day thereafter as maintenance.

The above products can be found in your local health food store. You can ask the health food store staff for assistance in choosing which products are the most convenient and cost-effective.

Pathogenic bacterial overgrowth

Bacteria that grow in the colon can be healthful or pathogenic. Salmonella, Shigella, Campylobacter, and Clostridium are examples of pathogenic GI bacteria that usually cause acute nausea, vomiting, abdominal pain, and diarrhea.

Other GI bacteria can be *mildly* pathogenic. These bacteria cause symptoms which are less severe. They include Klebsiella, Citrobacter, Staphylococcus, and Hemolytic E. coli. They produce mild-to-moderate symptoms, such gas, bloating, heartburn, and malodorous stools. When combined with other gastrointestinal problems such as fungal overgrowth, parasites, or the GI side effects from strong medications, mildly pathogenic bacteria may contribute significantly to an unhealthful intestinal state.

Unfortunately, most hospitals and private labs do not test for mildly pathogenic bacteria when processing a stool sample. Since these bacteria are not *always* associated with severe symptoms, especially in healthy people, most physicians and insurers do not believe they are worth culturing for. This is a classic example of modern medicine requiring a crisis to occur before intervention is felt to be warranted.

This is also an example of not seeing the forest for the trees. The big picture of intestinal health is missed when one seeks to attribute *1 cause,* or the presence of *1 organism,* to a problem. The occurrence of chronic fatigue, diarrhea, or malodorous gas is usually not the result of a single infection or medication side effect. It is most often a complex interaction of many factors which include your diet, activity level, and the overall healthfulness of your intestinal environment.

Richard

R ichard was asymptomatic until he started his first antiviral combination, D4T/3TC. Within 2 days he was complaining of severe nausea and diarrhea from the 2 antiviral medications which possess the least chance of causing GI side effects. A comprehensive stool analysis showed the presence of yeast, unhealthful bacteria, and 2 intestinal parasites including Giardia lamblia. After appropriate treatment, he was able to restart both medications without difficulty. If we had not gotten this test, these 2 medications would have been discarded forever due to intolerance. Richard has now been taking these same 2 medications for the past 2 years and tolerating them extremely well.

Fungal overgrowth

Fungal overgrowth of the GI system with Candida albicans and other species of mold can cause gas, bloating, abdominal pain, malabsorption, loose stools, and diarrhea. It can also contribute to chronic fatigue and weak immune function. Eradicating these organisms from the GI tract is essential if you are to maintain optimal health.

Overgrowth of the GI system with fungus and mold is extremely problematic in HIV(+) individuals due to the number of antibiotics they often need to take. Most physicians only treat fungal infections when they are present on visible areas of the body such as the skin, nails, tongue, or rectum. When observed in these areas, fungal infections are quickly treated with either topical creams or strong systemic medications.

However, overgrowth of the colon with fungus and mold is not a condition most standard physicians have been taught to treat. This is a classic case of "If you can't see it, it must not be causing a problem." This is not true. The GI system is a long, dark, hollow tube of enormous importance. A situation in which its walls are overgrown with mold needs to be addressed with as much if not more attention as if this infection were in a more visible place.

The biggest problem in treating intestinal fungal infections is that, if they are only treated with medications, they tend to recur. The long-term solution to fungal eradication is a combination of consuming less sugar, less alcohol, a healthful diet, and trying to avoid antibiotics as much as possible.

Medical history is replete with examples of the powers-that-be denying the existence of important disease factors and their effect on health. The importance of washing one's hands before surgery was once ridiculed; the bacteria Moroxella catarralis was once classified as a nonpathogenic organism (but now is known to be a cause of significant lung infections); and the presence of high cholesterol was once ignored as a risk factor for heart disease by medical scholars of the time.

It is important to look at your gastrointestinal environment as a complete ecosystem. When balanced, it efficiently digests food and eliminates waste in a healthful manner. When imbalanced, malabsorption can occur as waste products build up to unhealthful levels. In this environment, unhealthful organisms proliferate, and the immune system is forced to expend valuable energy which could more effectively be used elsewhere in its fight against HIV.

Ken

Ken is a 37-year-old restaurant operator who lives on the East Coast and tested HIV(+) in September 1994. Shortly thereafter, he was diagnosed with CMV (cytomegalovirus) colitis and was treated with 3 weeks of intravenous gancyclovir to suppress this infection. His normal weight was 205 pounds. After 3 months of CMV infection, he was down to 157 pounds, a loss of 25% of his normal body weight.

When Ken arrived in San Francisco for our initial visit in January 1995, he was having constant diarrhea (8 to 10 bowel movements per day) and was terribly fatigued. His doctor, in fact, had just told him to make his final arrangements because he probably had no longer than 3 months to live.

Ken and his sister sat in my office hoping for redemption but also not wanting to "expect too much." "This is the last place we have to turn, Dr. Kaiser," his sister said. Ken added, "I really want to live Dr. Kaiser, but all my doctors back East have told me I only have a few months left. Is there anything you can do?"

My first intervention was to tell Ken that he needed to keep believing that surviving beyond 3 months was possible. I needed to reinstill in him a sense of hope that the possibility of continued survival and actual improvement was real. Once this change in attitude was established, we could begin going over the details of how to make it happen.

Our first order of business was to address Ken's medical needs. First, I started him on gancyclovir in oral form, 4 capsules 3x/day to continue suppressing his CMV infection while at the same time allowing him to stop his daily IVs. Second, I retested Ken's stool for cryptosporidium and other parasites that might be contributing to his diarrhea. Third, I prescribed 3x/week injections of Neupogen to raise his white blood cell count to a safer level. Fourth, I started him on digestive enzymes to lessen the stress on his gastrointestinal tract and make it easier for him to digest his food. Fifth, I recommended that he start combination antiviral therapy with AZT/DDC. (This was before protease inhibitors and NNRTIs had become available.) Sixth, I put Ken on a strong prophylaxis program for PCP, MAC, and fungal infections. Last but not least, I made dietary recommendations designed to decrease his diarrhea by eliminating hard-to-digest foods such as fats and oils, uncooked foods, and dairy products. These recommendations achieved good results. Finally, I recommended to Ken that he "fire the doctor" that told him he only had 3 months to live.

After 6 months on this program, Ken's diarrhea was gone. His energy level improved significantly, and he was exercising 4x/week with weights. His CD4 count had climbed from 30 to 200 cells/mm3, and his viral load decreased from 179,000 to 39,000 copies/ml. We continued to adjust his antiviral medications, leading to further decreases in his viral load and improvements in his overall condition.

Despite all this good news, Ken periodically experienced a

recurrence of his psychological depression. There is no doubt that his healing program required a lot of work. However, he was good about picking up the phone and talking with me about it. Usually, after one of our conversations, he would feel a renewed sense of hope and a more positive attitude toward the future. In November 1995, I switched Ken's antiviral medications to AZT/3TC/indinavir, and his viral load finally became undetectable. I also prescribed testosterone and DHEA supplements to optimize his hormone levels, and these helped continue his steady return to a normal weight.

In June 1996, 18 months after our first meeting, Ken and his sister again returned to San Francisco for a visit. I almost didn't recognize the person sitting in front of me. After starting at 147 pounds, Ken was now a healthy 212! He resembled a Greek god. He was healthy, happy, and working full-time. His blood counts were stable and he was asymptomatic. Dramatic and satisfying results had been achieved utilizing an aggressive program of natural therapies, a triple combination of antivirals, and lots of very hard work. My most recent visit with Ken in June 1998 revealed a picture of continued stability, obvious good health, and a definite healing of HIV in progress.

SUMMARY

1) Multiple factors contribute to the quality of your intestinal health. These include the food that you eat, the amount of exercise you get, your stress level, and the number and kind of drugs you are taking.

2) Mild symptoms such as gas, bloating, and loose stools should never be ignored for long periods of time. They signify an unhealthful intestinal state and should be evaluated with a comprehensive stool analysis.

3) Overgrowth of the colon with mildly pathogenic bacteria, mold, and intestinal parasites is *never* normal. It is crucial to eliminate all gastrointestinal infections to prevent their stimulating increased HIV activity that will ultimately lead to a shorter duration of response from your antiviral drugs.

Chapter Eight

Intestinal Parasites

Intestinal infections have been described as constituting the greatest single worldwide cause of illness and disease. Numerous studies have shown that the incidence of intestinal parasite infections may approach 99% in countries of the developing world. In the United States, intestinal infections are the third leading cause of illness and disease.

Although most Americans have grown up with modern sanitary conveniences, parasitic infections are still more common than we think. A survey of public health laboratories in the U.S. reported a 15.6% incidence of intestinal parasites among all samples checked. In my practice, *greater than 50% of asymptomatic HIV(+) individuals test positive for at least 1 intestinal parasite when screened.* Fortunately, many physicians are becoming more aware of the incidence of intestinal parasite infections and their relationship to chronic disease states.

The reason these organisms are called "parasites" is that they injure their hosts. By definition, *nonpathogenic parasites do not exist.* The only variable is the intensity of the effect caused to the host. Some parasites, such as Entamoeba histolytica, cause acute abdominal pain and profuse diarrhea. Others, such as Giardia lamblia, are more commonly responsible for malodorous gas and bloating. Still others, such as Blastocystis hominis, may produce a state of chronic fatigue as their only noticeable effect. However, all parasites cause stress to the immune system and can stimulate HIV to be more active.

The classification of these organisms as pathogens continues to be in a state of flux. Only a few decades ago, Giardia lamblia, the leading cause of intestinal parasitic infections in the United States, was not considered a pathogen. In addition, Cryptosporidium, a well-known pathogen in animals, has only recently been classified as a human pathogen that can cause severe life-threatening diarrhea in children, pregnant women, and HIV(+) individuals.

Today, controversy continues to exist surrounding the status of Blastocystis hominis. Though often an asymptomatic inhabitant of the gut, B. hominis can cause acute diarrhea, chronic fatigue, increased HIV activity, flatulence, nausea, and rectal bleeding. Some 20 years ago, the Centers for Disease Control viewed Blastocystis hominis as an acute pathogen. Recently, it has retreated from this position and now classifies it as a "possible" pathogen.

Part of the problem in classifying parasites lies in the fact that the *overall health of the individual* is often a major determinant to the level of symptoms a parasite causes. In patients with poor diets and compromised immune systems, a mildly pathogenic organism may cause severe symptoms. In a patient with a healthy diet and normally functioning immune system, the same organism might be well tolerated and eliminated from the body in a relatively short period of time. In my practice, we view all intestinal parasites as placing significant stress on the immune system, and we treat them with a combination of natural and pharmaceutical means.

Parasite Transmission

Most intestinal parasites are transmitted through contact with fecal matter. That is, the organisms themselves, or their cysts, are expelled through the rectum of their host and find their way in some fashion to the mouth of their next host.

Fecal-oral transmission can occur in several ways:

Sexual behavior: Intestinal parasites are transmitted through sexual activity much more easily than HIV. Common safe-sex practices, including the use of condoms, is often insufficient at preventing their spread. If people remove contaminated condoms and then put their hands to their mouths, they cannot contract HIV, but they can become infected with intestinal parasites. Another common mode of transmission includes rimming, a sexual practice where the tongue is put in direct contact with the rectum of another person.

Contaminated food and water: The only way to completely prevent exposure to parasites through food and water is by cooking. Food prepared by individuals infected with parasites and who have not thoroughly washed their hands after using the bathroom may contain cysts and/or live organisms.

Unfortunately, not all waterborne intestinal parasites are killed by chlorine. Therefore, these organisms can exist in the water supply. Complete elimination can only be achieved by boiling (for at least 2 minutes), filtering with a 1-micron filter, or drinking distilled water. Bottled spring waters can vary greatly in their preparation methods but are usually safe. To find out about the safety of a specific brand of bottled water, call 1-800-WATER-11.

Household contacts: Individuals who present with recurring infections due to intestinal parasites, despite implementing careful hygienic measures, often live in households with infected members. Behavior as innocuous as using the same face towel previously used by an infected roommate can transmit these infections. If recurring infections with parasites are a problem, ask all of your sexual partners and household members to be tested. All infected individuals should be treated simultaneously, followed by a repeat test of all parties 1 month after the treatment cycle is complete. Surfaces in hot tubs, saunas, and bathhouses, where people sit naked, can also be a hidden source of exposure.

Common Intestinal Parasites

Blastocystis hominis: This organism is more prevalent than any other parasite, but often goes undetected due to poor laboratory technique. Next to fungal overgrowth, B. hominis is the most frequently observed pathogenic organism in the fecal samples of HIV(+) patients.

A significant weight of evidence supports treating B. hominis as a pathogen. Acute symptoms from this parasite can include abdominal pain, bloating, nausea, vomiting, weight loss, diarrhea, insomnia, dizziness, anorexia, and rash. Reports also identify it as a cofactor in many chronic conditions such as irritable bowel syndrome, chronic fatigue syndrome, autoimmune conditions, and arthritis. In my practice, it also appears to be responsible for reactivating HIV activity and may explain why some antiviral drug regimens fail prematurely. When treated appropriately, eradication of this organism is often associated with complete resolution of GI symptoms.

Dientamoeba fragilis: This organism commonly causes parasitic infections but often goes undetected also due to poor laboratory technique. It lives in the colon and is transmitted by direct ingestion through the fecal-oral route. Its symptoms may include diarrhea, fatigue, and abdominal bloating.

The Amoebas: Entamoeba histolytica, Entamoeba coli, Entamoeba hartmanni, Iodamoeba butschlii, and Endolimax nana: These organisms are cosmopolitan in their distribution. E. histolytica is most commonly linked to acute diarrhea and other GI symptoms. However, individuals may harbor E. histolytica without experiencing acute symptoms. The other amoebas have been associated with more chronic GI symptoms though they are not recognized to be pathogens. Variations in an organism's virulence and/or host resistance factors may explain differences in the severity of the observed symptoms. Amoebas are spread most frequently by ingestion of their cysts. As with all parasites mentioned in this section, *complete eradication* of these organisms from the GI tract must be the goal.

Giardia lamblia: Giardia lamblia most often resides in the small intestine. It attaches itself via a sucker to the mucosal cells of the intestinal wall and causes an inflammatory state to occur. When it detaches, it is swept into the fecal stream and transforms itself into a cyst before being expelled from the body. Infection is spread by the fecal-oral route, either directly or through food and water. Water-borne sources include mountain streams, well water, and even some chlorinated community water systems.

Diagnosing Intestinal Parasites

Diagnosing intestinal parasites depends upon the quality of the instruments, the technical skill of the examiner, and the number of samples examined. Laboratory procedures which may significantly affect detection rates include specimen collection and handling techniques, concentration procedures, and staining procedures. Many studies have also shown that detection rates increase from around 50% to more than 95% as sequential samples from the same individual are examined.

Since intestinal parasites may produce no obvious symptoms, I recommend that a yearly parasite screening be performed in all HIV(+) individuals. By discovering and treating hidden intestinal infections, a potential stimulus to increased HIV activity can be eliminated. By keeping your gut as healthy as possible, you may also improve your tolerance to antiviral and other medications.

An immunoassay technique known as immunofluorescence testing is also now available to detect E. histolytica, G. lamblia, and Cryptosporidium. This test can detect antigens (immune-activating chemicals) released by these parasites into the fecal stream and can raise the sensitivity of diagnosing 1 of these parasites to 95%.

Treating Intestinal Parasites

Once parasitic organisms have been detected, the goal is to eradicate them completely. Because antiparasitic drugs are powerful pharmacologic agents, they should not be taken without careful consideration. The most commonly prescribed antiparasitic medication, metronidazole (Flagyl), can cause a wide range of systemic side effects that include headache, nausea, dry mouth, dizziness, metallic taste, behavioral abnormalities, and peripheral numbness. These symptoms are more common in individuals who are especially sensitive to drugs.

Figure 8.1

COMMON DRUGS TO TREAT PARASITIC INFECTIONS (CDC Treatment Guidelines)

Infection	Drug (trade name)	Adult dosage	Adverse effects
Amebiasis, asymtomatic	iodoquinole (Yodoxin)	650 mg 3x/day x 20 days	Rash, acne, nausea, thyroid enlargement, diarrhea, cramps. Rare: optic atrophy, loss of vision, iodine sensitivity, peripheral neuropathy after prolonged use in high doses (months).
	paramomycin (Humatin)	25-30 mg/kg/day in 3 divided doses x 7 days	GI disturbances. Occasional: auditory or renal damage.
Amebiasis, symptomatic	metronidazole (Flagyl)	750 3x/day x 10 days	Nausea, headache, dry mouth, metallic taste. Occasional: vomiting, diarrhea insomnia, weakness, stomatitis, vertigo, paresthesia, rash, dark urine, urethral burning. Rare: seizures, encephalopathy, colitis, ataxia, leukopenia, peripheral neuropathy, pancreatitis.
Blastocysitis	metronidazole* iodoquinole**	750 mg 3x/day x 10 days 650 mg 3x/day x 20 days	See above See above
Dientamoeba	iodoquinole tetracycline	650 mg 3x/day x 20 days 500 mg 4x/day x 10 days	See above
Giardia	quinacrine (Atabrine)	100 mg 3x/day x 5-10 days	Dizziness, headache, vomiting, diarrhea. Occasional: yellow staining of skin, psychosis, insomnia, bizarre dreams, blood dyscrasias, urticaria, nail pigmentation, rash. Rare: hepatic necrosis, convulsions, severe dermatitis, ocular effects.
	metronidazole	250 mg 3x/day x 5-10 days	See above.

*Sources disagree on the proper dose for metronidazole. Some recommend 250 mg 3x/day which causes fewer side effects. Others recommend 750 mg 3x/d for more effective treatment, although there may be more side effects with the higher dose.

**Anecdotal reports suggest that iodoquinole may be more effective than metronidazole and may cause fewer side effects for the treatment of B. Hominus.

Reprinted with permission from *The Medical Letter* December 1993

Fig. 8.2

Dr. Kaiser's Intestinal Parasite Elimination Program

Extremely effective against: Blastocystis hominis, Endolimax nana, Iodamoeba butschlii, Entamoeba histolytica, Entamoeba coli

1) Paromomycin (Humatin)*	Frequency	Duration
2 capsules	3x/day	10 – 14 days
250 mg capsules		
and/or		
Iodoquinol (Yodoxin)*		
1 capsule	3x/day	10 – 20 days
650 mg capsules		

2) Psyllium seed husks		
2 teaspoons	3x/day	10 – 14 days
Add to water or juice		

3) Black walnut tincture		
2 droppersful	3x/day	10 – 14 days
Add to water or juice		

*Paromomycin and iodoquinol are prescription medications that are very effective and better tolerated than the more commonly prescribed metronidazole (Flagyl). If 2 or more parasites are present, which is frequently the case, I usually recommend taking both paromomycin and iodoquinol concurrently for 10 days, then continuing iodoquinol alone for an additional 10 days.

Add #2 and #3 to water or juice and take together with #1 on an empty stomach (one–half hour before or 2 hours after meals). All of the above must be taken together for maximum efficacy. It is essential that this program only be taken under medical supervision.

I usually attempt to treat intestinal parasites with alternatives to metronidazole such as paromomycin (Humatin) or iodoquinol (Yodoxin) plus several natural agents. By combining the effects of pharmaceutical agents *and* natural therapies, a high success rate and a minimum of side effects are achieved.

If only 1 intestinal parasite is present, I usually use a single pharmaceutical agent plus black walnut tincture and fiber supplementation (see Fig. 8.2). If 2 or more parasites are present, I recommend that paromomycin be taken for 10 days and iodoquinol be taken for 20 days concurrently. I also recommend taking black walnut tincture and fiber supplementation with this regimen as well.

A list of the standard treatment recommendations from the CDC for intestinal parasitic infections, as printed in *The Medical Letter* of December 1993, is reproduced in Fig. 8.1. My guidelines for the treatment of parasitic infections are printed in Fig. 8.2. Please consult your health-care practitioner to design the most effective and best-tolerated parasitic treatment program for your individual needs and sensitivities.

Important note: All treatments for intestinal parasites should be followed by a repeat stool examination 4 weeks after completing the initial treatment program. This ensures that the parasitic infection has been eradicated, not just temporarily suppressed.

SUMMARY

1) Intestinal parasites are a significant cofactor that may cause increased HIV activity.

2) All intestinal parasites are pathogenic to a host whose immune system is stressed and should be eradicated completely.

3) A yearly parasite screening is recommended for all HIV(+) individuals.

4) All treatments for intestinal parasites need to be followed by a repeat stool examination 4 weeks after completing the initial treatment program.

Chapter Nine

Body Cell Mass and the Immune System

B*ody cell mass* is the body compartment that includes skeletal muscle tissue, your internal organs, and a small percentage of metabolically active connective tissue. It replaces the older term, *lean muscle tissue,* and is responsible for generating the vast majority of the body's energy.

By increasing body cell mass (lean muscle tissue), you can boost the total amount of energy your body produces. Anything that increases your energy level in a positive, healthful manner ultimately facilitates a strengthening of your immune system. This can allow you to mount a stronger defense against HIV.

If your energy supply becomes compromised, your immune system is the first system of the body to suffer adverse consequences. Fatigue has been confirmed as an independent predictor for illness and opportunistic infection in people with HIV. This fact is supported by several important research studies.

Conversely, a boost to your energy level can greatly improve the functioning of your immune system. This fact is also supported by studies which show that the immune system is strengthened when malnourished patients are replenished with abundant amounts of energy-rich fuel.

With more energy, you experience less fatigue. You enjoy life more. You can exercise as much as you want and have more fun with your friends. You can even go back to work if you have previously been disabled.

By healthfully raising your energy level, you can improve your quality of life *and* strengthen your immune system. These goals can all be accomplished by *increasing your body cell mass.*

Measuring Body Cell Mass

Innovative technology has brought into clinical practice a device which accurately measures body cell mass in a matter of seconds. It's called bioelectrical impedance analysis (BIA), and it can usually be obtained at private clinics specializing in nutritional medicine or through the nutrition department of most hospitals and public health services.

The procedure is simple. It consists of lying down and attaching a set of electrodes to your wrist and ankle. Within seconds, a low-level electrical charge travels through the body and registers a set of numbers on a display. These numbers are then transferred to a computer program. At the end of the test you receive counseling from a health educator on the significance of the findings.

A BIA test measures the following parameters:

Body cell mass: This number tells you the exact number of pounds of metabolically active, energy-producing tissue on your body. It is important to obtain a baseline value as soon as you know that you are HIV(+), and then to follow it over time to see if there are any changes. Possible scenarios include stability, a drift downward which may signify the beginning of wasting syndrome, or a gradual improvement showing that your body cell mass is increasing.

State of hydration: The human body is normally about 60% water. By providing a measure of your state of hydration, the BIA test let's you know whether you are euhydrated (normally hydrated), dehydrated, or overhydrated. Body cell mass values from BIA testing are most accurate if you are in a euhydrated state.

Dehydration can cause fatigue and dizziness. Toxins and free radicals can also build up to dangerous levels. Adequate hydration is especially important if you are taking the antiviral drug indinavir (Crixivan), which can cause kidney stones to form if you do not consume enough fluid (3 liters/day).

If your BIA test shows that you are overhydrated, you may have edema, ascites, low sodium levels, or fluid overload from the overuse of anabolic steroids.

Body fat: Fat serves little purpose other than to provide long-term energy storage and to insulate you from the cold. In fact, too much fat can drain your energy due to the work it takes to carry it around. Excess fat provides a reservoir for drugs and toxins that should otherwise be excreted from the body. Fats also tend to become rancid over time and can be a source of oxidative stress to the immune system.

The ideal percentage of body fat in a healthy HIV(+) male is 12% to 20%. In a healthy HIV(+) woman it is 20% to 30%. These should be your target values.

Phase angle: The phase angle is a complex mathematical relationship between the reactance and the resistance of your body's tissues. In plain English, it is a summary of the density, and therefore the *healthfulness*, of the tissues of your body. It is also the body composition measurement which is *predictive of long-term survival from HIV disease.*

The normal range for the phase angle is between 4 and 12; however, the optimal value for an HIV(+) male should be greater than 5.6, and 5.0 for an HIV(+) female. This recommendation is based on a study published in 1995 in the *Journal of AIDS,* which showed that during a 3-year period, a phase angle of greater than 5.6 was a significant predictor of long-term survival in a group of male patients with advanced AIDS. Furthermore, it was more effective at predicting their long-term health than even their CD4 count. Based on these and other research findings, the following statement can be made.

The 3 Most Important Markers to Predict Long-Term Survival in HIV Are:

1) The viral load

2) The CD4 cell count

3) The phase angle

Keeping all 3 of these parameters in a healthful range *will ensure that your HIV condition does not progress.*

How Do I Improve My Phase Angle?

The target goal for body cell mass is to raise it to 100% of ideal for your height and weight. The target goal for your phase angle is to raise it above 5.6 for HIV(+) men and at least above 5.0 for HIV(+) women. Listed below are the 3 ways you can accomplish these goals:

1) Progressive resistance exercise
2) Increasing protein intake
3) Optimizing hormone levels

In this chapter, I would like to first discuss the most healthful ways to exercise. Optimizing your protein intake and hormone levels are covered in the next 2 chapters.

Exercise

Progressive resistance exercise, or PRE for short, is defined as the use of isometrics or weight-bearing exercises to add density and bulk to your body's musculature. PREs may include push-ups, pull-ups, and deep knee bends, but are even more effective when dumbbells, barbells, and exercise machines are used.

PREs do not include aerobic exercise, such as walking, jogging, biking, or swimming. While these are extremely healthful, they do not effectively increase your body cell mass. Aerobic exercise *does* improve the health of your heart, lungs, and skeletal muscles. It also promotes optimal circulation of blood and lymph, eliminates toxins, and decreases body fat.

As you may guess, the exercise programs I recommend to my patients are not limited solely to aerobics or PREs. They usually include a healthful integration of *both types of exercise* and are based upon the individual patient's individual BIA test results.

In general, I recommend doing some form of exercise at least every other day. Begin your workout with 10 to 20 minutes of stretching and mild aerobics to raise your heart rate, enhance the circulation, and warm up your muscles. Once you have exercised aerobically, you can then begin your resistance exercising. A second option might be to alternate the days on which you aggressively exercise aerobically or with weights (but always warm up with stretching).

I would like to provide an example of how to individualize an exercise program. If a patient is found to have a *low percent body fat* combined with a *low body cell mass,* can you guess what my exercise recommendation would be?

I would first recommend that this patient focus only on resistance exercises (supported by adequate protein intake and hormone supplementation) until the body cell mass and phase angle have normalized. Then, a gradual amount of aerobics would be added to the program for its general toning and circulatory system benefits. If another patient's BIA test were to show adequate body cell mass coupled with an abnormally high fat percentage, I would recommend that greater effort be put toward aerobics than resistance exercising. The only situation where I would recommend equal amounts of both is for general maintenance, when your body cell mass and percent body fat are both within the normal range.

There is a straightforward reason for avoiding aerobic exercise until your body cell mass is normalized: We all have limited amounts of energy. Our bodies use a large percentage of that energy for the vital processes of respiration, circulation, nervous system functioning, and mobility. The remaining energy is divided between fueling the immune system and allowing us to perform voluntary activities, such as exercise, traveling, working, and so forth. If you expend all of the energy available for exercise on aerobics, there will be very little left for resistance training to help improve your body cell mass. Since increasing body cell mass is more important for strengthening your immune function, resistance exercise must take precedence.

As you can see, there are no absolutes. That is why I advise each HIV(+) individual to obtain a BIA test every 3 to 6 months, and to work with a health educator to devise an integrative and individualized program of resistance and aerobic exercise. Once again, your primary goal is to maintain your body cell mass and percentage body fat as close to ideal as possible, and to keep your phase angle greater than 5.6 degrees for men and 5.0 for women. If your BIA results are maintained within these ranges, your chances of living a long and healthful life with HIV will be maximized.

SUMMARY

The more muscle you have on your body, the more energy you produce. Higher energy levels have been correlated with enhanced immune function and higher quality of life in HIV(+) individuals. A BIA test can quickly and accurately measure the amount of lean muscle on your body. A phase angle of greater than 5.6 has been shown to be a better predictor of long-term survival in men with advanced AIDS than a high CD4 count.

Chapter Ten

Protein and the Immune System

It has long been known that inadequate protein intake can cause depressed immune function. Examples include the occurrence of Pneumocystis carinii pneumonia in malnourished children, a high incidence of infection in burn patients, and increased mortality rates in malnourished individuals with AIDS. Numerous studies have also shown that enhancing the diets of these individuals with protein and caloric supplementation can significantly reverse their acquired immune system dysfunction.

Our bodies rely on protein to provide building blocks for many of the immune system's components. These include enzymes, antibodies, membrane receptors, chemotactic factors, and hormones. In fact, every cell depends on the presence of a vast array of intracellular proteins for its ability to function.

Most people do not realize that the amount of protein they need is based upon their level of health and activity. Patients with infectious diseases have long been known to require a greater amount of protein than that required by healthy individuals. It is therefore interesting that a significant number of HIV(+) patients, when seeing me for the first time, proudly proclaim that they have eliminated all animal products, including meat and dairy, from their diet. This change has usually been made with the goal of improving their health.

I generally do not support this strategy. A moderate amount of animal products in the diet provides many nutrients that HIV(+) individuals often lack. These include protein, calories, vitamin B₁₂, calcium, and zinc. While a vegetarian diet is preferable to prevent or reverse chronic ailments such as cancer, heart disease, and diabetes, it is often inadequate in the above nutrients to sustain an individual with a chronic infection for an extended period of time. If the above nutrients are consumed at below-optimal levels for several years, the immune system may experience a progressive decline that otherwise might have been avoided.

I encourage HIV(+) vegetarians who feel strongly about continuing this dietary style to consult a registered dietitian for expert guidance on how to meet their protein, calorie, zinc, and other nutrient needs.

How Much Is Enough?

In my first book on treating HIV infection, I printed a table listing the protein content of many commonly consumed foods. A similar table is reproduced at the end of this chapter. During the 5-year interval between this book and the last, I have increased the daily amount of protein I recommend that an HIV(+) individual consume. This new recommendation is based upon the past several years of clinical experience and research findings. I now recommend that an HIV(+) individual consume a minimum of 0.6 grams of protein/pound of body weight/day. For example, if you weigh 175 pounds (or your target weight is 175 lbs), you should consume *at least* 105 grams of protein per day (175 lbs X 0.6 gms/lb = 105 gms). Consuming more than this amount is not a problem as long as your kidneys and liver are functioning normally. The importance of consuming adequate protein is highlighted in the following patient story:

Ron

Ron is a 46-year-old self-employed businessman. Despite having been exposed to HIV in the early 1980s, he has successfully maintained his good health and stability without the use of antiviral medications. During the past 10 years his CD4 count has ranged from 450 to 650 cells/mm3, and his baseline viral load has recently been stable at between 20,000 and 40,000 copies/ml.

Though Ron is not taking antiviral drugs, he has not ignored the presence of HIV in his life. Ron meditates daily, gets regular exercise, belongs to 2 spiritually oriented support groups, takes vitamins and herbs, practices Chi gong, gets acupuncture, and follows a healthful nutritional program. Ron and I strongly believe that these strategies play an important role in maintaining his good health. He is even able to follow the above program while working full-time.

Approximately 3 years ago, Ron came in for his regular quarterly checkup. His only complaints at that time were a little fatigue and a recent weight loss of about 5 pounds. I asked Ron to get his blood tested and return in a week to go over the results. Disturbingly, Ron's CD4 count had fallen to 365 cells/mm3, his lowest level since discovering he was HIV(+). His viral load had also increased to 140,000 copies/ml.

I asked Ron, "What is going on here? Have there been any recent changes in your program? Are you under any unusual stress?" Ron said things were generally the same except that he was now following a macrobiotic diet. Macrobiotic diets typically include large amounts of grains, vegetables, and soy products with minimal fruit, sugar, and no animal protein. Upon further questioning, it appeared that Ron was getting only about half the protein his body needed to maintain a strong immune response to HIV.

"This is a serious situation," I told Ron. "I am strongly inclined to start you on antivirals today to prevent the loss of any more of your CD4 cells. Your viral load has gone up incredibly!" Ron was not happy to hear this, since he knew that once you begin antiviral therapy you are pretty much committed to staying on it for the foreseeable future and possibly the rest of your life.

"I'll tell you what," I said. "Let's take four weeks to try and turn this around. Meet with the dietitian, change your diet back to its original form, and begin taking protein supplements. I also want you to increase your resistance exercise and begin a course of testosterone supplementation to help replace the muscle mass you have already lost."

Ron was very satisfied with our comprehensive approach to treating this situation. It included dietary, hormone, and exercise interventions. Should our attempt be unsuccessful, it would be very important to Ron that we had exhausted all natural treatment options before he began antiviral therapy.

After aggressively following this program for 4 weeks, Ron returned to go over his new lab results. Miraculously, everything had improved to close to previous levels. His CD4 count was now back in the high 400s, his viral load had fallen by 50%, and his CD8 cells had increased as well. We both felt very fortunate that we were able to postpone his starting on antiviral medication at that time. Ron has continued to follow all of the recommendations I made, and *more than 3 years later,* his CD4 count is now over 500 cells/mm3 and his viral load has dropped to below 20,000 copies/ml. Ron continues to remain entirely asymptomatic, and he is still on no antiviral medication!

This patient's story describes a mutually satisfying physician-patient collaboration. We both approached the situation as equal partners with a common goal. It also highlights 2 additional points. First, the importance of maintaining adequate protein intake and second, the importance of not starting antiviral medication without first exhausting all efforts to identify the reason or reasons for the decline in your immune status.

High-Quality Protein Sources

Many HIV(+) individuals have lots of nutritional concerns to keep track of. These include:

- Did I remember to take my vitamins?
- Did I take my DDI on an empty stomach?
- Did I take my Crixivan on an empty stomach though apart from my DDI?

- Am I eating too much sugar?
- Is the dairy in my diet what's causing that awful gas?
- Did that glass of water contain any parasites?

I think you get the picture. If it can be avoided, I do not want to give my patients another dietary issue to worry about. Since many HIV(+) patients are already having trouble consuming all of the nutrients they need, my initial goals are that that they eat at least 3 highly nutritious meals a day, eat between meal snacks, and take all of their vitamins. I sound like a Jewish mother!

Given these concerns, I make 2 suggestions:

1) Do everything you can to optimize the protein you get from your food.

2) Add high-quality protein supplements to your diet.

Optimizing Protein Intake From Food

The following 5 suggestions can help enhance the protein you get from your diet:

1) Eat at least 3 meals a day that include a large portion of protein (> 20 gms/serving).

2) Eat between meal snacks.

3) Aim for 5 servings of protein each day.

4) Place "eat protein" reminder notes around your house.

5) Identify foods that are high in protein and keep a list of these foods in your wallet so you can refer to it when you go shopping.

High-Quality Protein Supplements

Taking protein supplements can allow many individuals to eat a normal diet, whatever's pleasing and appealing to them, without having to "worry so much" that they are consuming their requisite number of grams of protein per day. Once I learned how important it was to optimize protein intake in the treatment of HIV, I began to exploring the wide range of available supplement options.

There are many protein supplements on the market. They can be divided into the following 4 categories:

1) Protein powders
2) Snack bars
3) Fortified real foods
4) Premixed liquid drinks

Protein Powders

Choosing the best protein powder is not easy. There are several factors to keep in mind. First, it is important to determine whether the product is potent enough to supply you with the amount of protein you need. I recommend that any protein shake you use contain at least 25 grams of protein per serving. Some protein supplements mix up easily with a spoon in a small amount of water or juice, and their convenience justifies their lesser potency. You can refer to Fig. 10.1 for a comparison of the potencies, costs, and availability of many currently available, high-quality protein powder supplements.

The next important issue is the healthfulness of the product's ingredients. In my opinion, any protein powder that lists sugar, sucrose, dextrose, corn syrup, or fructose as 1 of its first 2 ingredients is detrimental to the heath of your immune system. The presence of a high concentration of sugar promotes the overgrowth of yeast in the GI tract and directly inhibits the functioning of your white blood cells. Don't be swayed if a protein powder that is high in sugar costs significantly less than its competitors. You get what you pay for! Other unhealthful ingredients to keep in mind are artificial flavors, colors, and sweeteners.

Some companies make special claims about the immune-boosting properties of their product's protein source. While there may be some validity to these claims, the evidence is insufficient at this time to suggest that 1 particular protein source provides a level of benefit that precludes the use of any other product. However, a few protein sources may offer some advantage.

Whey protein contains a significantly higher percentage of the amino acid cysteine than the more commonly utilized casein protein. Cysteine is used by the body to produce glutathione, an amino acid-like substance

Figure 10.1

PROTEIN POWDER COMPARISON CHART
(alphabetical order)

Product name	Protein per serving	Calories per serving	Cost per gram	Sugar content	Lactose content	Artificial ingredients	Product Availability	Phone number
Jarrow Formulas Function All	24 grams	240	.05	low	mod.	no	health food store	800-726-0886
MET-Rx Powder	37 grams	260	.04	low	low	yes	drug stores & mail order	800-396-3879*
Naturade Vegetable Protein	25 grams	100	.03	no	no	no	health food store	800-421-1830
Optimune	17 grams	120	.14	low	low	no	mail order	888-678-4644
OSMO Regeneration	30 grams	324	.04	low	low	no	mail order	800-219-2233
Proto Whey (hydrolyzed)	25 grams	152	.11	low	no	yes	mail order	888-494-2674*
The Ultimate Whey Designer Protein	18 grams	85	.05	low	low	no	health food store	800-468-6398
TwinLab Gainers Fuel	21 grams	531	.09	low	low	no	health food store	800-645-5626

* Medical discount program available

with immune-enhancing and antioxidant properties. A deficiency of glutathione can impair your body's ability to process free radical waste products and weaken the immune system over time. Glutathione levels have been shown to be depressed early in HIV infection and consuming whey protein may help raise them.

Some protein powders are formulated from rice protein. This protein source is hypoallergenic and may be beneficial to individuals with frequent allergic reactions and/or chronic diarrhea. Rice and soy are the most common protein sources found in supplements specifically formulated for vegetarians.

Some protein powders are enzymatically broken down (hydrolyzed) into very small molecules. This allows their amino acid building blocks to be more easily absorbed and metabolized. Because they are predigested, hydrolyzed protein supplements are often recommended for individuals with severely weakened digestive systems and chronic diarrhea. Try mixing hydrolyzed protein supplements with rice or soy milk for a good tasting, easy-to-digest source of protein supplementation.

Of course, palatability and taste are also important factors to consider. Consider asking yourself the following questions: Can I consume this product every day? Does it have a pleasant taste when mixed with water, or does it need to be mixed with juice or milk? Is the consistency of the product too filling, or can I also consume it with a meal? Since there are so many choices available, trial and error is often necessary to find the best protein powder for you.

Cost is also a major factor. The best way to evaluate a product's cost is to determine its price per gram of protein provided. At 5 cents per gram, you have found a very good bargain. A 30-gram serving would then come to $1.50. Since a 30-gram protein shake can make up the better part of a breakfast (though adding some fruit, toast, whole grain cereal, and/or eggs is still a good idea) this would be a fairly cost-effective benchmark. Some companies provide medical assistance programs (see Fig. 10.1), which supply their supplements to individuals with chronic medical conditions at a discounted cost. You can also check with a local buyers club for any protein supplements they may carry and sell at a discount.

Since many supplements on the market meet the above criteria, my suggestion is to choose a few and give them a try. Having several on your shelf at the same time will help prevent "burn out" on any 1 product and allow you to remain enthusiastic about their use well into the future.

Snack Bars

Snack bars provide another convenient way to supplement your protein. They are easier to consume away from home than powders and don't require a safe water source for preparation. There is just 1 caveat. In an effort to enhance the taste of snack bars, most companies use a sugar source as the first or second ingredient. Since large amounts of sugar promote the growth of yeast and depress immune function, I am not comfortable with a high concentration of sugar in the products I recommend. I am also not convinced that aspartame (NutraSweet) provides a very healthful alternative.

Since we all eat sweets at one time or another, and since a protein-fortified sweet is better for you than one which does not contain protein, a compromise can be made here. By substituting a protein-fortified snack bar for ice cream or cake of lesser nutritional value, you enhance your nutritional intake while at the same time satisfying your sweet tooth. A convenient but true rationalization.

You should also look for good taste, pleasant consistency, high potency (at least 5 to 10 grams protein per serving), and the minimization of artificial colors and sweeteners to help you choose the snack bar that best meets your protein-supplement needs.

Protein-Fortified Real Foods

Enhancing the protein content of the food you eat is another way to raise your protein intake. Currently available protein-fortified real foods include pancakes, pizza, and cheesecake (MET-Rx), instant packaged soups (Nestle's Clinical Nutrition), and protein-fortified decaffeinated coffee (Nestle's Clinical Nutrition). At the current time, MET-Rx fortified-foods are most readily available by mail order (800-396-3879), and Nestle's protein supplements can be specially ordered through your neighborhood pharmacy. As these foods gain more popularity, they will hopefully become easier to obtain.

Premixed Liquid Drinks

In my opinion, premixed liquid drinks are the least preferable way to supplement your protein intake. Almost all of them have sugar or corn syrup as their first ingredient after water. Furthermore, many of their other ingredients include oils, chemicals, synthetic vitamins, and artificial ingredients. They also tend to be very expensive.

Premixed liquid drinks have 1 saving grace. Some individuals on Medicaid (or other forms of government assistance) and private insurance can get premixed liquid drinks approved and paid for through these programs. If this is your only source of supplemental protein, by all means take advantage of it, but consume these beverages in moderation. Moderate use of these products is still better than no protein supplementation at all, especially if you are losing weight or unable to consume adequate amounts of solid food. In this case, I would try to limit your consumption to 2 cans per day while continuing to maximize the protein you consume from food. I would also ask a dietitian to prescribe 1 of the low-sugar varieties formulated for diabetics such as Choice AM (Mead-Johnson) or Resource Diabetic (Sandoz).

SUMMARY

Adequate consumption of protein and calories can make the difference between a healthy immune system and one that is in a progressive state of decline. Meeting with a registered dietitian can help you identify your target goals and find the right mix of foods and protein supplements.

In closing, there are many protein supplements on the market. Explore potency, quality, cost, and taste as key criteria when making your selection.

Figure 10.2

High-Protein Foods*

High-protein animal foods include:

Beef, 4 oz . . . . . . 28 gms	Chicken, 4 oz . . . . 28 gms	Halibut, 4 oz . . 24 gms
Ham, 4 oz. . . . . . 28 gms	Shrimp, 20 med. . . . . . 23 gms	Salmon, 4 oz . . 31 gms
Turkey, 4 oz . . . . 33 gms	Scallops, 4 oz . . . . 18 gms	Tuna, 4 oz . . . . 29 gms

High-protein vegetarian foods include:

Seitan, 1/2 c . . . . 28 gms	Garden burger . . . . 8 gms	Beans, 1/2 c . . . . 7 gms
Tempeh, 1/2 c . . 16 gms	Peanut butter, 2 tbsp. . 9 gms	Nuts, 1/4 c . . . . . 8 gms
Tofu, 1/2 c . . . . . 10 gms	Tahini, 2 tbsp . . . . 5 gms	Pasta, 1 c . . . . . . 5 gms
Lentils, 1/2 c . . . 9 gms	Soy milk, 1 c . . . . 7 gms	
Barley, 1/2 c . . . . 14 gms		

High-protein lacto-ovo foods include:

Milk, 1 c nonfat . 8 gms	Frozen yogurt, 1 c . . . . 4 gms
Cheese, 1 slice . . 6 gms	Egg, 1 large . . . . 7 gms
Cheese, 1 oz . . . . 7 gms	Cream cheese, 2 tbsp . 2 gms
Yogurt, 1 c . . . . . 8 gms	Cheese, 1/2 c cottage. . 12 gms

*Where relevant, all quantities are of cooked foods

Chapter Eleven

Hormonal Therapies

The word *hormone* is derived from the Greek word "to excite." Though hormones are released in very small amounts, they can have both wide-ranging and powerful effects. They influence sex drive, energy level, immune function, mood, metabolic rate, sleep, and appetite. Within 10 years, I predict the use of hormone-replacement therapy in men and women will play a very important role in standard medical practice.

Endocrine glands secrete hormones in response to stimulatory signals from the brain. The pituitary/hypothalamus region of the brain monitors the blood and decides when to stimulate hormone secretion by individual glands such as the testes (testosterone), the adrenal glands (DHEA, cortisol, epinephrine), the pancreas (insulin), the ovaries (estradiol), and the thyroid (thyroid hormone).

The endocrine system also affects the immune system both directly and indirectly. Hormones such as DHEA (dehydroepiandrosterone) and thymic factors have been shown to directly mediate immune system functioning by stimulating lymphocytes and other white blood cells. In contrast, testosterone's influence on mood, libido, and muscle mass has an indirect but significant effect on the immune system's functioning.

Many patients with chronic medical conditions, including HIV, experience a gradual decline in their quality of life which can extend over many years. Most of the symptoms associated with this decline are significantly influenced by hormones.

Listed below are descriptions of some of the hormones which can significantly affect the immune system; 2 of these hormones, testosterone and DHEA, are naturally produced by the body and need to be measured, monitored regularly, and supplemented if necessary.

Important note: When measuring serum hormone levels, the "normal range," as defined by the testing laboratory, is the average level found in the general population. In my experience, the normal range is not necessarily the "optimal range for healing," I define the optimal range as the hormone level found in 25- to 35-year-old adults who are at their peak of health.

Hormones and Body Cell Mass

As described in Chapter 9, maintaining a phase angle of greater than 5.6 for men and 5.0 for women, and a body cell mass 100% of ideal, is an important way to optimize the functioning of your immune system. Maintaining hormone levels within the optimal range can help ensure that these body composition goals are met.

Some physicians never test their patients' hormone levels. Others give all of their patients regular hormone injections whether they need them or not. As always, the key to maintaining good health is finding the right balance for each individual patient's situation.

Several hormones that build body cell mass are classified as steroids. This term refers to the physical structure of the molecule and not its function. Steroid hormones are essential to good health and exert a multitude of positive effects on the body. Estrogens soften the skin and stimulate the growth of the mammary glands. Androgens, such as testosterone, have masculinizing effects which promote hair growth, enlargement of the genitalia, and a deepening of the voice. Steroid hormones that increase muscle mass and protein utilization are termed anabolic steroids. Natural anabolic steroids, produced by both men and women for this purpose, are DHEA and testosterone. The anabolic hormones most commonly used in the treatment of HIV are listed below.

Anabolic Hormones Used to Treat HIV:

        1) Testosterone

        2) Oxandrolone

        3) Nandrolone

        4) Oxymetholone

        5) Recombinant Growth Hormone

        6) DHEA (dehydroepiandrosterone)

If you are experiencing progressive weight loss or a declining body cell mass, *do not hesitate* to use 1 or more supplemental anabolic hormones as part of your treatment program. They can greatly enhance both the quality and quantity of your future years. However, I do not support supplementing anabolic hormones just for the sake of appearance or for building body cell mass above 100% of ideal levels.

Testosterone

Testosterone is the hormone responsible for the masculinizing and tissue-building changes which occur in male adolescents. These include maturing of the genitalia and the development of secondary sexual characteristics such as hair growth. Women also produce testosterone, though only about 10% of that produced by men.

Several studies have shown that testosterone levels are frequently decreased in HIV(+) men. These studies suggest that approximately half of HIV(+) men with CD4 cell counts below 200 cells/mm3 have clear and demonstrable testosterone deficiency.

Research performed by Hellerstein and colleagues at the University of California, Berkeley, has also shown that the mean testosterone level of healthy, asymptomatic HIV(+) men is significantly lower than that of HIV-negative controls. His data suggests that suboptimal testosterone production in HIV(+) males is an extremely common occurrence. One can postulate from this and other studies that early hormone supplementation to restore an optimal testosterone level might play an important role in an HIV(+) individual's maintaining long-term good health and a high quality of life.

A recent study presented at the 2nd International Conference on

Nutrition and HIV in Cannes, France (1997), showed that in 14 asymptomatic HIV(+) men with hypogonadism (low testosterone levels), 79% developed an HIV complication within 15 months. In contrast, only 20% of the HIV(+) men with normal testosterone levels developed an HIV complication over a similar period of time.

Keeping your testosterone level in the optimal range is important for maintaining a healthful body cell mass as well as for preventing fatigue, depression, and diminished sex drive. As I previously stated, the *optimal range* for testosterone in HIV(+) men is not the same as the normal range commonly reported by most laboratories. The normal range for total testosterone in men is usually listed as 200–1000 ng/dl. The *optimal range* is 500–1000 ng/dl. This level is more effective at helping build and maintain body cell mass while still remaining within safe parameters.

Finally, testing the free testosterone level, as opposed to the total testosterone level, is much more expensive and usually does not provide additional benefit except in borderline or difficult-to-assess situations.

Testosterone Delivery Systems

Oral testosterone: Oral testosterone is cleared from the bloodstream by the liver within minutes of administration. As a means of overcoming this effect, several pharmaceutical companies have formulated synthetic forms of oral testosterone (i.e., methyl-testosterone). Although these products do a better job of raising testosterone blood levels, they also have been associated with significant liver toxicity. Oral administration of testosterone is therefore not a recommended delivery route option.

Injectable testosterone: Injectable testosterone is commonly used to treat testosterone deficiency. The injectable form, usually injected deep into the gluteus muscle every 2 weeks, ameliorates the underlying testosterone deficiency but can initially cause very high levels of testosterone in the blood. An injection of intramuscular testosterone usually results in a peak level above the limit of normal for several days followed by a gradual decline during the next 2 weeks. This promotes an increased risk of side effects such as headaches, anxiety, insomnia, irritability, mood swings, aggressive behavior, muscle tension, and testicular atrophy (shrinkage). This pattern of testosterone release is distinctly different from the body's normal testosterone release pattern, which provides a fairly steady blood level throughout the day. That is why testosterone patches (or creams), applied once daily, are currently the preferred testosterone delivery system in my practice.

Testosterone patches: There are 2 forms of testosterone patches currently available. The scrotal testosterone patch (Testaderm) is applied daily in the morning to a clean, dry scrotum which has been trimmed of hair. Company literature initially recommended shaving the scrotum every couple of days but trimming the hair with a small scissors works just as well. The scrotal patch comes in 2 sizes and can be itself trimmed for a more customized fit. The original Testaderm patch held to the scrotum without adhesive, but consumer feedback led to a reformulated, better-holding patch that now has thin lines of adhesive. The Testaderm patch effectively increases the testosterone level into the normal range in most individuals and is usually covered by insurance.

A second type of testosterone patch is applied to the upper body usually on the back, thighs, or anterior abdomen. At the present time, testosterone body patches are made by 2 companies. Alza Pharmaceuticals makes Testaderm TTS, which stands for testosterone transdermal system, and Smith-Kline Pharmaceuticals makes Androderm. Both patches are similar in their effect, but the Testaderm TTS patch is thinner, less bulky, and not as often associated with skin irritation. If skin irritation does occur, the application of triamcinalone 0.1% cream (available by prescription) underneath the patch can eliminate this side effect in most cases.

Testosterone patches may not be covered by some insurances, HMOs, and government programs because they cost more than testosterone injections. However, when the cost of an office visit every 2 weeks is factored into the equation, the cost is similar. The patches also put the control of this treatment into the hands of the patient and allow him to avoid the previously stated widely varying blood levels associated with testosterone injections.

Sublingual testosterone: Scheduled for release in 1999, the sublingual testosterone formulation allows natural testosterone hormone to be absorbed directly into the bloodstream through the blood vessels under the tongue. This mode of delivery effectively bypasses the liver clearance problem previously associated with oral administration. This new, high-tech delivery system can raise testosterone levels to normal within 20 minutes of administration and has been shown in several studies to be safe, effective, and well tolerated.

A study published in the *Journal of Clinical Endocrinology and Metabolism* in October 1996 looked at 51 hypogonadal patients who were withdrawn from their prior testosterone replacement therapy for at least 6 weeks. The 51 study subjects were then divided into 2 sublingual testosterone groups (2.5 mg and 5.0 mg 3x/day) and a testosterone enanthate injection group (200 mg every 20 days). The total treatment period was 60 days and evaluation of mood and quality of life parameters was performed at baseline and 3 subsequent intervals.

When compared to baseline, testosterone replacement in all groups led to significantly decreased anger, irritability, sadness, tiredness, and nervousness. In addition, energy level, friendliness, and sense of well-being were found to increase in all groups regardless of the type of testosterone supplemented.

These results were corroborated in a subsequent study in which 30 hypogonadal men were treated with sublingual testosterone at a dosage of 5 mg 3x/day for 6 months. All of these patients were also found to be significantly less nervous, more alert, friendlier, and more energetic during the 6-month treatment period when compared to their baseline while not on testosterone therapy.

The authors concluded that sublingual testosterone-replacement therapy in hypogonadal men is safe, effective, and improves multiple mood parameters when compared to treatment baseline. Of note, although testosterone delivered by intramuscular injections produced higher serum levels, no additional improvement in mood variables was seen.

Several additional studies have also shown that sublingual testosterone is also effective at increasing body cell mass, improving sexual performance, and increasing lower extremity muscle strength when compared to baseline and intramuscular testosterone injections.

Oxandrolone

Oxandrolone (Oxandrin) is a synthetic anabolic steroid hormone with approximately 6 times the muscle-building (anabolic) potency of testosterone. As a means of enhancing repletion of body cell mass in HIV(+) patients who continue to lose muscle despite optimal testosterone and DHEA levels, the administration of oxandrolone may be beneficial. Clinical trials have shown that oxandrolone is an effective therapy for promoting weight gain in a variety of other pathophysiologic conditions as well, including infectious diseases, trauma, and burns.

A significant benefit of oxandrolone therapy is its relative absence of significant virilizing or masculinizing effects. The ability to promote increased protein synthesis without masculinizing effects is due to changes that have been made to the molecular structure of this compound, thereby allowing it to be used in the treatment of HIV-associated weight loss in women.

A study presented at the 2nd International Conference on Nutrition and HIV Infection in Cannes, France (1997), by Pharo and colleagues from Houston, Texas, found that oxandrolone therapy produced a significant increase in body cell mass in HIV(+) positive women with no adverse side effects. In this study, 20 HIV(+) women were randomly assigned to 1 of 2 dosage groups in addition to a supervised resistance exercise training program. All of the women were also provided a protein drink and vitamin supplements. Evaluation of their nutritional status was performed at entry and at the end of the study using bioelectrical impedance analysis testing (BIA). After 7 weeks on the study, all of the women showed significant increases in body cell mass with no adverse side effects. Clinical trials conducted with greater than 450 men and women have shown that *99% of all patients* experience no masculinizing side effects from oxandrolone.

Another benefit of oxandrolone therapy is the fact that this compound has relatively few adverse effects on the liver when used as directed. The chemical structure of oxandrolone has been modified to allow the majority of an oral dose to be excreted by the kidneys relatively unchanged. This enables oxandrolone to bypass extensive hepatic metabolism and avoid placing significant stress on the liver.

In fact, the effect of oxandrolone on liver function was carefully scrutinized during its initial investigations. Its low potential for liver toxicity was demonstrated in a study comparing oxandrolone versus placebo in 273 patients with alcoholic hepatitis. In this group of patients with severe liver disease, there were no complications attributed to oxandrolone even when used at 80 mg/day, a dose 4 times what is normally recommended, during a period of 3 months. When statistically analyzed, no difference was found between the incidence of any complications of liver disease in the oxandrolone group versus the control group. In addition, in patients who were deemed moderately malnourished, oxandrolone decreased the mortality rate during the first 6 months of the study by sevenfold (4% treatment group vs. 28% placebo group).

Oxandrolone has also been shown in extensive clinical trials to have a positive impact in men on the treatment of HIV-related weight loss and wasting syndrome. A study of 63 patients with HIV-related wasting who received either oxandrolone (5 mg/day or 15 mg/day) or placebo showed that patients on the higher dose of oxandrolone experienced significant weight gain while on the therapy. Throughout the 16-week study, those receiving 15 mg/day of oxandrolone gained weight, those on the 5 mg/day dose maintained their weight, and those receiving placebo experienced continuing weight loss. Participants on the 15 mg/day dose also had increased appetite and activity levels when compared to those receiving placebo. There were no significant differences in adverse effects between the 3 groups. Oxandrolone was well tolerated by all patients enrolled in the study.

Data recently presented at the 12th World AIDS Conference in Geneva (1998) by Hellerstein and colleagues showed that when oxandrolone 10 mg 2x/day was combined with exercise and testosterone replacement in HIV(+) patients with wasting syndrome, a mean increase of 15 pounds body cell mass was observed after 8 weeks. This compared to an increase of only 7 pounds in the exercise and testosterone only group during a similar period of time. A gain of 15 pounds of body cell mass in 8 weeks is extremely impressive and illustrates the enhanced benefit that can be obtained when exercise, testosterone supplementation, and oxandrolone are combined.

Further evidence of the safety and efficacy of oxandrolone in treating HIV-related weight loss and wasting syndrome was demonstrated in a Phase IV Open Label Study that collected 12 months of data on 572 HIV(+) men and women. The dosage tested was 10 mg 2x/day. The data currently shows significant increases in weight and body cell mass in addition to significant improvements in appetite and activity levels in the majority of study participants. At the 12-month evaluation point, there was an average total weight increase of 13.9 pounds as well as a mean 7.9 pound increase in body cell mass among the participants. Oxandrolone was well tolerated in over 90% of the individuals participating in this study.

Several side effects are listed on the package insert included with an oxandrolone prescription. If you read it closely, however, you will notice that this document describes all of the adverse reactions that have been associated with use of the entire anabolic steroid class. No serious or life-threatening adverse effects have been associated to date with oxandrolone's use in clinical practice.

The most recent study to look at the potential side effects of oxandrolone administration was performed by Grunfeld and colleagues at the University of California, San Francisco. Preliminary results presented at the 12th World AIDS Conference in Geneva (1998) indicate that oxandrolone is extremely effective and well tolerated at a dosage of 20 mg/day. The 40 mg/day dosage appears to provide additional increases in weight and body cell mass, though there was a trend toward increased side effects as well. The side effects most commonly observed at this dosage were increased AST and ALT liver enzyme levels. At present, the 80 mg/day dosage is not recommended due to a significant incidence of these effects.

The use of synthetic anabolic steroids such as oxandrolone and nandrolone (see below) is meant to be complementary in nature to a strong antiviral and nutritionally oriented program. The duration of their use should depend on the response seen. Regular body cell mass evaluations (BIA testing or skin fold measurements) should be utilized to monitor their effects and the therapy is best discontinued as soon as reasonable goals are met.

The usual adult dosage of oxandrolone is 10 mg 2x/day. A course of therapy for 12 weeks is usually adequate to raise body cell mass to acceptable levels. The duration of this therapy should depend upon the individual patient's response and may be repeated as necessary.

For those without adequate insurance or the financial resources to afford oxandrolone therapy, a compassionate use program has been set up by the manufacturer, BioTech General Corporation (BTG). Information on this program can be obtained by calling 800-741-2698.

Nandrolone

Nandrolone (Deca-durabolin) is a synthetic anabolic hormone that is only available in injectable form. Although nandrolone has few masculinizing side effects when compared with testosterone, it is less anabolic and more masculinizing than oxandrolone.

In a study performed by Strawford and colleagues at the University of California, Berkeley, 2 doses of nandrolone were tested in comparison to placebo in men with AIDS, hypogonadism, and wasting syndrome. Subjects were monitored for 21 days on the metabolic ward, where they were fed diets of identical nutritional composition. Body composition, strength, endurance, and quality of life were measured. Nitrogen balance, total weight, and lean body mass were found to increase significantly in the nandrolone groups while the placebo group patients continued to lose weight. The response to nandrolone was related to the dosage used. Improvements in strength, endurance, and quality of life paralleled body composition changes. The authors of this study concluded that supplementation with nandrolone in hypogonadal HIV(+) men with wasting syndrome has significant positive effects on body composition and exercise endurance.

Nandrolone is given as a deep intramuscular injection in the gluteus muscle. It can be mixed with injectable testosterone, as both are suspended in an oil matrix that gradually releases the active hormone over approximately 2 weeks. The most common dosage of nandrolone given to men is 200 mg administered every 2 weeks.

Nandrolone, similar to oxandrolone, should only be used in supplementary fashion once optimal blood levels of the body's natural anabolic hormones (testosterone and DHEA) have been achieved. In my opinion, there are only 2 specific instances in which nandrolone is preferable to oxandrolone. The first includes patients who are overwhelmed by the number of pills they have to take and prefer a biweekly injection. The second is in individuals who have little or no private insurance and are forced to use nandrolone therapy because of an inability to pay for oxandrolone.

Oxymetholone

Although not officially approved for the treatment of HIV-related weight loss, oxymetholone (Anadrol) is being aggressively marketed to the HIV(+) community as another anabolic steroid for the treatment of HIV-related weight loss.

This compound was originally studied and approved during the 1960s for the treatment of anemia due to low red blood cell production. The treatment of anemia was the original indication given to the entire anabolic steroid class of medications. Since oxymetholone is known to also possess anabolic (muscle building) properties, Unimed Pharmaceuticals, Inc., is trying to position oxymetholone as another treatment for HIV-related weight loss.

In the only study of oxymetholone performed in HIV(+) individuals to date, Hengge and colleagues assessed the weight-promoting activity of oxymetholone alone or in combination with ketotifen, a tumor necrosis factor inhibitor.

In a nonblinded, controlled study, 60 HIV(+) patients were randomized to the following 3 groups:

1) Oxymetholone 50 mg 3x/day: 14 patients
2) Oxymetholone 50 mg 3x/day plus ketotifen: 16 patients
3) Untreated controls (not taking a placebo): 30 patients

Weight gain of at least 4.4 lbs was observed in 23 of 27 patients in the treatment groups and in only 1 of 29 patients in the control group. The average weight gain at week 20 was 18 lbs in the oxymetholone group, and 13.4 lbs in the combination treatment group. There was an observed weight loss of 4 lbs in the untreated control group. The treatment in all study arms was well tolerated.

Though this data suggests that oxymetholone has potent anabolic activity in HIV(+) individuals, it is a single small study that was not blinded to either the patients or investigators. It also did not include a placebo arm. The study is therefore inadequate to support recommending the use of this compound for the treatment of HIV-related weight loss.

Also, though liver toxicity is an effect associated with the entire class of oral anabolic steroids, individuals on long-term therapy with these agents appear to be the most at risk. Accordingly, there have been several recent reports of hepatotoxicity associated with long-term oxymetholone treatment. Atlay and coworkers reported on hepatotoxicity in 65 Turkish patients who had undergone *long-term therapy* with oxymetholone. Peliosi hepatitis (dilation of hepatic sinuses) occurred in 4 patients and hepatic cancer developed in 1. Kosaka and colleagues also documented the occurrence of hepatic cancer in a 35-year-old woman on long-term therapy with oxymetholone. The authors of this study recommended that routine ultrasound or CAT scan screening of the liver be performed in all patients taking long-term anabolic steroid therapy.

Oxymetholone has been used by the bodybuilding community for many years as well. Michael Mooney in *Medibolics: The Power Program for Wellness Restoration* newsletter (fax: 310-659-1597), describes the general experience with oxymetholone among bodybuilders. While acknowledging that these reports are anecdotal, Mooney states that oxymetholone is known to be highly potent as an anabolic agent but is also associated with a high frequency of side effects. These reportedly include hair loss, impotence, fatigue, high blood pressure, prostatic enlargement, and mood swings.

Recombinant Human Growth Hormone

Human growth hormone (hGH) is a hormone normally produced by the pituitary gland in the brain. It aids growth and maintenance of strength by increasing lean body mass, decreasing fat, and improving immune function. Some of these actions occur through the release of insulinlike growth factor (hIGF-1, or somatomedin), which is produced in the liver and other areas of the body.

In the 1980s, advanced biotechnology led to the ability to manufacture recombinant human growth hormone (rhGH). Since that time, rhGH has been safely administered to thousands of adults and children with pituitary disease and other growth hormone deficiency syndromes.

A number of clinical trials have also demonstrated that rhGH (Serostim) administered at 0.1 mg/kg/day (approximately 6 mg/day) significantly increases total weight and body cell mass in HIV patients with wasting. It has also been shown to reduce fat, improve physical performance (measured by treadmill), and improve the quality of life of patients with wasting due to AIDS.

In a multicenter, double-blind, placebo-controlled study of rhGH, 178 people with AIDS-related wasting syndrome were randomized to receive either human growth hormone at 0.1 mg/kg/day subcutaneously or placebo for 12 weeks. Patients in the hGH-treated group showed an average total weight gain of 3.5 pounds. Their gain in *body cell mass* was even greater, at 6.6 pounds. This greater increase in body cell mass occurred because the hGH-treated subjects lost fat at the same time that they gained muscle. All forms of weight gain in the treatment group were found to be statistically significant. A proportionate increase in the amount of intracellular water was also recorded in the hGH-treated group. This indicates that the hGH-treated individuals were producing metabolically active tissue. Considering that these patients were severely immunocompromised at study entry with an average CD4 count of 87 cells/mm3, these results are very impressive.

In a second multicenter, double-blinded, placebo-controlled study, 177 people with AIDS-related wasting syndrome received human growth hormone at a dose of 6 mg/day administered subcutaneously compared to placebo for 12 weeks. Assessments at weeks 6 and 12 showed that the increases in total body weight in the GH-treated group were significantly higher than increases for patients in the placebo group. Changes in body cell mass were not monitored in this investigation.

Side effects associated with rhGH (Serostim) in these trials included joint pain and stiffness, and tissue turgor or puffiness. These results were reported as mild and resolved spontaneously with over-the-counter analgesics or dose reductions. Mildly elevated blood sugar levels (hyperglycemia) were also seen in patients during these and other clinical trials. Elevated blood glucose levels can occur in HIV-infected individuals due to a variety of reasons. Most recently, there have been reports of hyperglycemia associated with the use of protease inhibitor antivirals. Patients with significant risk factors for glucose intolerance such as obesity, a family history of diabetes, or protease inhibitor use, need to be monitored closely while receiving growth hormone therapy.

At the 12th World AIDS Conference in Geneva (1998), Torres and colleagues reported in a case series that rhGH (Serostim) reduced "buffalo hump" (dorsocervical fat pads) and truncal obesity in 4 patients with HIV-related lipodystrophy syndrome. Clinical trials are currently underway to further investigate the safety and effectiveness of prescribing rhGH for this condition.

The main goal for using anabolic hormone supplementation for the treatment of HIV-related weight loss is to build and maintain body cell mass (lean muscle tissue), as measured by BIA or skin fold testing. If your body cell mass is low, and the levels of your *natural* anabolic hormones (testosterone and DHEA) have been optimized, supplementation with anabolic hormones is probably necessary to help you build your muscle mass to 100% of ideal. This intervention will help support your immune system's functioning and keep your quality of life high.

I believe human growth hormone is an effective therapy to use for this purpose. As an anabolic agent, it is relatively fast, safe, and reliable. It achieves peak lean body mass increases within 6 to 12 weeks, and these are often retained for long periods off therapy. It does not *require* exercise to increase body cell mass, but a combination of the two may work even better. It has no virilizing (masculinizing) side effects and is therefore is an excellent option for women who need to build muscle. It may even help build muscle when other agents have proven ineffective. However, which anabolic agent performs the best is an open question since head to head comparisons of rhGH (Serostim) to other anabolic agents (oxandrolone and nandrolone) have not been performed.

The above properties make rhGH (Serostim) best suited as an acute 6 to 12 week intervention rather than for chronic therapy. Approximately 95% of the patients who use rhGH do not require therapy longer than 12 weeks to obtain maximum body cell mass. Its cost also makes long-term use prohibitive.

The decision of which anabolic agent to use is ultimately up to the patient and his or her physician. It is best based upon factors such as access to the drug, tolerability of the treatment, and whether or not individual patients are more comfortable taking pills (oxandrolone) or giving themselves injections (rhGH, nandrolone).

Serono Laboratories, the makers of rhGH (Serostim), have capped the price of their product at $36,000/year in an effort to be more competitive with the other products indicated for the treatment of HIV-related weight loss. They have also developed an extensive patient support program called SeroCare, which provides free, confidential reimbursement services to both physicians and patients. You can speak to a Serono SeroCare reimbursement specialist by calling 800-714-2437.

DHEA (dehydroepiandrosterone)

The adrenal glands produce several hormones that help protect the body from stress. Adrenaline helps protect the body from short-term stress. For instance, if you happen to be crossing a street and notice a car is about to hit you, adrenaline is immediately released and within a split second you have the ability to move out of the way more quickly than would otherwise be possible. With the help of adrenaline, the stressful situation has been successfully corrected.

Other adrenal gland hormones, such as cortisol and DHEA, help protect the body from long-term stress. The levels of these hormones rise when the body is faced with the initial stress of an illness. However, as the illness or long-term stress continues, adrenal gland production of these important hormones sometimes begins to decline. As their protective effects are lost, a chronic inflammatory state begins to develop. This chronic inflammatory state is like a smoldering fire whose effects can weaken the body over time.

DHEA production is normally most abundant when people are in their twenties and thirties. Its production declines about 10% per year thereafter. Coincident with this decline is an increased incidence of such diseases as cancer, heart disease, and diabetes. Is this merely a coincidence? Many scientists currently involved in DHEA research think not.

DHEA levels also commonly decline as HIV progresses. In fact, most HIV(+) individuals have far below the optimal level for this hormone. In addition, DHEA supplementation can improve many of the symptoms associated with HIV disease such as fatigue, muscle loss, and depression. It is also available without a prescription, well absorbed orally, and virtually nontoxic.

Measuring DHEA Levels

There are 2 forms of DHEA in the body. DHEA is the active form, while DHEA-sulfate is the storage form. Both can be measured with a blood test. DHEA-S is the least expensive of these 2 tests because there is more of it to measure. The units are ug/dl for DHEA-S and ng/dl for DHEA. The optimal range for DHEA-S (which is present when people are at their peak of health) is between 300–600 ug/dl for HIV(+) men and 100–300 ug/dl for HIV(+) women. Sometimes DHEA-sulfate levels are reported in such a way that you need to move the decimal point 2 places to the right (when reported as ug/ml). For instance a level of 3.0 ug/ml would then be read as 300, and 4.2 ug/ml would be read as 420. Ignore the normal range values the laboratory uses because they are usually too wide or have been adjusted for age, which is not what you want.

It is best to use the same test and the same laboratory when tracking DHEA or DHEA-S values. This ensures the greatest level of consistency when monitoring your test results.

The Rationale for Supplementing DHEA

There are 2 basic reasons I recommend maintaining an *optimal level* of DHEA in your blood:

1) Extremely positive clinical effects that I have seen in my HIV(+) patients who maintain optimal levels of DHEA.

2) Several recent studies which have shown significant benefits from DHEA in HIV treatment with no adverse side effects.

Clinical Experience

Since 1994 I have prescribed DHEA to hundreds of HIV(+) individuals in order to bring their levels into the optimal range. By keeping their DHEA levels in this range, this and the other supportive measures of the Healing HIV program have enabled their immune systems to continue functioning optimally.

My experience with DHEA has been extremely positive. Patients feel better, have more energy, and are far less susceptible to the negative effects of stress. In addition to using healthful nutrition, vitamin therapy, and aggressive antiviral strategies, DHEA supplementation has helped the vast majority of my patients maintain complete stability for very long periods of time. Coincidentally, wasting syndrome and dementia are virtually unknown in my practice.

I am amazed at the large percentage of HIV(+) individuals whose DHEA-S levels are low. I estimate that about 80% of HIV(+) men have DHEA-S levels below 200 ug/dl. As described above, the optimal range for a HIV(+) man is between 300 and 600 ug/dl. The optimal range for an HIV(+) woman is between 100 and 300 ug/dl. I have treated dozens of women with DHEA and see the same beneficial results that I see in men with virtually no androgenic (masculinizing) side effects. Occasionally, it can cause acne.

Utilizing DHEA in this fashion, a large number of my patients have been able to eliminate fatigue, alleviate depression, and improve their level of well-being beyond anything they have *ever* experienced. DHEA supplementation is safe, beneficial and nontoxic *as long as blood levels are monitored regularly.* I highly recommend its use as an integral part of optimal HIV care.

Bryan

Bryan is a 40-year-old HIV(+) individual with 550 CD4 cells/mm3. He has experienced chronic depression since he was a teenager. Bryan's initial DHEA-S level was 142 ug/dl. After starting DHEA at 200 mg 1x/day, his DHEA-S level increased to 545 ug/dl (optimal range: 300–600 ug/dl). Bryan told me that since starting DHEA, his depression has completely resolved, and he no longer needs to take the antidepressant medication he has been taking for years.

In addition, Bryan's energy level and sense of well-being are now excellent, and his general level of health has never been better. Bryan attributes all of this improvement to his starting DHEA. He has been on DHEA for over a year now with no side effects, and he continues to experience good health.

Recent Research Studies with DHEA

DHEA Levels Decline in HIV(+) Individuals

In this section, I discuss recent research studies related to DHEA and HIV(+) patients (complete citations for these studies can be found in the References section). An observational study published in the 1993 *American Journal of Medical Science* looked at the relationship of serum DHEA-S levels and CD4 cell counts in people with HIV. Blood tests were done in 98 HIV(+) adults. The authors found that DHEA-S levels declined in parallel with CD4 cell counts. They did not see a decline in serum cortisol levels. The authors concluded that when the study participants were analyzed by clinical subgroups, those with the lower DHEA-S levels were more commonly found to have advanced disease. These data show a positive relationship between the immune status of people with HIV-related illness and DHEA-S levels, leading to the hypothesis *that the presence of a deficiency in the hormone DHEA may contribute to a declining immune status.* (*American Journal of Medical Science*, 1993)

Another study published in the *Journal of AIDS* showed that DHEA levels declined as HIV(+) individuals became more symptomatic. The authors concluded that declines in several steroid hormone concentrations during the development of HIV infection, including DHEA and testosterone, may have negative effects on immune responsiveness in patients, and *that DHEA may form part of a complex network of immunomodulatory factors.* (*Journal of Acquired Immune Deficiency Syndrome,* 1992)

Low DHEA Levels as a Predictor of HIV Progression

A cohort study was performed in 1992 at the University of Amsterdam, The Netherlands, Department of Infectious Diseases. It investigated serum DHEA levels in 41 patients with asymptomatic HIV disease who progressed to AIDS within 5 years after entering the study. These were compared to 41 HIV(+) individuals who remained asymptomatic during the 5-year period *and* 41 HIV-negative controls. Upon entering the study, DHEA levels among the HIV-negative controls were higher than in either of the HIV-positive groups. *DHEA levels in the progressors were consistently found to be lower than in the nonprogressors. The authors concluded that low DHEA levels were an independent risk factor for HIV disease progression.* (*Journal of Infectious Diseases,* 1992)

Jacobson and colleagues at San Francisco General Hospital looked at blood samples taken from HIV(+) men followed prospectively since 1984 in the San Francisco Men's Health Study. Among 108 HIV(+) men who had CD4 counts between 200 and 499 cells/mm3 at study entry, serum DHEA levels *below the normal range* (less than 180 ng/dl) were predictive of disease progression after controlling for hematocrit levels, age, and CD4 counts. This was the first large prospective cohort study in which an endocrinologic variable was shown to be independently predictive of HIV disease progression. These observations suggest *that HIV(+) patients who maintain a normal DHEA level possess a survival advantage when compared to those with lower DHEA levels.* (*Journal of Infectious Diseases,* 1991)

Another study presented at the 2nd International Conference on

Nutrition and HIV in Cannes, France (1997) looked at the correlation between low DHEA and DHEA-sulfate levels, and the occurrence of weight loss and loss of body cell mass in 38 HIV(+) men. The results of this study showed a highly significant correlation between low DHEA and DHEA-sulfate levels and the occurrence of HIV-associated malnutrition. The authors suggest *that supplementation of DHEA might help improve the quality of life and survival rates of HIV(+) individuals.* (2nd International Conference on Nutrition and HIV, 1997, Oral presentation 05)

DHEA's Effect on Viral Activity

A study of DHEA's effect on HIV replication in cell cultures showed a dose-dependent inhibition of HIV's cytopathic effect, as measured by reverse transcriptase activity. At very low concentrations, DHEA reduced AZT-resistant HIV replication by over 50%. This study provides evidence that DHEA can independently inhibit the replication of AZT-resistant, as well as wild-type, HIV. Combined with its immunoregulatory properties, the authors suggest *that the use of DHEA may have a much broader spectrum of activity than originally anticipated.* (*Biochemical and Biophysical Research Communications,* June 1994)

A 1992 study at the Temple University Department of Microbiology and Immunology revealed that the exposure of human lymphocytes to DHEA resulted in down regulation of HIV replication as measured by syncytia formation, release of p24 antigen, and reverse transcriptase activity. DHEA also reduced syncytia formation in HIV(+) lymphoblasts. The conclusion was that DHEA, previously shown to have antiproliferative effects, *appears to also directly suppress HIV replication. DHEA could therefore become an alternative and/or adjunctive treatment for HIV infection.* (*AIDS Res Hum Retroviruses,* 1992)

DHEA'S Effect on CD4 Counts

An abstract presented by the Houston Immunology Institute at the 1994 International Conference on AIDS in Yokohama, Japan evaluated the use of DHEA supplementation, in addition to standard antiviral and prophylactic OI therapy. In the study, 12 patients received an average DHEA dose of 75 mg per day. CD4 and CD8 counts were obtained at baseline and at monthly intervals. Baseline values were CD4<50: 2 patients, CD4 50-100: 6 patients, and CD4 101-200: 4 patients. The patients were followed for 4 to 12 months, with a mean duration of 8 months. The results showed that, although there were 2 deaths during the 12-month study period, 9 of the surviving 10 patients showed an increase in CD4 cell counts; 5 of the 9 patients (56%) had more than a 25% increase in CD4 cells; and 8 patients (68%) experienced an increase in CD8 cell counts as well. Since increases in CD4 and CD8 cell counts may be clinically significant and are associated with long-term survival, this paper concluded *that a randomized clinical trial of DHEA supplementation was warranted.* (International Conference on AIDS, 1994, Abstract #PB0322)

Most recently, Sanusi and colleagues at the Nassau County Medical Center in New York performed a prospective, randomized, double-blind study to look at DHEA's effects on clinical laboratory markers in women with AIDS. In the study, 29 HIV(+) women were administered either DHEA 50 mg 1x/day or a placebo. All of the study participants were taking a stable triple-combination antiviral regimen during the duration of the study. Subjects receiving DHEA supplementation showed improvements in the following categories when compared to placebo: total weight, energy level, physical functioning, cognitive abilities, emotional well-being, and CD4 count (DHEA group (+) 111 cells/mm3 vs placebo group (-) 11 cells/mm3). There was also a trend to a greater decrease in viral load in the DHEA group. The authors concluded *that oral administration of DHEA for 6 months in HIV(+) women produced beneficial effects in CD4 count, weight, and several other subjective health parameters without producing side effects.* (12th World AIDS Conference, Geneva, 1998, Abstract #42373)

DHEA's Effect on Mental Health

A double-blind, placebo-controlled study randomized 32 men to either DHEA 50 mg 1x/day or a matching placebo group for a period of 4 months. Clinical data, virologic, and immunologic markers, DHEA-S levels, and mental health/quality of life scales were recorded every month during follow-up. DHEA-S levels rose in the treatment group. A significant improvement in mental health/quality of life scores was observed in the DHEA-treated group when compared to the placebo group (p=0.01). No changes in CD4 counts were noted, and no side effects of DHEA occurred. The authors concluded *that administration of DHEA in advanced HIV(+) patients resulted in a beneficial effect on mental health and quality of life scores.* (12th World AIDS Conference, Geneva, 1998, Abstract #42326)

Side Effects of DHEA

A phase 1 dose escalation study was performed to evaluate the safety and pharmacokinetics of DHEA in people with symptomatic HIV disease and an absolute CD4 count between 250 and 600 cells/mm3. In the study, 31 subjects were evaluated and monitored for safety and tolerance. DHEA was given orally 3x/day in doses ranging from 750 to 2250 mg/day for 16 weeks. This is an extremely high dosage range. The supplement was well tolerated and no dose-limiting side effects were noted. Although this study was not designed to specifically evaluate the immunologic effects of DHEA, no sustained increases in CD4 cell counts were noted during this brief study. (*Journal of Acquired Immune Deficiency Syndrome, May* 1993)

Common Sense and DHEA

If found to be below normal levels by a blood test, hormones are generally supplemented in an effort by physicians to restore normal homeostatic balance to the body. Insulin, estrogen, testosterone, growth hormone, cortisol, and thyroid hormone are all supplemented if their levels are found to be low. Yet just because we haven't fully documented all of the subtle beneficial effects of DHEA, or found that a deficiency of it causes an acute short-term problem, we assume that supplementation is not necessary. How shortsighted we physicians can be!

Because the beneficial effects of DHEA are subtle, and it does not significantly improve CD4 cell counts or decrease HIV viral load by itself, studies to identify its benefit should look for a lessening of symptoms, a maintenance of healthful weight and muscle mass, and an improvement in quality of life over the long term. They should also look for improved trends in disease progression and mortality as markers of its overall effect. These studies should utilize the dosage necessary to optimize blood levels, not pick an arbitrary dosage that assumes everyone's need for DHEA is the same.

Taking DHEA

It is important to make sure that your DHEA supplement is pure and effective. Health food store products claiming to be DHEA are not always of the concentration and purity necessary to treat a medical condition. Buyers' clubs or compounding pharmacies are often a more reliable source. Always ask if an independent lab has confirmed the product's purity before taking this hormone for medicinal purposes.

The dosing guidelines for DHEA are fairly straightforward. For HIV(+) men, a 200 mg supplement 1x/day is taken if the DHEA-S level is below 100 ug/dl. A 100 mg supplement is taken 1x/day if the DHEA-S level is below 200 ug/dl, and a 50 mg supplement 1x/day is taken if the DHEA-S level is in the 200–300 ug/dl range. *If you are taking a protease inhibitor antiviral, cut the recommended dosages by half.* HIV(+) women should take 25–50 mg/day if their level is below 100 ug/dl.

I advise obtaining a repeat DHEA-S level 4 to 6 weeks after starting DHEA therapy or changing your dosage. Once on a stable dosage, I strongly recommend regular monitoring at 6-month intervals.

Anabolic Hormone Guidelines

An aggressive prevention-oriented philosophy that includes good nutrition, vitamin supplements, regular exercise, stress reduction, and effective antiviral therapy is clearly the best way to prevent HIV-related weight loss. The use of anabolic hormonal therapies in a stepwise, escalating fashion, gives the patient and practitioner powerful weapons to counteract wasting if prevention-oriented measures begin to fail. The supplementation of anabolic hormones, such as oxandrolone, nandrolone, or recombinant human growth hormone should be considered in the following situations:

1) When your body cell mass is less than 100% of ideal (as measured by BIA testing) despite optimal levels of testosterone and DHEA.

2) When your phase angle (as measured by BIA testing) is less than 5.6 in or 5.0 in women, despite optimal levels of testosterone and DHEA.

3) When significant fatigue or weight loss is present which has not responded to other treatment measures.

SUMMARY

Early intervention with a multifaceted program that includes healthful nutrition, intelligent vitamin supplementation, optimizing testosterone and DHEA levels, and effective antiviral therapy is highly effective at preventing HIV-associated weight loss and maintaining strong and stable immune function. If additional intervention is necessary, anabolic hormones such as oxandrolone, nandrolone, or recombinant human growth hormone can be extremely beneficial when used in supplemental fashion. Periodic monitoring of DHEA-S and testosterone blood levels, with supplementation as necessary to maintain them in the "optimal range," is an important and necessary part of first-class HIV care. There are a wide variety of testosterone delivery options. The goal should be to mimic your body's normal physiologic release of this hormone as closely as possible with patches (or creams) unless injections are your only option due to cost or availability.

I would now like to briefly summarize the information presented in the past several chapters:

1) Consume adequate protein from healthful sources. You can calculate your minimum protein requirement by multiplying your body weight in pounds times 0.6. This gives you your minimum daily protein requirement in grams.

2) Exercise with weights at least 3x/week or as tolerated.

3) Optimize your natural anabolic hormones. These include testosterone and DHEA. See the material in this chapter for a detailed

discussion on the best ways to monitor and supplement these natural hormones.

4) Utilize synthetic anabolic hormones such as oxandrolone, nandrolone, and recombinant human growth hormone as necessary to increase your body cell mass to 100% of ideal levels. Obtain regular body composition testing to monitor your progress. This will ensure that your immune system is functioning at peak strength and that you are maximizing your chances of remaining healthy and stable well into the future.

Chapter Twelve

Preventing and Treating Fatigue

Fatigue is more than just feeling tired. It is tiredness that does not go away with rest. It is important to eliminate fatigue for 2 reasons. First, the immune system is the most sensitive system of your body to your energy level. If your energy is low, it has a diminished ability to function effectively. Second, several studies have shown that patients with ongoing fatigue experience quicker progression of HIV to infections and death.

Your body can generally communicate with you in 2 ways. It can speak with pain or with tiredness. This is how your body tells you that something is wrong with a pattern in your life and lets you know that changes are necessary. *Fatigue is your body's way of sending an early warning that something is not right.*

For example, if you go to the gym to work out, and your right elbow starts to send you pain, you could interpret that pain as your body's way of sending you a message. It is most likely telling you that it has become slightly injured and you need to stop what you are doing for a while. This allows it time to heal.

In essence, an unhealthful pattern occurred, the body communicated the problem to you with pain, you interpreted the message correctly, and you took the appropriate corrective measures. The body can now return to its original state of healthful balance.

Fatigue presents a similar situation. However, most people do not interpret fatigue as well as they interpret pain. People often become unhappy with their bodies for being tired without searching for the deeper causes behind this symptom. Fatigue is your body's way of communicating to you that there is something wrong. It can either be with your body, your medications, or with your life's current patterns. It may be as simple as not getting enough rest. However, it also may be more complicated. Whatever the cause, it needs to be addressed, not ignored, and certainly not treated by taking increased amounts of stimulants such as caffeine or testosterone.

If you ignore your body's initial warning signs, louder and more problematic messages will usually follow. These louder messages can include opportunistic infections or an increase in your viral load. One of the keys to long-term health and stability if you are HIV(+) is to identify and address minor imbalances early, so that you can avoid more serious ones later on.

Think about it. When you are tired, your eyes don't go blank, your heart doesn't stop beating, and your muscles don't stop moving. But if you are pushing yourself too hard and not resting when you are tired, your immune system will become drained, and the opportunity for developing infections (such as sinusitis, pneumonia, thrush, and herpes) increases.

There are 2 large studies which support the above comment. They both show that fatigue is a marker for the development of opportunistic infections and progression to AIDS. This correlation is true, independent of patients' CD4 counts or whether they are taking antiviral medications. Therefore, fatigue should be treated as an early warning sign that, if ignored, can progress to a more serious situation.

The 6 Causes of Fatigue

Fatigue in HIV(+) individuals can be caused by 1 or more of the following 6 factors:

1) Nutritional deficiencies
2) Hormone imbalances
3) Anemia

4) Concurrent infections

5) High-level HIV activity

6) Depression

Although any of these factors can cause fatigue independently, several can be present concurrently.

A medical evaluation of HIV-related fatigue requires a collaborative approach between patient and physician. It is extremely important to inform your doctor of the extent of the fatigue you are experiencing. If you want your health practitioner to appreciate what you are saying, you need to describe how significantly it impacts your quality of life. The better your physician understands how debilitating your fatigue is, the faster he or she can implement any necessary evaluation and treatment.

Typical laboratory testing includes a complete blood count (CBC) to identify anemia, a blood chemistry panel to look for liver problems, a stool sample to screen for intestinal parasites, and an HIV viral load. Other tests, when medically indicated, may include a chest x-ray and blood cultures.

Nutritional Deficiencies

When the body is under significant stress, it requires additional amounts of high-quality fuel. If fuel intake is low, fatigue may develop. For optimal nutrition, it is important to consume a diet rich in both macronutrients (calories and protein) and micronutrients (vitamins and minerals).

Macronutrients are burned 8% to 40% faster by HIV(+) individuals than in those who are HIV negative. Since protein is a vital macronutrient for supporting immune function, consuming protein supplements may help ensure you get all that you need. I strongly urge every HIV(+) individual to consult with a registered dietitian to evaluate your diet, identify your nutritional needs, and help you set realistic, healthful goals.

Micronutrients are also depleted more quickly if you are HIV(+). Several studies have shown that vitamin and mineral supplementation can have a strengthening effect on the immune system and prevent the progression of HIV. In Appendix 9 and in Chapter 15, I list my current recommendations on micronutrient supplementation for individuals who are HIV(+).

Herbs can also help improve your energy level. Licorice, damiana, astralagus, and ginseng help increase energy and improve circulation to organs such as the bone marrow (where red blood cells are formed), the liver (the organ that helps detoxify drugs), and the spleen (the body's largest lymph gland). Maintaining the optimal health of these organs is critical to avoiding energy depletion. Consulting a skilled herbalist or acupuncturist experienced in treating HIV(+) individuals may help you formulate an herbal regimen that appropriately meets your body's needs.

Hormone Imbalances

The levels of cortisol, thyroid hormone, testosterone, and DHEA (dehydroepiandrosterone) can be profoundly depressed in HIV(+) individuals. If fatigue is present, each of these hormone levels needs to be evaluated and supplemented if necessary. Please refer Chapter 11 for information on how to evaluate and supplement testosterone and DHEA. The measurement and supplementation of cortisol and thyroid hormone are more straightforward and your standard physician can help you with this. It is your responsibility to make sure that all of these hormone levels have been checked if you are suffering from severe fatigue.

Anemia

The main function of red blood cells is to deliver oxygen throughout the body. The more oxygen delivered to your cells, the healthier you will be. If your red blood cell count begins to fall, the cells of your body receive less oxygen. Still, many physicians let the red blood cell counts of their patients drop substantially before intervening with treatments that can reverse this process.

Anemia can be diagnosed by measuring the hemoglobin or hematocrit level in a simple and inexpensive blood test. The normal hemoglobin range is 12 to 15 g/dL. The normal hematocrit range is 39% to 48%; levels below 11 g/dL for the hemoglobin and 33% for the hematocrit signal serious anemia and can often be reversed with appropriate intervention.

Anemia may be caused by a number of factors that include bleeding from the bowel, medication side effects, bone marrow infections, vitamin deficiencies, and/or a deficiency of the hormone erythropoietin, a red blood cell growth factor produced by the kidneys. An easy-to-read flow chart to help you identify potential causes of fatigue and anemia is shown in Fig. 12-1

Figure 12.1

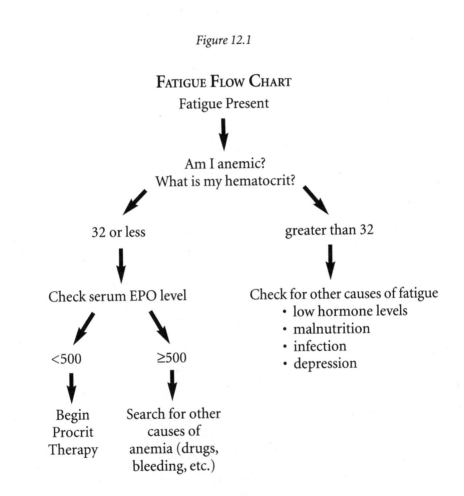

Your serum erythropoietin hormone level can be measured and, if low (less than 500 ug/mL), can indicate the need for timely and preventive supplementation to correct anemia. Otherwise, your red blood cell count may continue to fall, worsening your fatigue and causing the eventual need for a transfusion.

Whereas transfusions are definitely necessary if anemia is acute and severe, recent studies have shown an association between transfusions and increased HIV progression. It is important to point out that this association has been identified only in preliminary studies which still need to be replicated; a definitive link has not been established. If your anemia is severe, a transfusion may be necessary and beneficial. However, proactive monitoring of your hemoglobin and hematocrit levels, with subsequent supplementation of the hormone erythropoietin if necessary, may help prevent the need for transfusions.

You can self-administer erythropoietin supplementation by injection, usually at an interval of 3x/week. Since erythropoietin is a natural hormone, side effects are rare. Please consult your health-care practitioner for more specific guidelines based on your individual needs.

Concurrent Infections

Hidden infections with pneumonia or MAC (Mycobacterium avium complex) may cause fevers, night sweats, cough, and diarrhea, as well as severe fatigue. If these symptoms are present, it is important that your doctor perform a thorough medical evaluation that includes a chest x-ray, blood culture, sputum culture, and any other lab tests which might be indicated, such as a gallium scan. Infections such as these are serious; their prompt identification and treatment are extremely important.

Infection with intestinal parasites can often be asymptomatic, but their most common presenting symptom is fatigue. As you might imagine, parasites are not the first thing your doctor thinks of when you complain of fatigue. All HIV(+) individuals in our practice are screened for intestinal parasites yearly. We often see a significant cause-and-effect relationship between the eradication of parasites and the improvement of a patient's fatigue symptoms. Other seemingly unrelated effects from infection with these organisms include allergies, skin rashes, and rectal bleeding. If you have never been checked for intestinal parasites and have any of the above symptoms, you need to be tested soon.

Mark

Mark first visited with me in March of 1996. After 10 years, he had developed full-blown AIDS and now had a CD4 count of 8 cells/mm3. He was also experiencing frequent fevers and night sweats due to an infection with MAC (a chronic infection similar to tuberculosis). Mark's viral load was 176,000 copies/ml despite taking AZT/3TC for 6 months prior to our visit. Additional symptoms included diarrhea, weight loss, and extreme fatigue. Mark also had severe, chronic low back pain due to a previous injury.

Admittedly, Mark did not look or feel well. His fatigue, low back pain, and very low CD4 count significantly contributed to his depressed state and diminished hope for living. This was probably an appropriate response to his present situation.

Our most important initial intervention was to change Mark's antiretroviral program. To rebuild his immune system, we would need to completely suppress his viral load. After a few tries, we were able to institute a well-tolerated regime consisting of D4T/3TC/indinavir. Mark began to feel better almost immediately. With the further addition of DHEA 250 mg 1x/day and erythropoietin injections 3x/week (Procrit) to treat his anemia, Mark began to gain ground. Some 2 months after his initial visit, Mark's CD4 count was up to 65 and his viral load had become undetectable.

Although everything was moving in the right direction, Mark's liver function tests began to rise. This meant that his liver was beginning to become inflamed due to his antiviral medications. In order to help his liver handle the stress of taking these drugs, I recommended that Mark start on my Liver Support Program, which includes Lipotropic Factors at a dose of 3 capsules 3x/day between meals (see Appendix 9). Within 1 month, Mark's liver function tests had significantly improved, and the rebuilding of his immune system was able to continue without the need to switch medications.

In July 1996, 4 months after our first consultation, Mark's CD4 count had risen to 129 cells/mm3. His viral load also continued to remain undetectable. His energy level and sense of well-being were vastly improved, and his anemia, diarrhea, and severe fatigue had all resolved. His CD4 count continued climbing during the next several months to 165 cells/mm3.

Mark's story illuminates the tremendous benefits that can be obtained by integrating standard and complementary therapies. His chronic symptoms and liver inflammation were successfully treated with a natural therapies program. This allowed him to continue taking antiviral medications that were working. His immune system is rebuilding itself with an extremely potent and well-tolerated triple-combination regimen. Mark and I are continuing to fine-tune his program so that his good health and stability continue for a very long time.

High-Level HIV Infection

Increased HIV replication, manifested by a high viral load, can place a significant drain on the body's resources and contribute to fatigue. If this is a significant problem, all measures should be taken to bring your viral load down to an undetectable level. These measures include the elimination of all the cofactors that may stimulate HIV activity (see scenario #5 in Chapter 6) and the use of highly effective antiretroviral therapy.

Depression

Most people would agree that living with HIV can be very stressful. It is therefore possible that, as a result of this chronic stress, a decrease in neurotransmitter levels in the brain may occur. This is the exact medical definition of depression. This condition can cause chronic pain, difficulty sleeping, changes in appetite, and chronic fatigue.

You can use several natural remedies to treat depression. These include psychotherapy, regular exercise, support groups, and herbal therapies such as St. John's Wort. If these are unsuccessful, or in addition to them, the use of one of the newly released antidepressants, such as Prozac,

Zoloft, Paxil, Serzone, Wellbutrin, or Effexor, may help raise your neurotransmitter levels into the normal range, thereby eliminating many of the psychological and physical symptoms of depression. It is very important that you work with a primary-care doctor or psychiatrist who is comfortable prescribing these medicines if depression has become a significant factor in your life. It is also important to check with your pharmacist regarding potential drug interactions if antidepressant are being prescribed in conjunction with protease inhibitor or NNRTI antiviral medications.

SUMMARY

1) Fatigue is a *multifactorial condition.*

2) Monitor your hemoglobin, hematocrit, thyroid, testosterone, and DHEA levels. Be sure they remain solidly within the normal and/or optimal ranges.

3) Treating anemia with erythropoietin supplementation may help prevent the need for transfusions.

4) Natural therapies (diet, vitamins, exercise, and stress reduction) all work best as preventive therapies. Begin them early to ensure that your long-term-health remains strong.

4) Being proactive is the easiest way to make sure that you never have to treat severe fatigue.

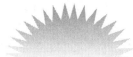

Chapter Thirteen

Preventing and Treating Neuropathy

Peripheral neuropathy is usually described as pain, numbness, or tingling in the hands or feet. It can occur as a direct effect of HIV infection on the peripheral nerves, or more commonly as a side effect from certain medications.

The most common medications that can cause neuropathy are the antivirals D4T (Zerit), DDC (Hivid), and DDI (Videx). Neuropathy can occur less commonly from AZT, IV pentamadine, and a multitude of other medications. (Ritonavir, a protease inhibitor, can cause numbness and tingling around the mouth 1 to 2 hours after dosing. This is not true neuropathy since it is temporary and not secondary to nerve damage).

Prevention

Since peripheral neuropathy is D4T's most common side effect, whenever it is prescribed I recommend consuming 3 nutrients to help protect the nerves. These nutrients and the dosages I recommend taking are shown below. When combined with the careful use of antiviral medications, they will protect the nerves and enable most HIV(+) individuals to avoid experiencing the pain and discomfort of peripheral neuropathy. They are also a part of my new daily supplement recommendations (see Appendix 9).

Nutrients That Help Prevent Neuropathy

Calcium .... 500 mg 2x/day

Magnesium .... 250 mg 2x/day

Vitamin B$_6$ ..... 100 mg 2x/day

Treatment

If a person is already experiencing symptoms of peripheral neuropathy, a reduction in the causative medication's dosage, or stopping it completely, can cause the symptoms to diminish or resolve over time. In addition, adding the above nutrients to your supplement program plus increasing the vitamin B$_6$ dosage to 200 mg twice daily may also have a significant positive effect. I have had many clients report back to me either complete resolution or a very significant decline in their symptoms within a couple of weeks after beginning the above regimen.

In cases of advanced neuropathy, where severe or prolonged injury to the nerves has occurred, it may take several months of an aggressive combination of remedies to effect improvement. Nerves take time to heal. Therefore, even if you put together the perfect program of remedies, it might still take a couple of months before improvement begins. Don't give up!

In addition to the nutrients listed above, the following list of additional measures can greatly enhance your success at preventing and treating neuropathy. Remember, the dosage of vitamin B$_6$ to treat neuropathy that is already present should be 200 mg 2x/day.

In closing, it is very important that you understand the following statement: *Where your attention goes, your energy flows.* The presence of your healing energy is essential to bring about healing change to any part of your body. If a part of your body is in pain, don't get angry with it. Don't ignore it. It is in distress, and it needs your attention now more than ever.

Additional Measures to Treat Neuropathy

Acupuncture: By performing acupuncture along various lower extremity meridians, a skilled acupuncturist can encourage healing energy to flow downwards to the affected peripheral nerves. When performed regularly, this practice can often reduce pain and hasten the resolution of this condition.

Massage: Although regular massage by a skilled practitioner can have a wonderful and generalized healing effect, my strongest recommendation is that you perform self-massage twice daily on any part of your body that is sending you pain. Just take a few minutes to get into a comfortable position, choose a massage oil that has a pleasant aroma, and begin massaging your extremities in whatever fashion feels the most pleasant and soothing.

Sometimes your hands or feet may be so sensitive that it initially feels as if you are making them worse. Don't worry. This can be fairly common at the beginning and does not mean that you should stop. It just means that you need to be more gentle. You may first need to place your hands *above* the area that is sensitive and just wait. Wait until it feels okay to touch the area. And then just touch it. Remember, these nerves have been injured and traumatized. Though it may seem difficult at first, they need to be reassured and nurtured. By reconnecting to the part of your body that is hurting and sending it love, you maximize your chances for healing. *Everyone's hands* have the power of healing touch!

Alpha-lipoic acid: This natural substance is a powerful antioxidant which possesses potent liver-strengthening and detoxifying qualities. If extremity pain does not resolve after several months of taking the 3 nutrients mentioned above, adding alpha-lipoic acid at a dosage of 200 mg 2–3x/day may bring with it additional benefit.

Amitriptyline (Elavil): This drug was originally used as a treatment for depression. However, when taken in extremely low doses, one-fifth to one-tenth of that normally used to treat depression, it effectively blocks the brain from receiving chronic painful stimuli. It is taken once a day before bedtime and can also help promote deeper, calmer, and more restful sleep. The key is to start at the lowest dosage level, 10 milligrams, and then work up by 10 milligrams every 3 days until a beneficial effect is realized.

Unlike natural remedies, amitriptyline's effect is felt very quickly because it is not attempting to heal the nerves, only to make you less aware of the pain. Potential side effects are morning grogginess, blurry vision, dizziness, and urinary hesitancy. These are all more prominent at higher dosages and sometimes resolve after 1 or 2 weeks of continued use.

Pain management: Supplementing the above measures with non-narcotic or narcotic pain medications can help relieve whatever residual discomfort still remains. A good choice might be a long-acting remedy such as naproxen sodium (Naprosyn) which you take every 8 to 12 hours (known as Aleve in its over-the-counter formulation). You can also use shorter-acting preparations such as ibuprofen (Motrin and Advil).

Nerve growth factor: Currently in clinical trials, nerve growth factor appears to be effective at diminishing the chronic pain associated with peripheral neuropathy. Several patients in my practice have been using this treatment with good results. It is given twice weekly as an injection. Although this treatment is designed to promote the regeneration of peripheral nerves, stopping therapy is often associated with a rebound of symptoms. Finally, many patients describe nerve growth factor injections as being particularly painful at the site of injection. More data on this promising new therapy will hopefully be forthcoming.

SUMMARY

1) Prevention with nutritional supplements is extremely important.

2) Be judicious with medication dosages. Take only as much antiviral medication as you need.

3) Use a combination of measures, including nutrients, acupuncture, massage, and medications to achieve the optimal result.

4) Be patient. Nerves take time to heal.

Chapter Fourteen

Preventing and Treating Kaposi's Sarcoma

Kaposi's Sarcoma (KS) is primarily a disease that mostly affects gay and bisexual men with HIV. It is, however, rare in people who were infected with HIV through intravenous drug use, by transfusions, and through blood products, such as hemophiliacs. In addition, women have been observed to be at much lower risk for developing KS than men.

Due to these epidemiological trends, researchers have searched for a viral agent that could be responsible for contributing to the transmission of KS. New studies have recently indicated that human herpes virus 8 (HHV8) may be this agent. This virus is now known as Kaposi's sarcoma herpes virus (KSHV). This research explains a significant amount of KS's epidemiological characteristics.

Recent reports indicate that the overall incidence of KS has decreased dramatically. There are several possible reasons for this decline. If KS is transmitted sexually, changes in sexual behavior, such as practicing safe-sex techniques, may be responsible. Other possibilities include suppression of HIV activity by protease inhibitor drugs and a clear improvement in the general health and immune system strength of many HIV(+) individuals.

At the start of the AIDS epidemic, KS was the leading cause of AIDS and often occurred in people with relatively high CD4 counts. At that time, a KS diagnosis was associated with a significantly increased risk of death. Today, KS usually affects HIV(+) individuals who have very low CD4 cell counts and are in poor health. It is also now a much less common contributing cause of death.

KS Pathogenesis

KS lesions are the result of small blood vessels called capillaries that grow out of control. When this occurs, a thick, purplish mass can appear on any external surface of the body. KS lesions also occur internally, most commonly in either the intestines or the lungs.

Several cytokines and growth factors are believed to play a major role in the growth of KS lesions. Fibroblast growth factors are naturally produced substances which have been associated with stimulating the growth of new blood vessels. These factors have also been associated with KS lesions. Inflammatory cytokines such as interleukin-1 (IL-1), IL-6, and tumor necrosis factor alpha (TNF-alpha) have also been shown to indirectly stimulate the growth of new blood vessels within preexisting KS lesions.

Clinical Features

KS lesions can appear in a variety of colors and shapes and are usually described as macules, nodules, papules, or plaques. Macular lesions are small in size and can be pink, purple, or red. Papular lesions and plaques are often found on the extremities of the body. Larger plaques and nodules can also be found on the elbows and around the knees. These plaques and nodules can be associated with pain and edema (tissue swelling).

KS lesions can also occur in the mouth. Oral lesions are sometimes asymptomatic but can result in difficulty swallowing and oral pain. They are usually treated with local injections of tumor-inhibiting medications (see below).

The most serious form of KS, which can be life threatening, is found in the lungs. Patients with pulmonary KS can have problems breathing, relentless coughing, and hemoptysis (coughing of blood).

Diagnosis

Although an experienced clinician can recognize the distinctive appearance of a KS lesion, a biopsy of the lesion is commonly performed to confirm the diagnosis. This is a simple procedure, with the results available in about 2 days. A bronchoscopy, gallium scan, or x-ray is usually needed to detect pulmonary KS. Biopsies of pulmonary lesions are usually not performed, as there is a high risk of bleeding from pulmonary KS lesions. KS lesions in the gastrointestinal tract are usually diagnosed visually during an endoscopy procedure and can be confirmed with a small biopsy without significant risk.

Prevention

The incidence of KS has declined dramatically during the past several years. A possible reason for this is that a highly suppressed HIV infection allows the immune system to remain strong thereby keeping other potential viruses and cancers in check. This hypothesis would support my recommendation that your immune system needs to be strengthened and supported as much as possible for KS to be effectively prevented. Effective prevention includes finding the best possible combination of aggressive natural therapies and standard HIV medications. You can use the information contained throughout this book to help you accomplish this goal.

Treatment

The treatment of KS is best individualized based on the size and extent of the lesions. There are differing views on whether people with relatively few KS lesions should be treated immediately. However, some researchers believe that all people with KS should be treated to prevent further KS from spreading. Others believe that routine monitoring to determine the course and aggressiveness of the condition is more appropriate. Not surprisingly, I recommend a highly aggressive program of prevention with gradually escalating pharmaceutical intervention as necessary.

Local Therapies

Liquid nitrogen cryotherapy: This treatment is often used for small, lightly pigmented lesions especially those found on the face, neck, and hands. Liquid nitrogen freezes the lesion until it begins to fade and can usually achieve attractive cosmetic results. However, because this type of therapy results in hypopigmentation (a flat white scar), it may not be suitable for people with dark skin. This form of therapy also does not result in a killing of KS cells, as it merely freezes the top layers of skin. Lesions treated in this fashion can blister and then form a crust. It is therefore best to keep the frozen site covered until it is completely healed.

Cryotherapy usually results in resolution of the treated lesion that lasts for 6 weeks to 6 months. It may be necessary to have repeated cryotherapy in order to keep the KS lesion from reappearing.

Intralesional chemotherapy: This has also been shown to be effective for treating small numbers of KS lesions. Intralesional chemotherapy can be used to shrink raised, bulky lesions while cryotherapy is best used to treat flat lesions.

A drug known as vinblastine (Velban) is commonly injected below the skin at a dose of 0.1 mg/mm2 of lesion. Some pain may be associated with these injections, which can last for a 1 or 2 days.

It is important to exercise caution when using intralesional vinblastine near the eyebrows and around the hairline, as this may lead to shedding of the hair follicles. In addition, caution is required when using intralesional vinblastine around large peripheral nerves (in the arms and legs) to avoid producing neuropathy.

Radiation therapy has been used for many years to treat localized KS. However, it appears that HIV-related KS does not respond to radiation therapy as well as non-HIV-related KS (KS occasionally occurs in HIV-negative individuals). Using a dose of 400 rads once a week for 6 weeks, people with non-HIV-related KS had a median duration of response for 48 months, whereas people with HIV-related KS had remission for as short as 6 months but as long as 3 to 4 years. Radiation therapy is often indicated when the KS lesions are localized to a specific area of the body, such as the foot, groin, legs, or back.

Experimental Intralesional Therapies

A small study of recombinant platelet factor-4 (rPF-4) found that this drug has anti-KS activity when used intralesionally. However, there were only responses in the lesions that were directly injected with little activity in lesions that were separate from the injection site.

A study of intralesional tumor necrosis factor (TNF-alpha) showed some anti-KS activity as well. This treatment also achieved a response in the lesions directly treated but had no activity in the noninjected lesions. Unfortunately, there were also significant side effects. These included fevers, rigors, and chills. It is unlikely that intralesional TNF-alpha will play a major role in the treatment of KS in the future.

A dose-escalation study of human chorionic gonadotropin-beta (beta-HCG), a hormone produced in high amounts during pregnancy, demonstrated anti-KS activity at all doses, with the higher doses showing better activity. The doses studies were 250, 500, 1000, and 2000 units/10 ccs. The treatment was well tolerated at all doses. Resolution of the surrounding lesions was reported in some early studies. Additional research is currently ongoing using this highly promising intralesional therapy.

There are numerous other local therapies, including surgical excision, photodynamic therapy, radiotherapy, and synthetic retinoid application. In addition, there are a number of intralesional therapy studies looking at myeloid colony stimulating factor and sclerosing agents. None of these is currently showing a high degree of promise.

Systemic Therapies

Chemotherapy is the most widely used systemic therapy for treating KS. There are a variety of these agents available to treat KS. Most of them are also used to treat other kinds of cancers.

Drugs used as single agents to treat KS include bleomycin (Blenoxane), liposomal daunorubicin (DaunoXome), doxorubicin (Adriamycin), liposomal doxorurbicin (DOXSL or Doxil), etoposide (VP-16 or VePesid), teniposide (Vumon), vinblastine (Velban) vincristine (Oncovin), and paclitaxel (Taxol). Commonly prescribed combination regimens include bleomycin/vincristine, bleomycin/vincristine/doxorubicin, bleomycin/

vinblastine/doxorubicin, methotrexate/vinblastine, and bleomycin/ doxorubicin/etoposide/vinblastine.

It is not known whether any of these drugs or combinations is more effective than the others since only a few studies directly comparing these treatments have been conducted. In addition, the response criteria and patient populations in each of these studies have been different. Many physicians use alternating treatment regimens to reduce the risk of side effects. G-CSF injections are often used to enhance white blood cell counts before and during KS chemotherapy.

There are numerous side effects associated with systemic chemotherapy. Most chemotherapy agents can cause nausea, hair loss, neutropenia, anemia, thrombocytopenia, and peripheral neuropathy. In addition, each individual drug may have its own specific side effect. The availability of drugs such as ondansetron hydrochloride (Zofran) and granisetron hydrochloride (Kytril) has resulted in a decreased likelihood of nausea when taking chemotherapy drugs. The choice of specific chemotherapy agents is usually based upon a patient's wish to minimize certain side effects and by the various efficacies of the different regimens. Often, a failing treatment may be replaced by a different drug regimen that once again achieves a therapeutic response.

Liposomal therapy is a novel treatment strategy that takes advantage of "stealth technology" as applied to pharmaceutical agents. In this type of chemotherapy, the medication is encapsulated in tiny vesicles called liposomes. Though significantly smaller than blood cells, liposomes resemble them chemically and are therefore allowed by the immune system to circulate throughout the body until they come in contact with tumor cells. Since the blood vessels that supply tumor cells are usually more porous than the blood vessels supplying normal tissue, the drug-containing liposomes leak into the tumor, are taken up by the cancer cells, and release their drug inside them. This destroys the tumor cell. Studies have shown that the concentration of liposomal drug in normal tissues of the body remains very low. This technology allows the chemotherapy treatments to be given less frequently and minimizes side effects such as fatigue, hair loss, and peripheral neuropathy.

Liposomal daunorubicin (DaunoXome) has been approved by the FDA as first-line therapy to treat individuals with advanced KS. The dosage of this medication most commonly used is 40 mg/m2 every 2 weeks. A clinical study showed that liposomal daunorubicin when used alone was as effective as adriamycin/bleomycin/vincristine.

Liposomal doxorubicin (DOXSL) has been approved as second-line treatment for recalcitrant KS. The dose of liposomal doxorubicin is 20 mg/m2 every 3 weeks. A study comparing liposomal doxorubicin to adriamycin/bleomycin/vincristine showed that individuals receiving liposomal doxorubicin had a better response than people receiving the triple combination. There were also fewer side effects reported among people receiving the liposomal doxorubicin. A second study comparing liposomal doxorubicin to a combination of bleomycin/vincristine also showed that people receiving liposomal doxorubicin had a better response rate compared to those receiving bleomycin/vincristine.

Paul

In 1996, when Paul first came to see me, he was in very poor shape. Kaposi's sarcoma lesions had extended into his lower extremities and were causing him severe swelling and pain. Paul had been HIV(+) since the early 1980s and currently had a CD4 count of 65 cells/mm3. His other symptoms included chronic fatigue, depression, and weight loss. Fortunately, he had no opportunistic infections other than KS.

Paul had taken many antiviral drugs during the past decade. Recently he had begun his first triple combination consisting of AZT/3TC/saquinavir. Though he was tolerating this regimen fairly well, he still had significant symptoms as well as a low CD4 count and a viral load of 26,000 copies/ml. Clearly, there was significant room for improvement.

My first suggestion to Paul was that he begin treating his KS with systemic liposomal therapy. Liposomal therapy consists of chemotherapy medication that is surrounded by small, membrane-like vesicles. These vesicles are called liposomes. The body does not recognize liposomes as foreign. However, when tumor cells consume them, the medication is released, killing the tumor cell in the process. This treatment enables the patient to avoid several common side effects which are associated with more standard forms of chemotherapy. These include hair loss and peripheral neuropathy. Liposomal therapy is infused once every 2 to 3 weeks and spares most of the body's normal tissues from severe toxicity.

After starting liposomal therapy, Paul's KS stabilized and began to recede. With the addition of massage, physical therapy, elevation of his lower extremities, and regular exercise, Paul's legs healed from KS to the extent that he could return to work full-time as a hotel concierge, a job which requires many hours of standing. I remember reassuring Paul that, as long as he kept his faith and worked hard, his legs would heal. I admire his courage and applaud his hard work. It certainly has paid off.

The next change I made to Paul's treatment program consisted of modifying his antiviral medications to include a new triple combination. The reasons I changed his regimen were 1) his viral load was still significantly elevated and 2) his CD4 count, though stable, was not improving. The goal of the Healing HIV program is to raise the CD4 count to above 300 cells/mm3 no mater where you start from. Once you are above this level, your immune system functions relatively normally.

I therefore recommended that Paul switch his antiviral medications to D4T/3TC/indinavir, a very potent regimen. Paul took this particular combination until August 1997. During this time, his CD4 count climbed from 65 to 312 cells/mm3, and his viral load also became undetectable. Paul started DHEA and testosterone-replacement therapy to optimize his hormone levels. He also continued to receive regular massage therapy, exercised regularly, took vitamin supplements, and followed a daily practice of meditation and other spiritual healing techniques.

Though doing quite well, Paul subsequently complained of persistent gastrointestinal discomfort. A work-up for infection, intestinal parasites, and other digestive imbalances proved negative and a trial switch of his protease inhibitor, from indinavir to nelfinavir, improved his GI situation significantly. It also helped raise Paul's CD4 count even further, to 435 cells/mm3!

Paul's story is a good example of how an individual with a CD4 count less than 100 cells/mm3, significant fatigue, and other systemic symptoms, as well as severe Kaposi's sarcoma, can work his way back to full functional status and a normally functioning immune system. As you can see, Paul combined diet, vitamin therapy, exercise, massage, stress reduction, antiviral medication, as well as chemotherapy, to successfully accomplish a profound healing of his condition. Paul's treatment program illuminates the central tenet of the Healing HIV program: The most successful treatment of any health condition is one which incorporates a truly holistic approach to the problem — one that combines natural, psychospiritual, and standard medical treatments.

Another systemic KS therapy known as Interferon-alpha has also been extensively studied during the past 8 years. The Food and Drug Administration (FDA) has approved 2 different versions of interferon-alpha for the treatment of KS: interferon-alpha-2a (Roferon-A) and interferon-alpha-2b (Intron A). Both are approved to treat KS in people with greater than 200 CD4 cells and are given as either an intramuscular or subcutaneous injection.

The exact mechanism by which interferon inhibits the growth of KS lesions is not completely understood. It is thought to inhibit angiogenesis (the formation of new blood vessels). Laboratory studies have also shown that interferon-alpha has direct, although weak, anti-HIV activity.

Clinical studies have shown that high-dose interferon is capable of inducing tumor regression in about 30% of participants when their CD4 count is at least greater than 200 cells/mm3. In addition, laboratory and animal studies have shown that there is synergy between interferon and AZT, DDI, and DDC. In human clinical studies, people who received AZT plus interferon had better response rates against KS than people who received interferon alone. Several studies of interferon at lower dosages have also shown activity against KS. Most of these studies involved the use of interferon-alpha in combination with antiretroviral therapy. It is probable that combining interferon with the triple-combination antiviral regimens currently in use will work at least as well.

There are several side effects associated with interferon therapy. These include a "flu-like syndrome" (fevers, chills, malaise, and myalgia), headache, confusion, neutropenia (low white blood cell count), and anemia. Colony-stimulating factors such as G-CSF are often used with interferon (especially when it is used in combination with AZT) to raise the white blood cell count.

Experimental Systemic Therapies

A few studies of paclitaxel (Taxol) have shown that this drug is active against KS even in people who have been on extensive prior chemotherapy. In laboratory studies, paclitaxel has been shown to have anti-angiogenesis activity.

Another class of compounds that are in study for both the treatment of KS and HIV are the camptothecin derivatives. These include topotecan (Hycamtin) and irinotecan (Camptosar). In laboratory studies, these compounds have activity against various kinds of cancers as well as inhibiting the integrase enzyme of HIV.

Several compounds that have shown anti-angiogenesis activity in laboratory studies have shown little anti-KS activity in small clinical studies. These compounds, which include TNP-470 and DS-4152, are continuing to be studied to determine if there is better activity using higher doses of these drugs.

A study is also planned for cidofovir (Vistide) to determine its activity against KS. Laboratory studies show that cidofovir has potent activity against HHV8, which is now considered the causative agent for KS. Cidofovir is currently used to treat another viral infection, cytomegalovirus. Although it only needs to be administered once every 2 weeks in an IV infusion, its use is limited due to a fairly high incidence of toxicity to the kidneys.

SUMMARY

Our improved understanding of the pathogenesis of KS continues to lead to more effective prevention and treatment methods. Highly active antiretroviral therapy has already had an enormous effect on decreasing the incidence of KS by suppressing the replication of HIV in the blood. Anyone with currently active KS should strive to get their viral load as low as possible, preferably to an undetectable level. This is the first step in effective KS treatment. Thereafter, local versus systemic therapy can be decided upon based on the number, location, and occurrence rate of your lesions. Interferon therapy is indicated for the treatment of KS only when the CD4 count is greater than 200 cells/mm3 and should be combined with highly active antiretroviral therapy for best results. Liposomal therapy can be used at any CD4 count, is infused once every 2 to 3 weeks, and has been shown to be less toxic than traditional KS chemotherapy regimens.

Chapter Fifteen

Aggressive Natural Therapies

••••••••••••••••••••••••••••••••••

"Nature can do more than physicians."

••••••••••••••••••••••••••••••••••

— Oliver Cromwell

I often use analogies from nature when describing ways in which people can heal. For example, if a plant is subsisting in a stagnant environment, without enough water, light, or nutrients, it cannot grow or be healthy. If that same plant were moved into an environment that was too bright or too wet, it would still remain unhealthy. It is important that all of us find the right balance of rest, stimulation, and climate for our optimal growth and development to occur.

A patient came into my office the other day and asked me if I thought a promotion he was trying to get would be too stressful and therefore detrimental to his health. I answered that it was important for *him* to determine this. If the new position was going to be stimulating and a source of joy, it would eventually be healthful. If it was stressful and overwhelming, it would soon become unhealthful. He answered that he was really looking forward to the increased responsibility and that the new job would enhance his work environment. The right choice for him to make then became clear.

The environment you live in and the daily patterns you follow help determine your level of health. The hectic pace, noise pollution, air pollution, artificial light, and amount of concrete present in the average urban environment block our ability to connect to the subtle but powerful healing rhythms of nature. These natural rhythms provide signals that keep our bodies functioning healthfully. They include cycles of light and dark that stimulate the pituitary and pineal glands to secrete hormones, scents which signal the brain to produce pheromones, and natural sounds which promote inner peace and calm.

Deepak Chopra, the well-known physician and philosopher, recommends that we regularly affirm the following: "I will take time each day to commune with nature and to silently witness the intelligence within every living thing. I will sit silently and watch a sunset, or listen to the sound of the ocean or a stream, or simply smell the scent of a flower. In the ecstasy of my own silence, and by communing with nature, I will enjoy the life throb of the ages, the field of pure potentiality, and unbounded creativity."

Healing is a process that occurs when the body, mind, and spirit move to a state of greater balance and strength. Naturopathy is the study of how to use natural therapies to facilitate this process. They include dietary changes, vitamin supplementation, stress reduction, exercise, acupuncture, herbs, massage, breathwork, and others. They can be used to revitalize and rejuvenate the flow of energy between our bodies and our environment.

I recently visited the virgin redwood forests of Humboldt county, Northern California. During my first evening in the forest, I camped in a campground not far from the highway. The clean air, high concentration of oxygen, and beautiful surroundings were relaxing and serene. However, it wasn't until I hiked 5 miles into the depth of the virgin forest that I truly felt connected to the powerful healing energy I am attempting to describe. The concentrated healing energy that can be found deep within pristine natural environments is potent and profound.

Within this environment, your entire being begins to harmonize with nature's vibrations and rhythms. There are no phones, no alarms, no deadlines, no schedules. There are no lights, no radios, no newspapers, no mechanized vehicles. There are no errands, no chores, no "to do" lists, and no clocks. All that exists are trees, plants, animals, the earth, the sun, the stars, and the moon. You awaken when your body feels like it. You eat when you are hungry. The only things you need "to do" are sleep when you are tired, eat when you are hungry, and explore the forest for exercise. In this laid-back, unstructured environment, a human being's energy can become recharged and rebalanced.

To heal and prevent disease, it is very important that each of us get out of the city on a regular basis. You may want to plan a day in the country once a month. Or at least take a walk in a park or on a beach every couple of days. These natural environments can affect us in subtle but powerful ways. We need to access them as much as possible if we are to retune, rebalance, and heal ourselves back into a state of harmony and strength.

This philosophy does not preclude healing within an urban environment. But you must have your priorities straight. Patterns often need to be adjusted so stress and muscle tension are reduced as much as possible. This can be accomplished through a regular daily practice of meditation, deep breathing, chi gong, prayer, or yoga.

Your diet is also very important and needs to consist primarily of natural, unprocessed foods. As I say on many occasions, "True healing does not come out of little bottles; it comes from within."

In the absence of living deep within a virgin redwood forest, many holistic practitioners, acupuncturists, and naturopaths employ the assistance of "natural supplements." These supplements, found on the shelves of health food stores, utilize technology to extract and concentrate the healing properties of nature into tablets, capsules, tinctures, and powders. When taken within, these supplements release their healing power in a variety of ways. When used correctly, they can detoxify, rebalance, and reinstill vital energy that can then be used by your body for its healing process. Natural supplements help your body reestablish the strength, integrity, and balance of good health.

To summarize: prayer, quiet time, meditation, acupuncture, massage, chi gong, regular exercise, a healthy diet, and regular periods of rest and relaxation are essential for health and healing to occur. Spend as much time as possible in natural settings such as parks, beaches, and forests to help you stay connected to the powerful healing rhythms of nature.

Figure 15.1

Healing HIV Program
SUMMARY OF NATURAL THERAPY RECOMMENDATIONS

1) Diet
   Immune Enhancement Diet

2) Vitamins and Nutritional Supplements

AM: High-potency multiple vitamin . . . . . . 1 tab   (with breakfast)
    High-potency multiple mineral . . . . . . 1 tab   "
    Vitamin C 1000 mg . . . . 2 caps   "
    Vitamin E 400 iu . . . . 1 cap   "
    Vitamin B₆ 100 mg . . . . 1 cap   "
    Coenzyme Q-10 30 mg . . . . 1 cap   "
    N-acetyl cysteine 500 mg. . . . . 1 cap   "
    Acidophilus . . . . 1 cap   "

PM: High-potency multiple vitamin . . . . . . 1 tab   (with dinner)
    High-potency multiple mineral . . . . . . 1 tab
    Vitamin C 1000 mg . . . . 2 caps   "
    Vitamin E 400 iu . . . . 1 cap   "
    Vitamin B₆ 100 mg . . . . 1 cap   "
    Coenzyme Q-10 30 mg . . . . 1 cap   "
    N-acetyl cysteine 500 mg. . . . . 1 cap   "
    Acidophilus . . . . 1 cap   "

3.) Herbs
   Consult a skilled naturopath, herbalist, or acupuncturist for the most individualized herbal treatment program. Consider rotating to different tonic formulas every several months. Herbs are best used in a preventive fashion to help keep you balanced.

4) **Exercise**

Obtain at least 30 minutes of exercise 3 to 5x per week. In general, it is healthful to split your time and energy 50/50 between aerobic and resistance exercise. Exercise recommendations are best individualized based on body composition testing.

5) **Stress Reduction**

Include 15 to 20 minutes of deep relaxation (relaxation tapes, prayer, meditation, yoga, chi gong, self-massage, etc.) twice daily.

AGGRESSIVE NATURAL THERAPIES

Nutrition and HIV

••

"Let thy food be thy medicine, and thy medicine be thy food."

••

— Hippocrates

Eating is an activity that we practice several times a day. Based on the composition of each meal, different hormones are secreted into the bloodstream. These hormones affect the way we feel and how our bodies function. For us to feel good and possess abundant energy, our diets need to be healthful.

There is no shortage of controversy when it comes to what constitutes a healthful diet. In this chapter, I will present to you a diet that can strengthen and balance your immune system. It is important to understand that a healthful diet constitutes the central foundation of the Healing HIV program; I call it the Immune Enhancement Diet because it will help keep your immune system strong and healthy. If you follow its recommendations, every other part of my program will work better.

I have tried to make this diet easy to integrate into the average person's lifestyle. You can go to your favorite restaurant, attend your best friend's dinner party, and continue to feel that you are a valid, participating member of society. You can stay within the healthful boundaries of this program and still continue to enjoy every moment of your life. If you cannot enjoy your life on this diet, *it will not work well!*

So what constitutes a healthful diet? First, your food must be natural and minimally processed. This allows your body to digest and absorb the correct concentration of nutrients. It also prevents the body from being exposed to artificial chemicals that may negatively affect its functioning. Second, because the body has unusually high metabolic needs in the presence of an HIV infection (8% to 40% greater), your diet must contain an abundance of vitamins, minerals, calories and protein. Meeting these requirements will help support and strengthen your immune system for the long haul.

The Immune Enhancement Diet: General Principles

1) Increase your consumption of *whole grains* (brown rice, oats, cracked wheat, barley, corn, rye, millet, quinoa, and buckwheat). Always prepare more than you need. You can keep the leftovers in the refrigerator for a week. Add them to soups and other dishes. Attempt to have a portion of cooked whole grains at least once a day.

2) Increase your consumption of *vegetables* (fresh, steamed, stir-fried or juiced). Eat as many of them as you can. They provide plentiful amounts of fiber, vitamins, and minerals.

3) Increase your consumption of *fresh fruit.* Use them as snacks and as a natural pick me up instead of processed sugar products.

4) Increase your consumption of *natural soups, teas,* and *warm beverages.* Optimal beverages include water, herb teas, fruit juices, and roasted grain coffee substitutes such as Inka, Caffix, and Postem. These are nutritious beverages as opposed to sugar-laden soft drinks. Mineral water is fine. Do not drink anything that is ice cold. Your body will have to expend energy to warm it up. This depletes energy that could otherwise be utilized by your immune system. Quick, inexpensive, and extremely nutritious soups are found in dried form in most supermarkets and health

food stores.

5) *Eat a nutritious breakfast every day.* Hot whole-grain cereals are an important part of an optimal breakfast. High-fiber breads, toast, and cold cereals made from whole grains are the next best choice. Healthful breads made from whole grains are high in fiber and low in additives and sugar. A high-quality breakfast provides strength and good nutrition at the very beginning of the day. Include a cup of hot tea or roasted grain beverage with your morning meal to help promote efficient digestion.

6) Eat plenty of *onions, garlic,* and *ginger* .

7) The best oils to use are high-quality *canola, olive,* and *sesame.*

8) Eat *locally grown, seasonal foods* — organic, if possible.

9) Make sure that your diet provides you with *abundant protein.* Recommended protein sources include fish, poultry, legumes, beans, tofu, tempeh, seitan, whole grains, and an occasional portion of red meat.

10) *Limit your dairy consumption* to approximately 10% of your total diet. Most people have a limited tolerance for dairy products (milk, butter, cheese, yogurt, etc.). When you exceed this limit, this can cause the production of excess gas, loose bowel movements, and even fatigue. This situation is not optimal for the efficient functioning of your digestive system. If dairy products are limited to 10% of your dietary intake (by volume), you will lessen the likelihood of experiencing these symptoms.

11) *Avoid sugar, alcohol, and caffeine.*

12) *Avoid raw foods* such as clams, oysters, marinated (uncooked) fish, sushi, very rare meats, and "runny" eggs. These can contain infectious bacteria and intestinal parasites.

13) *Combine and balance foods properly.* Do not eat vegetables and fruits at the same time. When eaten together, they promote inefficient digestion due to the different enzymes and digestive time that each requires. Rest for at least 10 minutes after each meal to promote healthful digestion. Try not to eat and run.

Health Levels of Various Foods

The following list assigns foods to different levels. Health level #1 contains a list of foods that possess especially high nutrient and antioxidant levels.

Health Level #1

Consume unlimited quantities (at least 60% of your diet).

Tofu	Tempeh	Seitan
Carrots	Garlic	Avocados
Sprouts	Shitake mushrooms	Bananas
Broccoli	Brown Rice	Apples
Onions	Barley	Oranges
Buckwheat	Oatmeal	Strawberries
Vegetarian soups	Lentils	Berries
Sunflower seeds	Bulgur wheat	Grapes
Almonds	Shoyu (aged soy sauce)	Raisins
Beans	Ginger	Peaches

Other lightly steamed or stir-fried vegetables, including cabbage, spinach, red cabbage, celery, red chard, Swiss chard, cauliflower, beets, etc.

Health Level #2

Consume unlimited quantities (at least 20% of your diet).

Vegetable juices	Yogurt	Eggs
Meats	Potatoes	Peanuts
Whole-grain breads	Fish	Corn
Sprouted-seed breads	Papayas	Cashews
Whole-grain pastas	Lemon	Olive oil
Nut butters	Herb teas	Spring water
Fruit juices*	Yams	

* Fruit juice is best diluted with an equal amount of water due to its high acid content.

Health Level #3

Nutritional Supplements

Supplements are used to enhance the diet. They are not meant to replace a healthful selection of foods. Please refer to the section on nutritional supplements later in this chapter for more information regarding their appropriate selection and usage.

Health Level #4
Minimize consumption of these foods or substances.

Coffee	Desserts	Ice cream
Honey	Dry cereals	Cookies

Health Level #5
Avoid these foods or substances completely.

Smoked meats	Alcohol	White sugar
Canned vegetables	Drugs	White flour
Frozen foods	Pesticides	Black coffee

Breakfast

Breakfast is the most important meal of the day. In the morning, most people immediately begin expending energy at a high rate. We leave for work, perform errands, and quickly begin to face the day's stresses. Accordingly, it is important that we provide our bodies with high-quality fuel right from the start. When we skip breakfast, or just have a quick cup of coffee, we are not providing our bodies with enough fuel to start the day.

The following is an important statement to keep in mind: *Your immune system is the most sensitive system of your body to your energy level.* When you are stressed, your heart beats faster and your muscles work harder. Your mind becomes stimulated, and adrenaline is released into your bloodstream. Energy is diverted away from your immune system and preferentially used for other bodily functions. Eating breakfast ensures that abundant energy is available at the very beginning of the day to help prevent a depleted state from occurring if you become stressed.

The ideal breakfast contains protein, fiber, carbohydrates, and fat. The protein and fat can come from eggs, milk, nuts, and/or yogurt. Protein supplies the building blocks for cell regeneration and repair. Carbohydrates are best found in hot whole-grain cereals, granola, whole-grain pancakes, waffles, toast, and fruit. High-fiber foods provide a matrix in which other nutrients can be healthfully digested. They tonify and improve the circulation to the digestive system. It is also helpful to have a warm drink in the morning to help "stoke your fire" and get the digestive processes going after a long night's sleep (consumption of caffeine is *not* necessary).

Protein

For the immune system to remain strong, it is extremely important to consume an adequate amount of protein. Inadequate protein intake results in lowered resistance to infection, poor wound healing, weight loss, and a general lack of vigor. If you do not consume adequate protein, your immune system will gradually weaken over time.

The amount of protein I recommend for an individual who is HIV(+) is 0.6 grams per pound per day. This amount reflects a 50% increase over what I recommended 5 years ago in my previous book, *Immune Power*. The new recommendation is based on more recent research which underscores the importance of building and maintaining a high percentage of body cell mass (muscle tissue). Muscle tissue produces more energy than any other tissue of the body. This energy is used to fuel a strong immune response. Adequate protein is also necessary to help the body produce abundant amounts of CD4 cells and antibodies, both important components of a strong and healthy immune system.

A 170-pound individual would therefore require a daily intake of 102 grams of protein (0.6 grams per pound). In Fig. 15.2 you can find many common foods and the amount of protein they contain. Estimate your daily protein intake based on your target weight. This will provide enough to begin adding muscle to your frame. Remember, it's also important to get the right amount of exercise, and to maintain optimal levels of testosterone and DHEA, to fully achieve these goals. Other anabolic hormones, such as oxandrolone and recombinant human growth hormone, may be added as supplements if you have still not achieved your ideal weight.

If you are not getting the recommended amount of protein for your weight, locate the foods in Fig. 15.2 that provide a large amount of protein, such as fish, chicken, seitan, tempeh, tofu, cheese, beans, seeds and nuts, and increase them in your diet. Also, refer to Chapter 10 for a complete description of the many types of available protein supplements.

The debate about the benefits of vegetable protein over animal protein is a long-standing one and will surely not be settled here. The most important points I would like to make are that your protein consumption should be varied, of adequate quantity, and combined with appropriate amounts of other healthful foods in your diet (i.e., whole grains, fresh vegetables, fruits, etc.)

Figure 15.2

PROTEIN SOURCES
(Minimum requirement: 0.6 grams per pound of body weight)

Source	Quan.	Protein
Meat		
liver	4 oz	30 grams
hamburger	4 oz	25 grams
steak	4 oz	28 grams
lamb	4 oz	20 grams
chicken	4 oz	28 grams
fish	4 oz	28 grams
Vegetarian		
seitan	4 oz	28 grams
tempeh	4 oz	16 grams
tofu	4 oz	10 grams
red beans	1 cup	14 grams
soy beans	1 cup	14 grams
chick peas	1 cup	14 grams
lentils	1 cup	16 grams
black beans	1 cup	12 grams
alfalfa sprouts	1 cup	5 grams
green beans	1 cup	2 grams
potato	(baked)	4 grams
Nuts		
peanuts	1 cup	32 grams
almonds	1 cup	25 grams
cashews	1 cup	15 grams

Source	Quan.	Protein
Dairy		
cottage cheese:		
creamed	1 cup	31 grams
uncreamed	1 cup	44 grams
cheese:		
cheddar	4 oz	28 grams
Swiss	4 oz	28 grams
milk	1 cup	8 grams
yogurt	1 cup	8 grams
egg	one	7 grams
Grains		
most grains	1 cup	3–5 grams
brown rice	1 cup	5 grams
white rice	1 cup	4 grams
oatmeal	1 cup	5 grams
bread	1 cup	2 grams
Seeds		
sesame	1 cup	42 grams
sunflower	1 cup	24 grams

*All quantities are of cooked foods.

Vegetables

You cannot eat too many vegetables. They provide your body with large amounts of vitamins, minerals, and fiber. Raw, steamed, stir-fried, or juiced, they are among nature's most nutritious and healthful foods. They are especially healthful when added to soups so that the nutrients contained within the cells can dissolve into a warm and easily digestible broth. The absorption of nutrients from soups and juices requires very little expenditure of digestive energy and is therefore an optimal way to obtain beneficial nutrition.

Whole Grains

A lack of whole grains is one of the biggest deficiencies in the standard American diet. Whole grains provide fiber, vitamins, and trace minerals that are extremely important to keep the immune system healthy. For years, large food producers tried to convince us that their bleached white flour products were as healthy, if not healthier, than those made from whole-grain flour. Remember how the Wonder Bread television commercial stated that it contained all the vitamins and minerals necessary to build strong bones and healthy bodies? White bread has such minimal fiber that it indirectly contributes to heart disease and colon cancer by substituting for other foods in the diet that contain higher amounts of fiber. Only during the past 10 years has fiber become enough of a health issue that we are adding whole grains back to our diets in adequate amounts.

One important health benefit of fiber is the stimulation of immune-enhancing cells in the linings of the intestines called Peyer's patches. When stimulated, these cells help activate and strengthen the immune system by producing antibodies that are the body's first line of defense against disease in the intestinal tract. Whole grains provide large amounts of fiber that stimulate the blood flow to these cells, thus enhancing their ability to function.

Another reason that fiber is so healthful is that it helps cleanse the colon of toxins, such as fats and bile acids, by absorbing them and carrying them out of the body. Abundant fiber also helps to prevent intestinal infections such as parasites and fungal infections.

Soluble vs. Insoluble Fiber

There are 2 types of dietary fiber, soluble and insoluble. Soluble fiber dissolves in water. It has a binding effect and slows the passage of food as it moves through the gut. In cases of diarrhea, you would do well to consume large amounts of soluble fiber because of its ability to soak up excess water and oil. This decreases irritation to the gastrointestinal tract and helps the colon form stool. Foods high in soluble fiber include oatmeal, white rice, oat bran, barley, bananas, beans, apples, apricots, peaches, and strawberries. Crushed psyllium seeds and oat bran powder are soluble fiber supplements that can also be used to enhance the amount of soluble fiber you consume. Remember, *soluble fiber helps the colon form stool.*

Insoluble fiber *does not dissolve in water.* It therefore has a stimulating and sometimes irritating effect on the colon and can cause foods to move faster through the system. Foods high in insoluble fiber include corn, dried fruits, raw fruits, nuts, seeds, popcorn, wheat bran, vegetables (except those listed above under soluble fiber), and grains (except oats, barley, and white rice). By cooking fruits and vegetables, their insoluble fiber becomes softer and easier to digest. Remember, insoluble fiber promotes *faster movement of food through your system.*

The Intact Whole Grain

I would like to make an additional point regarding whole grains and fiber. There is an important distinction between the consumption of flour products made from whole grains and the consumption of the *intact whole grain itself.* Intact whole grains such as oats, brown rice, cracked wheat, barley, corn, rye, quinoa, millet, and buckwheat have a strengthening effect on the digestive system. *The consumption of flour products is not equivalent.* The digestion of *the intact whole grain* enables the entire digestive system to get a tonifying workout. If you were trying to strengthen your muscles, you wouldn't give them a workout with 2-pound weights. You would progressively increase your workout to keep your muscles strong. That is why *intact* whole grains are so strengthening to the digestive system. Flour products are like 2-pound weights while intact whole grains provide a much more stimulating and strengthening workout that helps keep your digestive system tonified and healthy.

One of the simplest ways to consume an adequate amount of intact whole grains is to cook several day's worth of brown rice, barley, cracked wheat, or quinoa, and store the leftovers in the refrigerator. Just combine a portion of the refrigerated whole grain with a small amount of simmering water or place them in the microwave for 2 minutes to reheat. You can then eat them as a hot cereal or side dish. They can also be added to soups, stir-fry, or other dishes quickly and easily.

Fruit

In general, fruit is an extremely healthy addition to your diet. Most fruits are high in vitamins, minerals, and fiber and add a healthful source of natural sweetness to your diet.

A frequently asked question concerns whether individuals who are trying to rebuild their immune systems should consume only organic produce. A study performed by researchers at Rutgers University showed that organic produce was, on average, 87% higher in minerals than nonorganic produce. Calcium, magnesium, potassium, manganese, iron, and copper were all found to be markedly higher in the organic produce. This occurs because commercial produce is usually grown in weaker, less nutritious soil.

While organic produce has been shown to have greater quantities of vitamins and minerals, it is also more expensive and sometimes difficult to obtain. Whenever possible, consider the use of organic produce to be superior in its healthful benefits to nonorganic produce. However, I do not believe that it is "required" to eat only organic produce for the Healing HIV program to be successful.

Make sure that you wash your produce with plenty of water. If there is a noticeable residue, use a small amount of mild dish-washing detergent. You may also want to get a soft brush to enhance this process. I am not in favor of washing fruits and vegetables in dilute chlorine bleach as some people recommend.

Even if your produce is organic, it is important to wash it thoroughly. Microorganisms from the soil can be a source of infection (mycobacteria, fungal diseases, or intestinal parasites) in individuals who are immunocompromised.

Fruit also contains a high concentration of natural sugar. Many HIV(+) individuals have noticed that even the sugar from fruit and fruit juice is enough to cause them to develop an overgrowth of thrush, a common oral infection caused by the yeast Candida albicans. Like anything that you eat, fruit's effect on you depends upon the quantity consumed. Too much fruit on a daily basis can cause thrush to become exacerbated or even appear for the first time. If you have any difficulty with thrush, processed sugar should be the first thing that you eliminate from your diet. If the problem continues, fruit and fruit juice should be eliminated as the next step. It is important to discuss with your doctor the appropriate use of topical antifungals (Mycelex troches, Nystatin pastilles, Fungisone oral suspension, etc.) as a short-term treatment.

During the past 10 years, it has been my experience that most individuals who are following the dietary recommendations of the Immune Enhancement Diet can eat fruit in unlimited quantities without developing thrush because they avoid consuming excessive amounts of the 3 substances listed below.

The Negatives: Sugar, Caffeine, and Alcohol

The dietary habits that cause the most problems to the immune system of HIV(+) individuals are the excessive consumption of sugar, caffeine, and alcohol. Unhealthful quantities of these 3 substances, especially if combined with skipping breakfast, high stress, and inadequate protein intake, will quickly weaken the immune system.

Sugar and the Immune System

Since 1973, there have been several scientific studies which have provided strong evidence of sugar's negative effect on the immune system's ability to effectively function. White blood cells, including CD4 cells, are adversely affected by excessive amounts of sugar in the bloodstream. A research study published in the *American Journal of Clinical Nutrition* in 1973 showed that when white blood cells were exposed to high levels of sugar in the bloodstream, they experienced a decreased ability to engulf bacteria (phagocytosis). The greatest effect occurred between 1 and 2 hours after a liquid sugar meal, *but their ability was depressed for up to 5 hours afterwards.*

In the above study, test subjects were divided into 5 groups. Group 1 received a placebo and acted as the control for the study. Groups 2, 3, 4, and 5 received a liquid drink containing 6, 12, 18, and 24 teaspoons of sugar, respectively. Blood samples were taken from these individuals at one-half, 1, 2, 3, and 5 hours after consuming the drink. The samples were then incubated with a suspension of staphylococcus bacteria, and were viewed under a microscope. The number of bacteria that were engulfed by each white blood cell was counted and averaged for each group.

The results of the study showed that the group which consumed no sugar had an average of 14 bacteria engulfed by each white blood cell. There was a progressive decline in the number of bacteria engulfed by each group's white cells as their sugar consumption increased. At 6 teaspoons of sugar, the average number of engulfed bacteria was 10 per white blood cell at 12 teaspoons of sugar, the average number was 5.5 per white blood cell; at 18 teaspoons, the average was 2 per white blood cell; and after 24 teaspoons of sugar, the average number of bacteria destroyed per white blood cell was only 1. Ingesting 24 teaspoons of sugar (the equivalent of 2 cans of soda) *produced a 92% decrease in the white blood cell's ability to engulf bacteria.*

Other studies performed at Rockefeller University in New York provide evidence that protein molecules, which are present in all cells, can be adversely affected by elevated levels of sugar in the bloodstream. High concentrations of sugar combine with protein molecules to form "advanced glycosylation end products" or AGEs. AGE particles act like glue, binding protein molecules together to form a rigid lattice network known as cross-linking. These large protein molecules can inhibit the functioning of the immune system, blur vision, and cause damage to the kidneys and lungs.

Ingesting large amounts of processed sugar also puts great stress on the body in general. The total sugar content normally present in your bloodstream is approximately 1 teaspoon. When a person consumes a can of soda or a bowl of ice cream (containing an average sugar content of *12 teaspoons*), the digestive system must work very hard to prevent this amount of sugar from entering the bloodstream all at once. To produce sufficient insulin for processing this amount of sugar, the pancreas must also work extremely hard. This stress is not healthy for your body.

Sugar can also act like a drug. As you *decrease* the amount you consume, you can experience withdrawal symptoms, including headaches, irritability, nausea, and anxiety. If these occur, it is best to completely eliminate processed sugar from your diet in "cold turkey" fashion. The symptoms will last for a few days, and then you will begin to feel much better. Drink a lot of clear fluids, such as water and herb tea, take plenty of B-complex vitamins (50 mg 3x/day) and vitamin C (2 grams 3x/day), and eat filling, nutritious meals consisting of whole grains and vegetables. You can also eat a small amount of fruit if you feel poorly. This is the best way to eliminate, or quickly diminish, your cravings for sugar.

Once you are free from sugar, you will probably notice that you feel calmer and more relaxed. Your thinking becomes clearer. Your stress level becomes lower, and you will begin to feel much more present in your body. Awareness of your body allows you to be more in touch with its needs. Also, your energy level will improve. This increase in energy can then be utilized by your immune system.

If your diet is basically natural and wholesome, and includes a healthful amount of whole grains, fruits, and vegetables, a small amount of processed sugar will not adversely affect your immune system. A *small amount* of processed sugar 1 to 3 times a week is allowed within the Immune Enhancement Diet.

Advertising Tricks

It is *imperative* that you read labels. On every package of processed food, check the label for sugar and other sweeteners. Ingredients are listed on food labels in order of greater to lesser weight. It is important to understand that the ingredients listed as numbers 4, 5, and 6, when added together, may outweigh ingredient number 1.

Sugar equivalents can also be listed under many different names. Corn syrup, dextrose, maltose, sucrose, glucose, and fructose are all highly concentrated sweeteners with the same negative effects on the immune system. If several of these are present, the cumulative amount of sugar makes the product unhealthful. *If only 1 ingredient is present, and it is not among the first 3 on the label,* it is safe to consume.

Since the consumption of sugar is so prevalent in our society (average consumption: 140 lbs/person/year or 1 lb per person every 3 days), I am frequently asked what sources of sugar are acceptable. The most healthful way to sweeten your food is by adding fruit to it. Foods that are sweetened with fruit juice are also acceptable. Small amounts of honey, pure maple syrup, and molasses can also be used as sweeteners. Keep in mind that the goal is to avoid *an unnaturally high concentration* of sugar. When you use fruit or fruit juice as a sweetener, you are providing your body with a natural concentration of sugar that it is able to process without causing stress to your system.

Figure 15.3 summarizes the best and worst choices for sweet foods.

Figure 15.3

SUGAR CONCENTRATIONS

Best   **Worst**

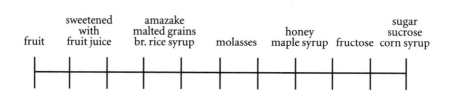

| fruit | sweetened with fruit juice | amazake malted grains br. rice syrup | molasses | honey maple syrup | fructose | sugar sucrose corn syrup |

Caffeine

A 1992 editorial in the *British Medical Journal* called caffeine "the world's most popular drug." The average American drinks approximately 32 gallons of caffeinated soft drinks and 28 gallons of coffee a year. This adds up to a total of 60 gallons of caffeinated drinks a year!

Healing occurs when the body is relaxed and its energy can be channeled inward. Regularly consuming caffeine impedes the body's ability to heal because caffeine blocks the cell's ability to regenerate its energy resources. No wonder you need a second and third cup of coffee to keep you going after the first one wears off!

Decaffeinated coffee is not as detrimental to the healing process as caffeinated coffee because it does not contain as much stimulant. However, it is not a healthful beverage, either. Instead of coffee, there are several healthful alternatives that may be consumed in the morning to help you get a good start on the day. These include tasteful and nutritious roasted whole-grain coffee substitutes, such as Inka, Caffix, and Postem. In addition, there are a variety of herb teas that you can drink as an acceptable alternative to coffee.

A moderate intake of caffeine (1 cup of strong coffee) a few times per week is allowed within the Immune Enhancement Diet.

Alcohol

When consumed in excess, alcohol is a poison to every system of your body. It depresses the nervous system, inhibits the bone marrow's ability to regenerate blood cells, is toxic to the liver, depletes B-vitamins, and is dehydrating.

If you are HIV(+), alcohol is best consumed in very small quantities or avoided altogether. This is especially true if you are taking a protease inhibitor, since these drugs already place a significant stress on the liver. Anyone who has chronic hepatitis B or C should completely avoid alcohol as well. Many individuals following the Immune Enhancement Diet have decided to avoid alcohol completely and are happy about their decision. They view it as another positive growth step that HIV has brought about in their lives.

The maximum amount of alcohol recommended by the Immune Enhancement Diet is 3 glasses of wine or beer per week. Avoid hard liquor entirely due to its higher alcohol concentration. It is a good idea to drink a lot of water before and after drinking alcohol to help dilute it and replace the fluids lost from its dehydrating effect.

Positive Motivation!

The process of eating a healthful, natural diet requires 2 things: 1) *Desire*, and 2) *Awareness*, the ability to see through slick marketing claims and identify exactly what makes up the products that you are consuming.

Another ingredient for success when it comes to improving your diet is a willingness to establish new habits and rituals. One of my patients pointed out that it wasn't the cup of fresh brewed coffee in the morning that he missed. It was the "ritual" of waking up to a hot, fresh-brewed beverage that helped him awaken his senses after sleep. He now substitutes a freshly brewed pot of herb tea or roasted-grain coffee as his morning ritual and is very satisfied.

Exercise is also a wonderful way to awaken your body in the morning and not feel the need for caffeine, nicotine, or sugar.

Allow yourself to begin incorporating some of the changes that I have outlined in this chapter on a daily basis. Start small. Eat breakfast every day. Begin avoiding caffeine, sugar and alcohol. Drink plenty of water. Buy some herb teas and find a favorite. These are some easy, healthful changes to begin with. Next, eat more fruits and vegetables. Make sure your protein intake is varied and substantial. Eat less junk food. All of these will help, and after a few weeks of combining these changes together into a program of healthful eating, you will begin to feel the difference! You will have more energy and feel stronger. You may also begin feeling better about yourself. Improving your diet is the right place to start. A healthful diet is the foundation of any healing program. Now is the time to start yours!

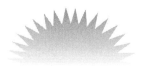

AGGRESSIVE NATURAL THERAPIES

Vitamins and Nutritional Supplements

There is an increasing amount of scientific evidence to support the use of vitamin supplements for both the prevention and treatment of disease. In spite of this, the medical establishment still discourages anything but their most minimal use. In this chapter, I hope to present data to support the use of vitamins and other nutritional supplements as an effective way to strengthen the immune system.

Although good nutrition is best obtained from your food, sometimes our diets are less than optimal. Dr. Howard Riddick, a researcher for the U.S. Department of Agriculture, confirmed in a conversation with me that *none of the 21,500 Americans surveyed* during the USDA National Food Consumption Study in 1984 consumed 100% of the RDA (Recommended Dietary Allowances) for the following combination of vitamins and minerals: Vitamins A, B_1, B_2, B_6, B_{12}, C, calcium, and iron.

In addition, it is well recognized that malnutrition plays an important role in the course and outcome of AIDS. Dr. Charles Halsted, chief of internal medicine at the University of California at Davis medical school, found that HIV attacks the intestinal cells that absorb vital nutrients *during the early stages of the disease.* He went on to state that "poor absorption of nutrients can be one of the early causes of malnutrition in AIDS patients."

A landmark study was also performed by Abrams and colleagues at the University of California, Berkeley, School of Public Health. This study looked at 296 HIV(+) men over a 6-year period to investigate how the intake of specific micronutrients might affect disease progression. After adjustment for baseline CD4 counts, HIV symptoms, and other risk factors, the risk of developing AIDS decreased as consumption increased for each of the 11 micronutrients studied. These included vitamin A, beta carotene, retinol, vitamin C, vitamin E, folic acid, riboflavin, thiamine, niacin, iron, and zinc.

Baum and colleagues at the University of Miami, and Tang and colleagues at the Johns Hopkins Medical School, have also conducted additional groundbreaking studies in the field of HIV nutrition during the past several years. At both the 2nd Conference on HIV and Nutrition in Cannes, France (1997) and the 12th World AIDS Conference in Geneva (1998), these researchers presented findings which highlight the wide range of micronutrient deficiencies frequently seen in HIV(+) individuals. The nutrients which have been directly linked to a more rapid progression of HIV include vitamins A, B_6, B_{12}, and E, and the minerals selenium and zinc. These studies also proved that ingesting supplements of several of these nutrients were associated with increases in CD4 cells as well as clinical improvement.

The goal of the supplement category of the Healing HIV program is to ensure that the body is provided with the nutrients necessary for the immune system to function optimally 100% of the time.

The government's RDAs (see Fig. 15.4) were initially arrived at by depriving army trainees of a single nutrient until they began to manifest symptoms of a deficiency disease. Vitamin deficiency diseases include rickets (vitamin D), beri beri (vitamin B_1), scurvy (vitamin C), and pernicious anemia (vitamin B_{12}). When these diseases occur, after months of absent or minimal intake, they constitute a total breakdown of many of the body's major systems, including the skin, blood, and nervous systems. The RDAs were established by the U.S. government as an arbitrarily "safe" margin above the level at which these vitamin deficiency diseases will occur. They are for the benefit of the general population and should not be considered adequate for individuals faced with illness or stress.

Although the RDAs prevent deficiency diseases from occurring, they are not designed to promote *peak performance* of the body. Applying the them to an HIV(+) individual is like taking a high-performance race car, in the middle of a grueling race, and giving it just enough octane in its fuel to keep it from breaking down. It may finish the race, but it is certainly not going to win it.

The following are 3 additional reasons why individuals who are HIV(+), or otherwise have depressed immune systems, can benefit from taking supplements of vitamins and minerals:

Figure 15.4

Recommended Daily Nutrient Allowances (RDA)

Nutrient	Adult Male	Adult Female
Vitamin A	5000 I.U.	5000 I.U.
Vitamin D	400 I.U.	400 I.U.
Vitamin E	30 I.U.	30 I.U.
Vitamin C	60 mg	60 mg
Thiamine (B_1)	1.5 mg	1.1 mg
Riboflavin (B_2)	1.7 mg	1.3 mg
Niacin	19 mg	15 mg
Folic acid	200 mcg	180 mcg
Vitamin B_6	2 mg	1.6 mg
Vitamin B_{12}	2 mcg	2 mcg
Calcium	800 mg	800 mg (> age 50: 1200 mg)
Phosphorous	800 mg	800 mg
Iron	10 mg	15 mg
Zinc	15 mg	12 mg
Magnesium	350 mg	280 mg
Iodine	150 mcg	150 mcg
Selenium	70 mcg	55 mcg
Pantothenic acid	10 mg	10 mg
Biotin	0.3 mg	0.3 mg

1) Vitamins and minerals are sensitive compounds that break down easily when food is cooked, exposed to light, or stored for long periods of time. Vitamins can also break down when food is handled roughly or processed. Much of the food that makes its way into urban supermarkets has been picked before it is ripe, transported long distances, and treated with waxes, fumigants, and other chemicals to preserve its flavor and appearance. Do you think this is the quality of food that nature originally intended for us to eat?

2) In addition, the soil in which most of our food is grown has been overworked by the widespread use of petrochemical fertilizers. No longer do farmers allow their fields to lie fallow for 1 year out of every 3 to rest and regenerate. Overworking the soil depletes it of essential nutrients and minerals that are necessary for the immune system to function effectively.

3) Modern living is stressful to our bodies. There is extensive pollution throughout the environment. The interaction of these pollutants with our cells often produces by-products known as free radicals. Free radicals are toxic to our cells and produce unhealthful changes that can weaken the immune system and promote cancer. Antioxidant compounds, such as vitamins A, E, C, beta-carotene, selenium, and zinc, circulate throughout the body and help it to neutralize toxic free radicals.

It is generally agreed that nutritional *deficiencies* have a negative effect on the functioning of the immune system. However, there continues to be increasing evidence that nutritional supplements *can enhance* the functioning of the immune system above the level that exists when no supplementation is provided.

A 1986 study, published in the journal *Contemporary Nutrition,* showed that the functioning of both T and B lymphocytes was enhanced by supplemental doses of vitamin A. Another controlled study, published in *Immunology Letters* in 1985, showed that after 1 week of beta-carotene supplementation, normal volunteers had increases in their CD4 counts while their CD8 counts remained the same.

Micronutrients and HIV Disease

Micronutrients include vitamins, minerals, and the class of compounds known as phytonutrients. They are necessary components of a healthy diet and contribute significantly to the achievement of optimal health. Micronutrients help to metabolize protein, fats, and carbohydrates; act as catalysts for thousands of important enzymatic reactions; and enhance the immune system's functioning by helping to neutralize free radicals and other toxins.

We often don't appreciate how many micronutrients become deficient very early in the course of HIV infection. Alice Tang and colleagues at

Johns Hopkins showed in a prospective study that low serum concentrations of vitamin B_{12} were associated with a 50% reduction in the time before the development of AIDS when compared to those with adequate vitamin B_{12} concentrations (median AIDS-free time was 4 vs. 8 years, respectively, p=0.004). In addition, Baum and colleagues at the University of Miami showed that normalization of vitamin A, vitamin B_{12}, serum zinc, and serum selenium levels in HIV(+) patients who were previously deficient, was associated with improved CD4 cell counts and clinical outcome. Dr. Baum has also reproduced Dr. Tang's finding that low vitamin B_{12} levels predict faster HIV disease progression and lower CD4 cell counts.

This data suggests that micronutrient deficiencies are integrally associated with HIV disease progression, as well as showing that normalization of their values may increase long-term stability of the immune system.

Given that there will be approximately 40 million HIV(+) individuals worldwide by the year 2000, the possibility that dietary changes plus micronutrient supplementation might delay the progression to AIDS has profound implications. Interventions that may enhance immune functioning, with or without antiviral therapy, strongly deserve further investigation. Most important, for the millions of HIV(+) individuals in developing countries unable to afford the expense of antiviral medications, the immune-enhancing effects of micronutrient supplementation could provide an extremely cost-effective start to their therapy.

The goal of the vitamin and nutritional supplement category of the Healing HIV program is to enhance the functioning of the immune system with intelligent and therapeutic nutrient supplementation. The daily program of nutritional supplements which I recommend to all individuals fighting a chronic viral infection is shown in Fig. 15.5. It includes a separate multivitamin and multimineral supplement both taken twice daily. The recommended dosages of the vitamins and minerals contained within the multiple vitamin and mineral tablets listed in Fig. 15.5 are specified in Fig. 15.6. You may want to shop around for the brand of multivitamin and multimineral that provides these dosages at the best price.

Figure 15.5

Chronic Viral Infection
Nutritional Supplement Recommendations

AM: High-potency multiple vitamin......1 tab   (with breakfast)

High-potency multiple mineral......1 tab   "

Vitamin C 1000 mg ....2 caps   "

Vitamin E 400 iu. ....1 cap   "

Vitamin B$_6$ 100 mg ....1 cap   "

Coenzyme Q-10 30 mg ....1 cap   "

N-acetyl cysteine 500 mg............1 cap   "

Acidophilus ....1 cap   "

PM: High-potency multiple vitamin......1 tab   (with dinner)

High-potency multiple mineral......1 tab

Vitamin C 1000 mg ....2 caps   "

Vitamin E 400 iu. ....1 cap   "

Vitamin B$_6$ 100 mg ....1 cap   "

Coenzyme Q-10 30 mg ....1 cap   "

N-acetyl cysteine 500 mg............1 cap   "

Acidophilus ....1 cap   "

The regimen in Fig. 15.5 achieves the following objectives:

1) It provides immune compromised individuals with an adequate dosage of all necessary vitamins and minerals.

2) It contains therapeutic amounts of several antioxidants (vitamins C, E, beta-carotene, and glutathione).

3) It is well tolerated by most individuals.

4) It is of moderate cost (approximately $75 per month).

Figure 15.6

Dosages to Be Obtained From Your Multiple Vitamin and Mineral Supplements

Multiple Vitamin Supplement	Total daily dosage
1) Vitamin A/Beta carotene	10,000-20,000 units
2) Vitamin B$_1$, B$_2$, B$_5$, B$_6$	50-100 mg
3) Vitamin B$_{12}$	500-1,000 mcg
4) Vitamin C	250-1000 mg
5) Vitamin E	150-400 units
6) Iron	9-18 mg
7) Zinc	10-25 mg
8) Calcium	50-250 mg
9) Magnesium	25-125 mg
10) Selenium	100-200 mcg

Multiple Mineral Supplement	Total daily dosage
1) Iron	9-18 mg
2) Zinc	25-50 mg
3) Copper	1-2 mg
4) Calcium	1000 mg
5) Magnesium	500 mg
6) Selenium	100-200 mcg

Almost all nutrients can cause unwanted side effects if taken at too high a dosage. However, an overdosage of some specific nutrients can cause severe toxicity. A listing of these nutrients and their maximal dosages is listed in Fig. 15.7.

Figure 15.7

Vitamins and Minerals
That Have Potential Side Effects

	Dosage	Potential Side Effect
1) Vitamin A	Greater than 100,000 units/day	Nausea, vomiting, liver damage
2) Vitamin C	Greater than 10 gms/day	Diarrhea
3) Vitamin E	Greater than 1200 units/day	High blood pressure, headaches
4) Vitamin B$_6$	Greater than 500 mgs/day	Peripheral neuropathy
5) Zinc	Greater than 100 mgs/day	Immune system depression
6) Selenium	Greater than 400 mcg/day	Immune system depression

The following additional information and research studies substantiate the use of vitamins and other nutritional supplements as part of a program to maintain a strong immune response to HIV.

Vitamin C

Michael Castleman, in his book, *Cold Cures,* reviewed the current medical literature on vitamin C and noted some interesting findings. Since 1945, 31 studies have tested vitamin C against the common cold; 15 showed no effect, and 16 showed significant benefit described as a 30 to 50% decrease in the severity and duration of symptoms. Why such different outcomes from these studies?

Upon closer inspection, the 15 studies that showed no effect from supplementing this vitamin all used low doses of vitamin C (250 mg or less) for short periods of time. All 16 studies that showed a significant benefit from vitamin C supplementation used high dosages (2000 mg or greater) and began supplementing the vitamin from the moment any symptoms appeared until they completely resolved. It appears that there is a threshold level above which vitamin C boosts the immune system against viral infections. Since HIV is a chronic viral infection, there is good reason to believe that the same immune-stimulating effect that vitamin C has against viral influenza might be of benefit in helping to combat HIV.

Steve Harakeh, Raxit Jariwalla, and Linus Pauling published a study in the *Proceeds of the National Academy of Sciences* in 1990 entitled "Suppression of human immunodeficiency virus replication by ascorbate in chronically and acutely infected cells." The results showed that continuous exposure of HIV-infected cells to nontoxic ascorbate concentrations (vitamin C) resulted in significant inhibition of both total virus and P-24 antigen formation. The ascorbate, in these concentrations, did not adversely affect either the host cell's metabolic activity or its rate of protein synthesis. Reverse transcriptase, the enzyme inhibited by AZT, showed a threefold to fourteen-fold decrease in activity when exposed to high concentrations of ascorbate.

This study provides evidence that vitamin C directly inhibits the growth and replication of HIV. Additional studies need to be performed in humans to look at its effect on such indicators as freedom from opportunistic infections, growth of viral cultures, and CD4 cell subset numbers. Hopefully, funding for these additional studies will be provided following these positive preliminary results.

Vitamin C is extremely helpful to the immune system in other ways as well. Additional benefits from vitamin C include enhanced proliferation of CD4-cells, increased levels of circulating IgA, IgM, and IgG antibodies, and improvement in the ability of white blood cells to engulf bacteria (phagocytosis). In fact, the intracellular concentration of vitamin C in white blood cells (lymphocytes specifically) has been shown to be greater than 10 times that in most other cells. Vitamin C also increases interferon levels and functions as a potent antioxidant.

Although Linus Pauling recommended dosages approaching 20,000 mg/day, most studies have shown significant antiviral benefit occurs at between 2000 and 6000 mg/day. It is also important to know that high doses of vitamin C can exacerbate or even precipitate loose bowel movements and diarrhea. As always, inform your primary-care practitioner of any new therapies that you are utilizing. Even if there is not total agreement, he or she can advise you as to whether or not your individual condition might warrant extra caution.

New evidence also indicates that vitamin C works synergistically with vitamin E. When these vitamins are taken together, they have a greater effect than if taken separately. Vitamin E scavenges for dangerous free radicals in cell membranes, while vitamin C attacks free radicals in biological fluids. These vitamins reinforce and extend each other's antioxidant activity; when supplementing one, you are wise to supplement the other as well.

Deficiency symptoms: Because the body cannot manufacture vitamin C, it must be obtained through the diet or taken as a supplement. Scurvy is the disease caused by vitamin C deficiency. It is characterized by poor wound healing, bleeding gums, edema, extreme weakness, and easy bruisability. Due to the consumption of vitamin C–containing foods, this condition is rare in Western society. More commonly seen are signs of lesser deficiency including gingivitis, increased susceptibility to infection, fatigue, poor digestion, and prolonged healing time.

Repletion information: Berries, citrus fruits, and green vegetables have the greatest concentration of vitamin C. Good sources include asparagus, avocado, broccoli, Brussel sprouts, cantaloupe, collards, grapefruit, kale, lemons, mangoes, mustard greens, onions, oranges, papayas, peas, sweet peppers, pineapple, radishes, spinach, tomatoes, Swiss chard, and strawberries.

For maximum effectiveness, it is important to take supplements of vitamin C twice daily. Esterified vitamin C (Ester-C) is an especially effective form of vitamin C for those suffering from chronic illness. It is created by complexing vitamin C molecules with a mineral such as calcium, magnesium, or zinc. This results in a form of the vitamin that is nonacidic and thereby less irritating to the stomach. Ester-C has been shown to enter the bloodstream and tissues 4 times faster than standard vitamin C and is retained by the tissues longer.

Vitamin E

Simin Meydani, a nutritionist for the Department of Agriculture, recruited 34 healthy volunteers and determined their level of immune response with standard skin tests and the measurement of white blood cell responses to foreign materials. Meydani then housed the 34 volunteers at the Department of Agriculture's Human Nutrition Resource Center in Boston for 30 days.

Group #1 was fed a normal diet containing 15 iu of vitamin E per day. Group #2 was fed the same diet plus daily supplementation of 800 iu of vitamin E. The study was designed so that neither the researchers nor the test subjects were aware which group was receiving the additional vitamin E until the study results were reviewed. After 30 days, the results of the study indicated that the group receiving the vitamin E supplementation had *a significant increase in their immune response* when compared to the unsupplemented group.

In addition, studies at Tulane University suggest that vitamin E increases the anti-HIV activity of AZT. It accomplishes this by making cell membranes more permeable, thereby increasing the diffusion of AZT into infected cells. Accordingly, lower doses of AZT might be more effective when combined with this vitamin. It is also believed that vitamin E may reduce the bone marrow toxicity caused by AZT.

Vitamin E has also been also shown to protect animals against radiation induced injury. In 1 study, 3 groups of rats were injected with 30, 60, or 120 units of vitamin E. Another 3 groups served as controls for the study. Then 2 hours after being irradiated with a single dose of 600 rads of ionizing radiation, researchers cut and sutured 2 5-centimeter incisions on the rats from all 6 groups. The average breaking strength of the wounds in the rats receiving no supplementation of vitamin E was 74% of normal. The average breaking strength of the wounds in the group receiving radiation plus an injection of 120 units of vitamin E was 95% of the nonirradiated animal's wound strength. The researchers postulated that the vitamin E promoted healing by neutralizing the free radicals formed by exposure to radiation. Free radicals and other by-products of toxins in the environment are known to cause cellular damage, which negatively affects both the ability of wounds to heal, and the immune system's functioning in general. Vitamin E supplementation can help prevent these negative effects.

Vitamin E comes in several forms. The optimal form of vitamin E supplementation is with the natural, oil-based D-alpha or D-mixed tocopherol form. This is the form of vitamin E that has the highest biological activity and the most potential for enhancing immune system functioning.

Deficiency symptoms: Vitamin E deficiency can result in damage to red blood cells and peripheral nerves. Signs of deficiency may include infertility (in both men and women), menstrual problems, nervous system impairment, anemia, and spontaneous abortions. Low levels of vitamin E in the body have also been linked to both bowel and breast cancer. An increasing lack of vitamin E in our diets has been linked to the overprocessing of our food.

Repletion information: Vitamin E is abundant in the following food sources: cold-pressed vegetable oils, dark green leafy vegetables, legumes, nuts, seeds, and whole grains. The largest concentration of vitamin E in whole grains is found in the germ of the grain. Whole grains that contain significant quantities of this vitamin are wheat, brown rice, corn, and oats. Eggs, milk, and sweet potatoes are also good sources of vitamin E.

Vitamin A and Beta-Carotene

Carotenoids make up more than 400 red and yellow pigments in nature. Beta-carotene is the carotenoid most plentiful in human foods. Beta-carotene is also known as "pro-vitamin A." It is converted to vitamin A in the gastrointestinal tract. The recommended dietary allowance (RDA) of vitamin A is 5000 iu for adults, and 2500 iu for children. There is no specific RDA for beta-carotene. This nutrient helps to maintain the integrity of the mucous membranes, fight infections, and detoxify air pollutants. It is required for the growth and repair of cells and is necessary for normal protein metabolism. It also serves as an antioxidant and helps protect the body against the growth of tumor cells.

A deficiency of vitamin A can cause anemia, neurologic degeneration, dry skin, an inflamed tongue, gastrointestinal disorders, and a loss of taste and smell. The need for this nutrient is increased if you are under stress.

According to the most recent survey by the United States Department of Health, Education and Welfare, about 60% of women and 50% of men have intakes of vitamin A below the RDA. Although supplementing vitamin A in large doses can be toxic, supplemental beta-carotene has not been shown to possess toxicity at any dosage level. When large doses of beta-carotene are ingested, the only side effect is a yellowing of the skin pigment, which is not harmful and is reversible by decreasing the dose. Smokers taking large doses of beta-carotene should be aware that a 1997 study showed an association between beta-carotene supplementation, smoking, and lung cancer. The results of this study have not been reproduced by other researchers.

Beta-carotene also possesses several positive effects not attributable to vitamin A. For instance, it has been shown to be more effective than vitamin A in promoting the formation of healthy skin cells. Its intake has also been shown to reduce the incidence of certain kinds of cancer, a discovery made by the Japanese more than 20 years ago. Since then, many studies have validated the fact that people who eat abundant amounts of fruits and vegetables rich in beta-carotene are less likely to develop cancer of the respiratory tract.

With the above information in mind, my advice to HIV(+) individuals is as follows:

1) Consume as much beta-carotene containing food in your diet as possible.

2) Obtain 10,000–15,000 units per day of beta-carotene in your multivitamin supplement.

3) Don't smoke cigarettes!

Deficiency symptoms: The following conditions have been attributed to beta-carotene deficiency: dry skin, poor growth in children, insomnia, fatigue, weight loss, respiratory disorders, and night blindness. Deficiencies of vitamin A are extremely rare given the large number of foods that contain it in significant quantities. A more common *potential* problem is vitamin A excess. Individual vitamin A supplements should be avoided because large doses of vitamin A can accumulate in the liver, causing toxic symptoms that may include abdominal pain, nausea, vomiting, hair loss, joint pains, and cracking of the lips and skin. Alternatively, beta-carotene supplementation does not result in toxicity because the body can easily excrete it. If you consume too much beta-carotene, your skin may turn a slightly yellow-orange color, especially on the palms of the hands.

Repletion information: The following foods contain significant amounts of vitamin A: animal liver, fish liver oils, and yellow and green fruits and vegetables. Foods containing significant amounts of beta-carotene include apricots, asparagus, broccoli, cantaloupe, carrots, collards, dandelion greens, garlic, kale, mustard greens, papaya, peaches, pumpkin, red peppers, spinach, sweet potatoes, Swiss chard, watercress, and yellow squash.

Vitamin B$_6$

Vitamin B$_6$ is a complex of 3 similar molecules: Pyridoxine, Pyridoxal, and Pyridoxamine. All are present in our food and converted into pyridoxal-5-phosphate by the body. This is the most active form of vitamin B$_6$. The functions of this vitamin include helping to metabolize proteins. By aiding in the metabolism of amino acids and proteins, vitamin B$_6$ is integrally related to the reproduction of CD4 and other immune system cells.

Vitamin B$_6$ also plays a critical role in nucleic acid synthesis, and its deficiency can significantly alter immune responses. Although isolated vitamin B$_6$ deficiency is rare in human beings, subgroups of individuals, such as those with chronic infections or the elderly, may be at increased risk. Marginal nutrient deficiencies, including that of vitamin B$_6$, may also contribute to the declining immune responses commonly observed in these groups.

Cell-mediated immunity, a function performed by CD4 cells, is profoundly affected by vitamin B$_6$ deficiency in animal models. Humoral immunity, which is responsible for antibody function, is adversely affected as well.

Human studies of vitamin B$_6$ deficiency have shown that the percentage of CD4 cells, as well as the concentration of several immunoglobulins, is lower in vitamin B$_6$-deficient individuals. Mariana Baum and colleagues have identified widely prevalent B₆ deficiency among HIV(+) individuals despite adequate dietary vitamin B₆ intake.

Deficiency symptoms: Early vitamin B₆ deficiency symptoms are peripheral neuropathy, generalized weakness, irritability, depression, insomnia, and anxiety. More severe vitamin B₆ deficiency can cause chronic dermatitis, nausea, vomiting, and occasionally convulsions. Carpal tunnel syndrome, premenstrual syndrome, and atherosclerosis may also be related to vitamin B₆ deficiency.

Repletion information: The following foods contain significant amounts of vitamin B₆: potatoes, wheat germ, nutritional yeast, legumes, bananas, and meats. In our practice, supplementation of vitamin B₆ has been found to greatly diminish symptoms of HIV-related peripheral neuropathy. However, supplementation of vitamin B₆ at a dosage greater than 500 mg per day for long periods of time has been associated in a few studies with *causing* peripheral neuropathy. In general, doses up to 500 mg daily have exhibited long-term safety. Persons with drug-induced neuropathy may tolerate and benefit from these higher than normal dosages of vitamin B₆.

Coenzyme Q-10

Coenzyme Q-10 is also known by the term *ubiquinone*. This name is derived from the fact that coenzyme Q-10 is ubiquitous among the energy-producing cells of the body. It is found in very high density in the mitochondria, which are the energy-producing organelles of mammalian cells.

Coenzyme Q-10 is intrinsically involved in cellular energy production and the phosphorylation of ATP (adenosine triphosphate). Deficiencies of coenzyme Q-10 have been shown in elderly and immunocompromised populations to be associated with coronary artery disease, congestive heart failure, hypertension, immune suppression, and periodontal disease.

Landmark studies have sparked international interest in coenzyme Q-10 as a treatment for heart failure. Hashiba and colleagues conducted a double-blind study involving patients with heart failure in 12 hospitals in Japan. In this study, 100 patients received oral coenzyme Q-10 (30 mg/day) and 97 received placebo. The study lasted for 2 weeks. Significant improvement in clinical symptoms, physical signs, and electrocardiogram parameters was shown in the study group.

A second double-blind study conducted at the same time as the Hashiba study was performed by Iwabuchi. He tested coenzyme Q-10 against a placebo in 32 patients with congestive heart failure. The coenzyme Q-10 group was shown to be superior to the placebo group when both objective and subjective measurements were analyzed.

You might ask why a treatment which shows benefit for congestive heart failure is mentioned in a book primarily dealing with immune dysfunction. The reason stems from the fact that coenzyme Q-10 stimulates energy production throughout the body. Since the immune system is the most sensitive system of your body to low energy, ensuring adequate energy supplies is of paramount importance.

There have also been several studies looking at coenzyme Q-10 supplementation in animals which show a cause-and-effect relationship between supplementation of this nutrient and improved immune function. Additional human studies are currently underway.

Research has also revealed that supplemental coenzyme Q-10 can also act as an antihistamine. It may therefore be beneficial for people with allergies, asthma, and other respiratory conditions. More than 12 million people in Japan are reportedly taking coenzyme Q-10 at the direction of their physicians for the treatment of heart disease, high blood pressure, and to enhance the immune system functioning. Its use in HIV disease may provide benefit but also needs further study.

Deficiency symptoms: Fatigue, irritability, headaches, decreased exercise tolerance, immune dysfunction, and shortness of breath.

Repletion information: Foods containing significant amounts of coenzyme Q-10 include mackerel, salmon, peanuts, beef, and spinach. The amount of coenzyme Q-10 present in the body declines with advancing age and increased stress. Supplementation should be considered in people experiencing these conditions. Coenzyme Q-10 is fat-soluble and best absorbed when taken with a fat-containing meal. It is also easily oxidized, and therefore it is important to store it away from heat and light.

Zinc

The presence of the mineral zinc is necessary to over 200 enzymatic reactions. It is also important for healthy prostate gland function, wound healing, and healthy immune system functioning. Adequate zinc levels are also necessary for optimal taste and smell acuity.

Zinc is also an essential component of the antioxidant enzyme superoxide dismutase (SOD). It has been found to enhance host defenses and provides a mild antiviral effect in the treatment of cold viruses. In our practice, one of the most common nutrient deficiencies found on nutrient blood level testing in HIV(+) individuals has been that of zinc.

Deficiency symptoms: Zinc deficiency may result in a loss of taste and smell acuity. It can also cause the fingernails to become thin and develop white spots. Other possible signs of zinc deficiency include acne, slow wound healing, fatigue, impotence, rash, increased susceptibility to infection, prostatitis, and recurrent viral infections.

Repletion information: Significant amounts of zinc are found in the following foods: brewer's yeast, egg yolks, fish, lamb, legumes, liver, meats, mushrooms, pumpkin seeds, sunflower seeds, and whole grains. The Healing HIV program recommends a total of 50–100 mg of zinc be consumed per day. It is generally not recommended to take more than 100 mg of zinc/day, since doses above this may cause depressed immune function.

Glutathione

Glutathione is a tripeptide produced in the liver from the amino acids cysteine, glutamic acid, and glycine. It is a powerful antioxidant that inhibits the formation of free radicals, highly charged molecules that are highly toxic to living cells. In so doing, it helps defend the body against damage from pollution, smoking, cancer chemotherapy, alcohol, and the harmful effects of many drugs.

Glutathione peroxidase is a key intracellular enzyme formed from the combination of glutathione and selenium. This enzyme provides our cells with the ability to detoxify many harmful free radicals. Glutathione peroxidase has also been shown to protect the brain, kidneys, liver, lungs, and skin against oxidative damage.

Glutathione deficiency has been shown to be prevalent in all groups of HIV(+) individuals, ranging from asymptomatic HIV(+) to full-blown AIDS. Lenin and Lenore Herzenberg and their colleagues at Stanford University Medical School have shown that a glutathione deficiency among CD4 cells is associated with markedly decreased survival rates in HIV-infected patients. This finding, combined with the fact that oral administration of N-acetyl cysteine clearly replenishes intracellular glutathione in these subjects, suggests that N-acetyl cysteine administration may improve survival in HIV(+) individuals. It also establishes that glutathione deficiency may be a key contributor to decreased survival in HIV disease.

Oxidative stress is a term which describes the negative effects free radicals can exert on the body. There are several mechanisms in which oxidative stress is believed to accelerate the progression of HIV disease. It encourages the production of nf-kappa B (nuclear factor-kappa B), which is a known activator of HIV replication within lymphocytes (CD4 cells). It is also known to increase the level of circulating tumor necrosis factor alpha (TNF-alpha), an inflammatory cytokine that can cause fevers, low appetite, and contribute to wasting syndrome. The production of these chemicals may be increased by depleted levels of glutathione in HIV(+) individuals. Intelligent antioxidant supplementation is a very cost-effective way to maintain the health and stability of HIV(+) individuals.

Deficiency symptoms: A wide range of human conditions such as aging, cancer, atherosclerosis, arthritis, viral infections, neurodegeneration, pulmonary diseases, and AIDS may be contributed to by high levels of free radicals (oxidative stress). The treatment of these diseases may therefore benefit from supplementation with antioxidants such as vitamin C, vitamin E, carotenoids, N-acetyl cysteine, zinc, and selenium. Patients with liver disease are favorably affected by treatments that increase intracellular glutathione as well.

Repletion information: Glutathione itself is poorly absorbed from the GI tract. Foods rich in this nutrient also do not significantly increase intracellular glutathione levels in immunocompromised individuals.

Cysteine appears to be the limiting amino acid in the intracellular synthesis of glutathione. Supplementation with cysteine itself is not recommended because it may cause GI side effects. Supplementation of up to 2000 mg daily of N-acetyl cysteine is safe and has also been shown to significantly raise glutathione levels. Foods rich in cysteine include meats, yogurt, wheat germ, and eggs. Whey-based protein supplements are also an excellent source of cysteine and have been shown to moderately raise glutathione levels.

Acidophilus Bacteria

One could call the bacteria that live in our intestines "the elixir of good digestion." As mentioned earlier, the intestinal tract of normal, healthy adults contains approximately 3.5 pounds of normal, healthy bacteria. Lactobacillus acidophilus is a major component of this community and helps to provide a beneficial environment for healthful digestion to occur.

Since the equilibrium of beneficial intestinal bacteria may be disrupted by stress and the use of antibiotics, supplementing the diet on a daily basis with acidophilus (and bifidus) bacteria is extremely helpful. Since the majority of HIV(+) individuals will manifest some form of digestive imbalance during their condition, acidophilus supplementation can help prevent these digestive problems from occurring.

Additional benefits of acidophilus supplementation include:

1) Production of significant amounts of B-complex vitamins, folic acid, and vitamin B_{12}.

2) Reduction of intestinal gas and diarrhea.

3) Improved digestion of dairy products due to the enhanced production of lactase enzymes.

SUMMARY

If the above reasons have not yet convinced you that there are significant benefits to supplementing your diet with vitamins and other nutritional supplements, consider the following:

1) Numerous studies have linked vitamin and mineral deficiencies to weakened immune system functioning. The most common deficiencies

are of vitamins A, C, E, B$_{12}$, B$_6$, zinc, selenium, and glutathione.

2) Many patients who have progressed to a diagnosis of AIDS have been shown to be deficient in both zinc and selenium.

3) AZT use has been linked to low zinc levels in AIDS patients when compared to those not taking this drug.

4) Malabsorption of vitamins and minerals from the digestive tract can occur due to antibiotic therapy, bacterial infections, intestinal parasites, and early HIV disease.

5) Multiple studies have shown that dietary supplementation of vitamins A, C, E, beta-carotene, and zinc enhances cell-mediated immune system functioning, which consists primarily of CD4 and CD8 cells.

6) CD4 cell function has been shown to be enhanced by antioxidants such as beta-carotene, vitamins C, B$_6$, E, zinc, selenium, and glutathione.

Since there is indisputable evidence that environmental stress combined with the presence of a chronic infection raises the body's needs for many nutrients, doesn't it make sense to add vitamin and nutritional supplements to your treatment program? In a study presented at the 12th World AIDS conference in Geneva (1998), 75% of HIV(+) individuals living in an urban environment subjectively believed vitamin supplements and other complementary therapies were moderately to extremely important for maintaining their health. Further research continues to highlight the benefits that nutrient supplementation can bring, and the hazards which nutrient deficiencies can cause, in the long-term management of HIV. Looking at the big picture, nutrient supplementation can be a very cost-effective way to increase the longevity of those living with HIV.

Yes, eating healthy and taking a lot of vitamins is hard work. But if you want to live and grow and remain healthy with HIV you must work a little harder than most average individuals to maintain your health. It has become your unique and special calling in life to learn how to stay healthy until a cure is found. You can do it!

AGGRESSIVE NATURAL THERAPIES

Herbs and the Immune System

Before the advent of our technologically based medical system, humans used an abundance of natural substances to aid in the healing process. These included echinacea and goldenseal as antibiotics, chamomile and valerian as sedatives, white willow bark and bayberry root for reducing fevers, and slippery elm and mint for curing indigestion and diarrhea.

Around the world, nature has provided an abundance of medicinal plants for healing. In fact, a 1975 survey showed that 74% of all prescription drugs worldwide were directly derived from plants. Major pharmaceutical manufacturers continue to scour the rain forests for active ingredients to make new drugs. The main difference between natural substances and synthetic drugs is that synthetic drugs produce a quicker, stronger effect. Although the quicker action of synthetic drugs may at times be lifesaving, they can also bring with them serious side effects. This is apparent when one considers that the amount of medication necessary to adequately treat HIV is often toxic to its host. This is a disturbing dilemma to anyone interested in a nontoxic approach to HIV treatment.

The Healing HIV program is designed to support the body's own ability to keep HIV suppressed. Medications are utilized only when necessary and in dosages that provide beneficial effects with a minimum of side effects. The addition of herbs to your program can help nurture and strengthen your body and your immune system.

In this section, I will present information to you that describes herbs from both Western and Asian schools of thought. Herbs can be utilized in 2 ways. First, they can be used as tonics. These are herbs that enhance the functioning of the immune system, promote beneficial circulation, restore energy and normalize physiologic processes. Second, herbs can be used as initial remedies for minor symptoms. *If the strength of your immune system is declining, herbal remedies should not be used as the sole treatment for an HIV infection.* An intelligent blend of both natural and standard medical therapies provides the optimal approach to treating HIV.

The following books may prove valuable to anyone interested in a more expanded and detailed discussion of herbal medicine:

1) *The Scientific Validation of Herbal Medicine,* by Daniel B. Mowrey, Ph.D., Cormorant Books, 1986.

2) *The Way of Herbs,* by Michael Tierra, C.A., N.D., Washington Square Press, 1983.

3) *The Male Herbal,* by James Green, The Crossing Press, 1991.

4) *The HIV Wellness Sourcebook,* by Misha Cohen, O.M.D., L.Ac., Henry Holt and Company, 1998.

Western Antibiotic Herbs

Western herbs that contain antibiotic and antiviral properties have been used for centuries by herbalists in the successful treatment of many types of bacterial and viral infections. These herbs possess many nutrients as well as antibiotic and antiviral components. They are excellent for general use as tonics or, in higher dosages, for the treatment of acute infections.

Echinacea

Echinacea angustifolia has been used in the Americas and Western Europe for hundreds of years to strengthen the immune system. Its major component, inulin, helps promote the movement of white blood cells toward an infection (chemotaxis). It also promotes the solubilization of antibody/virus complexes that need to be cleansed from the bloodstream. Echinacea also possesses a direct antiviral effect. Mammalian cells, treated with extracts of echinacea, have been shown to be 50% to 80% resistant to influenza, herpes and oral stomatitis viruses.

Recent pharmacological investigations also support the fact that echinacea is an immune-stimulating agent. A substance known as echinacin has been shown to be a lymphocyte and macrophage stimulator. It stimulates the production of interferon as well as other lymphokines.

Echinacea is probably the best detoxifying agent of any herb known to Western herbalists. Michael Tierra, author of *The Way of Herbs,* calls it "the most effective blood and lymphatic cleanser in the botanical kingdom." It is gentle and does not have any side effects.

Recommended dosage: 25–40 drops of high-quality organic echinacea tincture or 3–4 capsules of the dried herb, 3x/day. For acute ailments this dose is best taken every 1 to 2 hours for maximum benefit. *Side effects:* none.

Goldenseal Root

Goldenseal root is frequently used to help reduce inflammation and treat infections. It has been found to be effective for use as a restorative herb following protracted fevers. The alkaloids present in this herb, especially berberine and hydrastine, have been used to combat a wide variety of infections.

A study done in India showed that berberine has a protective effect against intestinal amoebic infections in rats. Other Indian studies demonstrated a similar but even more pronounced effect against cholera bacteria. Goldenseal extract has been shown to be effective against gram-positive bacteria, such as staph and strep, and against gram-negative bacteria, such as E. coli. In addition, the alkaloids in goldenseal root show the ability to inhibit the growth of tuberculosis organisms. It has been found to cure intestinal parasitic infections such as Giardiasis. This parasite has been a major problem in Africa and Asia, and is beginning to surface more and more frequently in Western countries, including the United States.

Goldenseal root is a powerful herb, and it should not be taken in large amounts or for prolonged periods of time. Excessive use of goldenseal can diminish B-vitamin absorption due to its antibiotic effect against favorable intestinal bacteria. Therefore, it is important that you supplement your diet with acidophilus bacteria if you are taking this herb. Taking 2 or 3 capsules a day of the dried root powder is generally considered safe and adequate for most conditions.

Recommended dosage: 2–3 capsules or 1–2 droppersful of organic tincture once a day. There are many beneficial combination formulas that contain goldenseal root. When taken in moderation, these combinations can be effectively used as general immune system tonics. You may increase the dosage for up to 1 week if any acute symptoms such as fevers, night sweats, or excessive mucous production are present. *Side effects:* nausea and inhibition of intestinal bacterial growth.

Garlic

The list of medicinal effects attributed to garlic is long and well documented. Garlic helps lower cholesterol levels, decreases high blood pressure, helps to prevent strokes, and inhibits the growth of many pathogenic microorganisms, including bacteria, fungi, and viruses.

The active ingredient in fresh garlic is called allicin. It is the key antibacterial and antiviral agent. It is also the chemical that gives garlic its notorious odor. Because onions, botanical cousins to garlic, also contain allicin, they possess similar properties. Dr. Byron Murray, head of the virus research laboratory at Brigham Young University in Utah, states that garlic, in high concentrations, kills viruses more effectively than alcohol, acetone, and most common disinfectants.

Garlic's antibacterial activity has been proven against numerous bacteria, including staph, strep, klebsiella, proteus, E. coli, salmonella, and Vibrio cholera. Of major significance are the antifungal studies that show garlic to be effective against Candida albicans, the organism responsible for thrush, and Tinea, the organism which causes athlete's foot and ringworm. At least 20 other pathogenic fungi are susceptible to either inhibition or destruction by garlic.

In addition, garlic is extremely nutritious and contains high levels of protein, vitamin A, vitamin C, thiamine, and many minerals including copper, zinc, iron, calcium, potassium, sulfur, and selenium.

In 1980, a study was performed in China with 11 patients who had contracted Cryptococcal meningitis. The patients were treated with garlic extract orally and by injection, either intramuscularly or intravenously, over a period of several weeks. Side effects were minimal and all 11 patients recovered successfully. This study was reported in the *Chinese Medical Journal* and was entitled "Garlic and Cryptococcal Meningitis. A Preliminary Report." Although this study shows that garlic has powerful anti-fungal effects, I would strongly suggest using it more for preventive therapy than as an acute treatment.

Recommended dosage: It is best to include an abundance of fresh garlic and onions in the diet. If desired, supplement your diet with garlic capsules taken 2 to 8 capsules per day. *Side effects:* indigestion, halitosis.

Digestive Aids

Chamomile

Chamomile is known in Europe as a "cure-all." Leading the list of its proven properties is an antispasmodic effect helpful in reducing irritable bowel symptoms. One of the most established properties of chamomile is its anti-inflammatory effect. It can be applied internally or externally to decrease inflammation. It can also be used on the gums to relieve swelling and pain.

Chamomile beneficially affects the nerves, stomach, kidneys, and liver. It is known as a diaphoretic (encourages sweating to help break fevers), and a potent sedative. It has antibacterial and anti-fungal effects and is also useful for treating dermatologic ailments. It has a mild stimulating effect on the liver.

Recommended dosage: A medicinal tea can be made by steeping one-quarter ounce of chamomile in a pint of boiled water for 10 minutes. Chamomile tincture can also be used 1 to 2 tablespoons at a time, 1–3x daily. Externally, chamomile can be applied to swellings, sore muscles, and painful joints as a poultice, a warm, moistened pack of herbs that is held to the skin by a clean cotton bandage. *Side effects:* none.

Slippery Elm

Slippery elm bark can be used internally and externally for soothing mucous membranes. This herb is extremely effective when used in teas for sore throats, bronchitis, and sinusitis. It is also very soothing to the digestive system.

Slippery elm was originally used by the American Indians and Western settlers to treat urinary and bowel irritation, scurvy, dysentery, and ulcers. It was applied externally as a poultice for tumors, burns, and open wounds. The active ingredient in slippery elm bark is mucilage. It is the soluble fiber responsible for its soothing action. For the treatment of HIV, slippery elm can be used to treat coughs, bronchitis, and any malabsorptive conditions of the digestive tract.

Recommended dosage: Slippery elm is best used internally in combination with other herbs. A traditional formula for treating colitis is one-half teaspoon of slippery elm bark powder added to a cup of chamomile/peppermint tea, then sweeten to taste with honey. Drink the tea slowly and repeat several times a day. *Side effects:* diarrhea and bloating if taken in excessive amounts.

Peppermint, Spearmint, and Catnip

Peppermint is probably the best known of the mints. Its use can be traced back to the beginnings of recorded history. Its essential oils enhance digestive action by stimulating the gallbladder to secrete bile. It has been shown to reduce intestinal gas and alleviate cramping. Recent research has attributed antiulcer and anti-inflammatory properties to peppermint. Peppermint has also been shown to inhibit and kill many kinds of bacteria and viruses that can cause digestive imbalances. Studies have been published showing peppermint's inhibitory effect on the following organisms: influenza A virus, herpes simplex virus, mumps virus, strep, staph, and pseudomonas bacteria, and Candida albicans yeast.

Peppermint is the most mentally stimulating of the mints and the best for improving digestion. Spearmint is more relaxing and has a diuretic action. Catnip, often called catmint, has many of the same properties as peppermint. It is soothing to the gastrointestinal tract and is often used to treat infant colic. Like peppermint, it has been shown to have antibiotic properties, although the research is not nearly as extensive. Catnip is sometimes called "nature's Alka-Seltzer," although this term is applicable to all of the mints.

Recommended dosage: One-quarter ounce of herb, steeped in 1 pint of boiled water, for 10 minutes. This produces an infusion (steeped tea) with the above-mentioned medicinal benefits. *Side effects:* none

Nervines

Nervines are herbs that strengthen and relax the nervous system. Since stress reduction is so important for a healthy immune system, these herbs can be a very beneficial part of your program.

The nervine family includes chamomile, hops, valerian, skullcap, and passion flower. These herbs work best when used in combination. They are taken as teas, capsules, or tinctures. Find the product that helps you relax the best. Use them to balance and strengthen your nervous system so that you can cultivate the inner calm necessary for good health and healing to occur. *Side effects:* none

Eastern Herbs

Chinese Tonic Herbs

Chinese tonic herbs have been used for centuries to protect the body from external disease and rebalance it if illness occurs. In addition to promoting strong immune function, Chinese tonic herbs help tonify and balance the "chi," or energy flow of the body.

Herbs have very potent effects when taken individually. However, the major benefit of most herbal preparations stems from their use in effective combinations. Combinations bring together herbs from different categories into effective, balanced formulas. A combination of different herbs often addresses the needs of the body more effectively than a single remedy.

Listed below are descriptions of 7 important Chinese tonic herbs found in many Eastern immune-supportive formulas. Extensive animal and human testing has been done with all of the herbs listed. Much of it substantiates them to be powerful natural substances possessing many immune-strengthening properties.

Unfortunately, medical research conducted in China and other foreign countries is often not accepted by American researchers. This is partially due to the fact that the Chinese medical system utilizes concepts and descriptive terms unfamiliar to most Western researchers (chi, meridians, energy flow, cooling and heating effects, etc.). I hope that as both the Eastern and Western schools of medicine share their findings, a truly universal system of medical treatment will begin to emerge that will be more effective than when either is used alone. This philosophy is already being utilized in China where Western drugs *and* herbal treatments are combined in the treatment of diseases such as cancer, heart disease, serious infections, and diabetes with excellent results.

The following description of Chinese tonic herbs and their properties was taken with permission from the work of Subhuti Dharmananda, Ph.D., the director of the Institute for Traditional Medicine and Preventive Health Care in Portland, Oregon. Much of it is from a paper he wrote entitled "Chinese Herbal Therapies for the Treatment of Immunodeficiency Syndromes" printed in the January 1987 issue of the *Oriental Healing Arts International Bulletin.* Dr. Dharmananda has been a pioneer for many years in the field of traditional Chinese herbal therapy and specializes in the treatment of HIV and other immunodeficiency syndromes. A list of practitioners who specialize in using Chinese herbs for the adjunctive treatment of immunodeficiency states is available by calling or writing the Institute for Traditional Medicine (ITM) 503-233-4907, 2017 SE Hawthorne, Portland, OR 97214.

Astragalus

Astragalus is the dried root of *Astragalus membranaceus,* a perennial attaining a height of about 2 feet and grown in northern China. This herb is now being commercially cultivated. After the roots are dug up, the outsides are briefly fired to remove the small rootlets, and the material is sliced diagonally to produce long, thin slats. The yellow color of the interior is used as a measure of the quality of the herb.

The following components are responsible for the active effects of astragalus: polysaccharides, gluconic acid, mucilage, amino acids, choline, betaine, folic acid, kumatakenin, and flavones including quercetin, isorhamnepin, and ramnocitrin.

Several specific fractions of polysaccharides are believed to be responsible for its major immunostimulating effects. These fractions, when injected into rats, increase the number of macrophages, enhance CD4 transformation (from CD8 to CD4), and increase phagocytosis. In mice, astragalus promotes the ability of the immune system to produce interferon and increases the clearance of toxins.

Human clinical trials have demonstrated that when astragalus is given to cancer patients receiving chemotherapy or radiation therapy, a substantial increase in 1-year, 3-year, and 5-year survival rates is observed. Astragalus has also been shown to increase certain beneficial antibodies (IgA and IgG) in the blood and to induce the production of interferon by white blood cells.

According to traditional Chinese medicine, astragalus is classified as a warm, sweet tonic that enhances the functioning of the Spleen and Lungs. It is recommended for general strengthening, to treat excessive perspiration, and for promoting the healing of damaged tissues. It is also commonly used in the treatment of edema, night sweats, skin ulcerations, and abscesses. Pure astragalus root is sometimes processed by cooking with honey, in order to enhance its effect and palatability. The cooked astragalus can be used for the treatment of lethargy, weak digestion, anemia, and poor appetite. Astragalus can also be taken as a decoction (the liquid fraction after boiling the root in water for half an hour) or combined with other herbs in powder form as pills, tablets, or capsules. The typical dosage of this combination formula is about 9 grams per day, of which astragalus traditionally comprises 15% to 20% of the total.

Schizandra

Schizandra is the ripe fruit of *Schizandra sinensis.* This plant is a woody vine that is generally found climbing treetops by twining around the trunks. It is native to the mountain forests of northern China. During the fall, the ripe fruit is collected and sun dried to prevent mildew. Schizandra is a stimulant herb, found to affect the central nervous system of both animals and human beings. Clinical evaluations have shown that it enhances energy level and mental acuity. It is thus helpful in overcoming stress, fatigue, and in enhancing one's performance at work.

Several studies involving schizandra were reported at an International Conference in Hong Kong in 1984. Schizandra extract was proven successful for the treatment of a number of hepatitis syndromes, including viral hepatitis. In animals, its effects include protection of liver cells from fatty degeneration and an enhancement of lymphocyte transformation. In patients with chronic hepatitis, schizandra has proven to lower the production of liver enzymes (ALT, ALT) in about 80% of the cases as well as producing overall improvement in a majority of clinical symptoms.

In traditional Chinese medicine, schizandra is regarded as a warm, astringent tonic. It is classically used as a chi tonic for the Lungs and Kidneys to treat edema, sweating, and chronic diarrhea. Schizandra is frequently combined with other herbs that nurture the Yin and essence in the treatment of exhaustion, weight loss, and thirst. The dosage for schizandra ranges from 3 to 20 grams per day depending on the condition to be treated. In pills, it usually comprises about 10% to 20% of the composition.

Ligustrum

Ligustrum is derived from the fruit of the *Ligustrum lucidium* plant, which is found throughout many parts of the Far East. In China, ligustrum is mostly collected throughout the Sichuan Province. The plant is an evergreen shrub that grows to about 13 feet in height, producing clusters of black berries. The fruit contains the following active ingredients: syringin, oleanolic acid, demanite, osolic acid, nueshenide, and oleuropenin.

Ligustrum has been used for several centuries in China as a tonic for the kidneys. Like astragalus, this herb is used as a good tonic when there has been a rapid deterioration of the body, such as occurs when the immune system is failing.

Ligustrum is a diuretic and cardiac stimulant. It inhibits the growth of bacteria and has been shown to raise the white blood cell count of patients undergoing cancer chemotherapy. As a measure of its ability to stimulate the immune system, mononuclear cells from 13 cancer patients were treated with ligustrum extract. The graft versus host reaction, a measure of the immune system's reactivity, converted from negative to positive in 9 of the 13 patients.

In traditional Chinese medicine, ligustrum is classified as a Yin tonic. It is used in the treatment of aging, dizziness, tinnitus, backache, and blurred vision. It has a sweet, bitter taste with cooling properties. It is usually prepared as a decoction. Alcohol extracts and tablets of this herb have also been used in clinical practice with success.

Ganoderma

Ganoderma is a mushroomlike fungus of the *Ganoderma lucidium* family. This family yields many important Chinese herbs and is also famous in Japan, where it is known as the Reishi mushroom. The fungus grows on old, broadleaf trees and often attains a weight of over a pound. Ganoderma is relatively rare and thus costly. Commercial cultivation has brought the price down considerably. The most useful form of the mushroom is the rare antler form, which has many branches and spores rather than a single cap. Recently a technique for growing high spore–content ganoderma has been developed in Japan.

Ganoderma contains polysaccharides that are known to enhance the functioning of the immune system. In laboratory studies, these polysaccharides suppress the growth of implanted tumor cells. The mechanism of action also involves an increase in T-cell and macrophage activity.

In the treatment of viral hepatitis, ganoderma has been shown to improve symptoms such as anorexia, insomnia, malaise, and liver swelling. In 1 study, the level of AST liver enzymes decreased (a sign of improvement) in 70% of the patients.

Ganoderma is a stress reducing herb effective in treating conditions such as stomach ulcers and high blood pressure. In persons suffering insomnia, it enhances the relaxation of muscles and increases sleeping time. It also reduces lipids and cholesterol in the blood.

Traditionally, ganoderma has been used in China as a chi tonic and sedative. The taste is sweet and slightly bitter. It is usually taken in doses of 9 to 15 grams prepared as a decoction, although doses as low as 4 to 6 grams daily have proven effective for the treatment of insomnia, nervousness, and chronic infections. It can be made into pills in combination with other herbs representing 10% to 20% of the combination. Liquid extracts of ganoderma have recently become available.

White Atractylodes

White atractylodes is the dried root of *Atractylodes macrocephala*. It is a perennial herb, growing 1 to 3 feet in height. It is generally found growing in the Zhejianj, Jiangxi, Hunan, Hubei, and Shanxi provinces of China. The wild plant is scarce. The herb on the market is derived from commercial cultivation. It is grown in sandy soil that is well drained and fertilized with organic material. White atractylodes is differentiated from "ordinary atractylodes," a less expensive herb of the Atractylodes family.

Important constituents of white atractylodes are found in the volatile oils which contain elemol, atractylol, and atractylon. It also contains vitamin A and has been proven useful in treating night blindness caused by vitamin A deficiency.

As an immune-stimulating agent, white atractylodes has been shown to be beneficial in enhancing the phagocytic functions of white blood cells and in increasing their numbers. It is an important component in several classic immune-enhancing formulas and is usually combined with astragalus and/or ginseng for maximum effect.

White atractylodes is a diuretic. In 1 study, a dose of 0.05 to 0.25 gms/kg of the decoction liquid injected intravenously into dogs resulted in excretion of urine nearly 9 times the level of controls and its effect lasted for more than 5 hours.

Laboratory experiments have demonstrated the tonic effect of white atractylodes. In oral administration of the decoction for 1 month, laboratory animals showed increases in body weight and enhanced physical endurance. It has also been shown to have a protective effect on the liver against damage by chemical toxins.

According to traditional Chinese medicine, white atractylodes is a sweet and bitter warming tonic for the Spleen and Stomach. It is used to rid the body of excessive moisture, improve digestion, increase appetite, and lessen fatigue. It has also been used for treating dizziness, diarrhea, and night sweats. The dosage used to make a decoction is 5 to 10 grams. It is also commonly combined with other herbs and commonly comprises 10% to 40% of the mixture.

Codonopsis

Codonopsis is the root of the *Codonopsis pilosula* plant. This plant grows in Northern China and is cultivated in the Sichuan and Hubei provinces. The perennial herb grows to approximately 3 feet in height. The roots, collected in the fall, are graded by size. The active constituents of this herb are saponins and alkaloids.

Codonopsis is used throughout China as a substitute for ginseng which is more expensive. It is considered to have nearly identical properties as ginseng, but to have less effect of "heating the blood." It is therefore the preferred herb for use in the treatment of HIV disease, a condition known for its excess heat and dampness. Codonopsis is also considered to be somewhat more active than ginseng on the lungs. It is in the same family as 3 other lung-active herbs: platycodon, adenophora, and lobelia. While ginseng has been amply tested and proven effective as an immune enhancer in both Korea and the Soviet Union, codonopsis has been evaluated only more recently. Like ginseng, it has shown to be beneficial in the treatment of laboratory animals and human patients undergoing cancer therapies.

Codonopsis stimulates the growth of red blood cells, enhances T-cell transformation, and stimulates phagocytosis. The combination of ganoderma, astragalus, and codonopsis has been shown to enhance phagocytosis and to promote lymphocyte transformation. In a study of its immune-stimulating effects, codonopsis was used as the main ingredient in combination with white atractylodes and hoelen. This mixture enhanced the rate of rosette formation of lymphocytes in the blood, a measure of their stimulation. It also increased the level of IgG antibodies in the bloodstream.

In traditional Chinese medicine, codonopsis is classified as a neutral energy, sweet chi tonic used for disorders of the Spleen and Lungs. It has been used in the treatment of heart palpitations, nervousness, menstrual disorders, and breast cancer. The usual dose is 9 to 15 grams taken as a decoction. It can also be used in pills, representing 10% to 25% of the mixture.

Licorice

Licorice is one of the most widely used herbs in Chinese medicine. It is derived from the root and lower stem of *Glycyrrhiza uralensis* and *Glycyrrhiza glabra*. Much of the Chinese licorice supply is from northern China, especially from Heilongjiang Province. The plant is a shrub that grows to a height of 2 to 3 feet. The dried root slices are frequently processed with honey to enhance it's chi-strengthening effect.

The principle active constituents of licorice are saponin glycosides. The sweet taste of licorice is due to glycyrrhizin, which is rated 50 times sweeter per unit weight than sugar. Glycyrrhizin has been shown to be effective in treating acute and chronic viral hepatitis. In 1 study, 85% of the patients receiving it experienced clinical cure and the remainder showed marked improvement. In contrast, only 35% of the 20-person control group, receiving a different therapy, were cured. In addition, glycyrrhizin has been shown to produce increases in IgG, IgA, and IgM antibody levels.

Licorice root's effects with regards to the treatment infections has been clearly substantiated. A study from China found that licorice root possessed antibacterial activity against several common gram negative intestinal bacteria. Later, in 1979, a team of Italian researchers reported a series of experiments in which they discovered several antiviral effects attributable to licorice root. These included the extracellular destruction of virus particles, the prevention of intracellular virus activation, and the impairment of the viral components to assemble. In China, experiments have revealed that licorice root activates the body's interferon mechanisms.

In the United States, a team of investigators has recently reported study results verifying licorice root's antimicrobial properties against staph and mycobacterium species. Mycobacterium organisms are responsible for MAC and tuberculosis infections, now the second leading cause of opportunistic infections in AIDS patients.

Licorice root is an important component of many Chinese herbal combinations and is classified as a sweet, neutral energy chi tonic. It may be used as a decoction, in doses of up to 24 grams for the treatment of laryngitis, coughing spasms, and severe pain. It usually comprises about 5% of a general tonic formula and works to potentiate other herbs in the combination.

Fu Zheng Therapy

Many Asian combination herbal formulas are based on a traditional Chinese form of healing known as "Fu Zheng therapy." Literally this means "to restore normalcy and balance to the body."

In practice, Fu Zheng therapy does not specifically treat an infective agent, but works toward rebuilding the resistance of the individual. Its goal is to enable the body to rebuild its strength and regain balance so it can more effectively contend with the disease.

Initial interest by Western medical researchers in Fu Zheng therapy can be traced back to research papers published by investigators at the Department of Medical Oncology at Beijing Cancer Institute in 1982. Clinicians there reported significant increases in the survival rates of cancer patients receiving a combination of Fu Zheng herbs and conventional therapies, such as radiation and chemotherapy. There was a notable decrease in the immunosuppressive effects of these therapies when Fu Zheng herbs were added to the standard medical regimen. Following the evaluation of several Fu Zheng combinations, 2 principal herbs were chosen for use as adjuncts to conventional therapies at the Beijing Cancer Institute. These were astragalus and ligustrum, 2 of the immune-enhancing herbs described above.

Studies in HIV(+) Patients

There have been several prior studies utilizing Fu Zheng herbs for the treatment of HIV. One of these studies was performed by U.S. herbalist

Subhuti Dharmananda in 1986. He and 2 other herbalists, Susan Black and Jay Sordean, developed a protocol for determining whether Chinese herbs might be helpful for persons with ARC or AIDS.

The Immune Enhancement Project treated 20 ARC patients for a period exceeding 3 months. Most of the participants were symptomatic and therefore able to report whether Fu Zheng therapy was helpful in diminishing their symptoms. The basic herbal combinations used in the Immune Enhancement Project consisted of an astragalus-based formula, known as Astra 8, designed by Dr. Dharmananda and a second formula prepared from shitaki and cascade mushrooms from Portland, Oregon.

Once a month, participants would fill out a questionnaire consisting of a lengthy checklist of symptoms. There was improvement in all 20 of the patients. Diarrhea and night sweats were virtually eliminated and energy levels were improved in all but 2 of the participants. There was no control group.

A second study utilizing Fu Zheng therapy was conducted by the Quan Yin Center for Healing Arts in San Francisco. This study, originally designed by herbalist Misha Cohen, also showed a decrease in symptoms and an overall improvement in most patients' energy levels. Some very ill patients were even able to return to work after adding Chinese herbs to their program of standard medical therapies.

Research performed at the University of Texas System Cancer Center, M.D. Anderson Hospital and Tumor Institute, by Drs. Chu, Wong, Mavligit and others, has shown that purified fractions of astragalus root possess potent immunorestorative activity both in the test tube and in rats. Dr. Chu and his coworkers have found that by incubating astragalus extract and white blood cells along with interleukin-2, a naturally produced immune-mediator, there was a tenfold increase in the white blood cell's ability to kill tumor cells. Since interleukin-2 is toxic when given to patients in high doses, the researchers hope that simultaneous use of astragalus purified fractions and interleukin-2 will allow smaller, less toxic dosages of interleukin-2 to be used yielding superior results.

In another paper from M.D. Anderson Hospital and Tumor Institute, Dr. Chu concluded that "a failing immune system in human subjects, manifested by deficient T-cell function from debilitating diseases such as cancer or AIDS, may be partially restored or augmented to a certain extent by various biological response modifiers.... Our data distinctly indicates that either the crude extract of astragalus membranaceus, or its column separated fraction #3, can completely restore a failing immune system and bring its T-cell's functioning, in vitro, to the normal level found among cells derived from healthy subjects. The properties possessed by this traditional Chinese medicinal herbal extract renders it an important biological response modifier which should be considered for clinical trials of immunotherapy in persons who suffer from primary or secondary immunologic deficiency and its associated serious complications."

Many of Dr. Chu's papers, including the above passage, were published in the *Journal of Clinical Laboratory Immunology* in 1988. As you probably know, there has not been a mad dash to begin studying the effects of astragalus and its purified fractions in AIDS patients, even as an adjunct to other antiviral therapies. Hopefully, as additional data surfaces to highlight the benefits that herbs can bring to HIV care, more research funding will be channeled in the direction of investigating these potent and beneficial medicines.

SUMMARY

I have discussed the benefits of many useful herbs in this chapter. Though I previously recommended daily use of a proprietary herbal combination called RESIST, I now prefer to recommend a program of herbs based on each patient's individual needs. Consulting with a naturopath, herbalist, or acupuncturist skilled in working with HIV(+) individuals is by far the best way to accomplish this goal. If you would like to experiment with herbs on your own, you can use this and other reference materials as guides. Remember, whenever you start a new herb or therapy, see how you feel on it and what your latest lab tests reveal. Most important, all herbs, similar to medications, eventually lose their effectiveness if taken continuously for long periods of time. Therefore, consider rotating to different tonic formulas every several months. This will keep your program fresh and your body strong.

It is also very important to realize that herbs comprise just *1 component* of an overall treatment program that includes a healthful diet, vitamins, exercise, stress reduction and, when indicated, standard medications. This type of overall approach will enable your herbal program to work much more effectively. The Healing HIV program employs a combination treatment approach. The immune-strengthening value of each of its components enables the entire program to be far more beneficial than the sum of its parts.

AGGRESSIVE NATURAL THERAPIES

Exercise

Check the box that applies to you:

❐ I make no effort to obtain regular exercise

❐ I live an active life and get my workouts from daily living activities, such as walking, climbing stairs, shopping, running for the bus, etc.

❐ I make a modest effort to obtain regular exercise (1–3x/week).

❐ I obtain regular exercise 3–5x/week (at least 30 minutes/session).

❐ I obtain regular exercise greater than 5x/week (at least 30 minutes per session).

If you checked the box stating that you live an active life but do not get any regular exercise, you are not providing your body with the stimulation it needs for the immune system to function optimally. Regular exercise is necessary *to enhance* the functioning of the immune system. The Healing HIV program recommends that an asymptomatic HIV(+) individual exercise 3 to 5 a week for at least 30 minutes per session. Symptomatic individuals should not exert themselves any more than they feel comfortable doing.

It is extremely important that you *enjoy* the exercise activities that you practice. If you enjoy them, you will look forward to them. Enjoyable exercise can become a wonderful outlet for stress, a source of personal satisfaction, and an invigorating physical release.

When deciding which exercises to make part of your treatment program, it is important that you achieve the following goals.

Deep breathing: During exercise, deep breathing helps to cleanse the lungs. It also acts as a pump for the lymphatic system. Lymph is a milky fluid made up of water, protein, antibodies, and white blood cells. It flows through the lymphatic channels which parallel the circulatory system. It passes through the lymph nodes and cleanses them. *It is the life blood of your immune system!*

Your lymph nodes can become swollen if they are congested with material that has been cleansed from your tissues. This can include dead cells, bacteria, and virus particles. To help relieve this congestion, lymph is pushed through the system by deep breathing and the pumping action of your muscles.

Imagine a stream that is moving sluggishly. The algae and waste products of the stream begin to build up and clog the system. This is an unhealthy situation. Only by removing the blockages in the stream, or increasing the force of its flow, does a healthful situation recur. Regular exercise, lasting at least 30 minutes per session, will help this occur.

Sweating. The next important goal to accomplish by exercising is to heat the body to the point at which sweating occurs. Viral replication is inhibited by high temperatures. Exercise can decrease viral activity by raising your body temperature.

Sweating serves another function. When the blood vessels of the skin dilate, the sweat glands act as tiny filters to remove toxins and waste products from the blood. The waste is then pumped to the surface of the skin as sweat. This cleansing action is very important to the body. It is also important that you shower off after you exercise so these toxins are not left on the surface of your skin.

A duration of at least 30 minutes. It is important to extend your circulation as much as possible to the deeper organs of your body. To achieve this, your exercise session must last at least 30 minutes. This allows enough time for the flow of blood to extend into the deep tissues of the spleen, liver, kidneys, lymph nodes, and bone marrow; bringing a fresh flow of oxygen and healthful nutrients to these organs.

When you are sedentary, white blood cells begin to stick to the walls of your blood vessels and become dormant. When aerobic exercise is performed, the white blood cells, including CD4 cells and macrophages, awaken and are swept back into the circulation where they can function at peak efficiency. This process is known as "demargination" and it occurs approximately thirty minutes into an aerobic workout. The benefits which occur as a result of this process will last for hours.

There are other activities that you can add to your program that produce many of the above benefits. These include dry saunas, steam rooms, jacuzzis, and hot tubs. These activities help to reduce your stress, improve circulation to your organs, and enhance your body's ability to excrete waste products. They can all be incorporated into your overall program.

If you feel overly tired or sore the day after you exercise, it is a sign that your session was too strenuous. If you feel invigorated, the intensity level was just right. This rule of thumb also goes for saunas, steam rooms, and hot baths. If you become dizzy or do not feel well when you finish, it was probably too vigorous for your system.

Remember: A powerful and harmonious *combination* of health-promoting activities is the goal of the Healing HIV program. Together they will suppress viral activity and enhance the functioning of your immune system. Continue to strive for *balance, moderation,* and *growth* in all of the treatments that you do. Review the information from Chapter 9 to help you find the best balance between progressive resistance exercise vs. aerobic exercise.

SUMMARY

1) Find exercise activities *that you enjoy.*

2) Exercise 3–5x/week for at least *30 minutes per session.*

3) Strive to promote *deep breathing* and *sweating.*

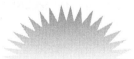

AGGRESSIVE NATURAL THERAPIES

Stress Reduction

What Is Stress?

I do not usually enjoy speaking about stress because, as the subject is discussed, people become tense! This is perfectly understandable. There is so much stress in our lives that it appears that we are becoming obsessed with finding ways to avoid it.

The dictionary defines *stress* as force, pressure, strain, or weight. These are not the conditions under which maximal healing occurs. Stress encourages just the opposite. It creates an environment that directly impedes healing, regeneration, and growth.

Deep Relaxation

I cannot overemphasize the importance of regularly practiced deep relaxation. When we relax completely, the baseline activity level of many of our bodily systems decreases. For example, our heart rate slows. Breathing becomes deeper and more regular. All of our muscles relax and utilize less energy. The mind also quiets and consumes less fuel. All of these effects directly contribute to a conservation of our energy. This energy can then be used by the immune system for healing.

Results of a 1992 study from the University of Miami Medical School reported that HIV(+) men who practiced regular relaxation techniques, or did regular aerobic exercise, had higher blood levels of CD4 cells than those who did not. In addition, over a 2-year follow-up period those who continued to practice relaxation and aerobic exercise regularly stayed healthier longer.

The participants of this study developed symptoms or died were among the least diligent in practicing relaxation and exercise, were the most distressed upon learning their diagnosis, and also tended to deny the need to take steps to cope with their situation. Researchers say the findings of this study suggest that HIV(+) individuals who are still healthy may benefit emotionally, as well as immunologically, from the regular practice of relaxation techniques and moderate exercise in addition to their other treatments. Dr. Mary Anne Fletcher, director of the Clinical Immunology Lab at the university stated that the increase observed in the study participant's CD4 cells "was about the same as you would expect in the same period if you gave the patients antiviral medication."

Regularly conserving energy is extremely important to a person who has a chronic infection. If an energy deficit is present, and persists over a long period of time in the presence of an HIV infection, the immune system will inevitably weaken. It is as if your energy checking account is constantly in the red. If this situation persists, energy bankruptcy will eventually follow.

Deep relaxation, practiced twice daily, allows your body to conserve energy which contributes to a more positive energy balance. In order to increase the chances that my patients practice deep relaxation regularly, I offer them cassette tapes containing prerecorded relaxation exercises. Each exercise lasts approximately 15 to 20 minutes, and I recommend that one be listened to twice daily. Approximately 15 to 20 minutes per session is the optimal length of time for a relaxation tape. In this amount of time, its benefit can be achieved without the technique creating stress by taking too much time out of the day. Prayer, yoga, and meditation are also good techniques that can be practiced regularly to promote deep relaxation.

Conserving your body's energy 15 to 20 minutes twice a day goes a long way to helping your body restore its energy balance. Energy stored during this time can be channeled toward the immune system. It can then be used by your body to regenerate cells, repair damaged tissues, rebuild the blood and, in general, shore up your defenses. It is similar to a cease-fire occurring twice daily in the midst of a battle; it allows you to repair equipment, feed the troops, rebuild embankments, and stay at full strength instead of constantly being worn down by the enemy.

In addition to the physical benefits that occur during deep relaxation, the mind is also encouraged to rest and become quiet. The relaxation tapes that I provide include positive affirmations to help promote a lessening of fear and a strengthening of positive attitude. The benefits of a positive emotional state are extensive and well worth achieving. They will be discussed in detail in the next chapter on emotional healing.

A second, more demanding, technique for establishing a positive energy balance is called "Your Healing Hour." This technique can be found in the next chapter. It is one of the most effective relaxation exercises I know of for helping a person return to balance.

Long-Term Stressors

Another important way to reduce your stress is by making positive changes in your life that focus on lessening your stress *in the long term*. These may include finding a new job, getting out of an unhealthy relationship (or into a healthy one), learning to establish healthy boundaries in your interactions with other people, or beginning to include a spiritual practice in your life. These activities might be called "making big changes in your life." They have the potential to significantly lessen your stress in the long run.

There is often a substantial amount of fear when it comes to making these changes. This is because a comfortable situation, even if it is an unhealthy one, often feels safer and less frightening than the unknown. In Chapter 16, I will introduce many techniques that will help you identify the positive changes that need to be made in your life to further your healing. These techniques are also designed to help you overcome fears that may be holding you back.

Honoring Your Illness

Some people say that being diagnosed with a major, life-threatening illness is your spirit's way of communicating the urgent need to make big changes in your life. It might be that you have been depressed and unhappy for so long, without taking any major steps toward improving your situation, that your mind/body/spirit is forced to send you a stronger message than plain old depression or unhappiness. It sends you a message that it hopes you will now heed; it sends you a physical illness to get you to stop and pay attention to what's going on.

The occurrence of a life-threatening physical illness may be the final straw that forces you to stop and reevaluate who you are, what you are doing, where you are going with your life, and whether this is the most healthful or skillful path for you to take. It may finally get you to notice how you are truly feeling.

Psychological distress has often been shown to precede the occurrence of a major physical illness such as a heart attack or cancer. It has also been shown to alter CD4 subsets and depress the overall strength of the immune system.

The majority of people with AIDS who have survived for greater than 5 years, as well as most individuals who have achieved complete remissions from other serious illnesses such as cancer, have *listened to their body's signals* and made major changes in previously out-of-balance lifestyles. Making big changes in your life takes you in a direction away from the cause of your stress (i.e., a bad job, an unhealthy relationship, a bad living situation, etc.) and toward new, potentially more positive experiences. At the very least, these new experiences can be invigorating and stimulating. Don't be afraid to make the big changes that you know deep inside you need to make. Who knows? Things could turn out better than you expect.

Being diagnosed with a major physical illness is not a sign that you will be broken forever. It is not a sign that you are a failure or that you are weak. But it may be a message from yourself that *now is the time to make some changes.* Change is the only constant in the universe. It is always occurring. Don't be afraid of the future if you change. Fear it only if you are constantly avoiding change and growth.

I hope that this chapter has not "stressed you out" too much. Instead, my goal has been to provide you with the motivation and confidence necessary to incorporate both deep relaxation and long-term stress reduction into your comprehensive treatment program.

SUMMARY
1) Keep your stress as low as possible.
2) Practice deep relaxation twice daily for 15 to 20 minutes.
3) Make changes in your life that will lessen your long-term stress.

Chapter Sixteen

Emotional and Spiritual Healing

....

"Mindfulness is a willingness to be in this moment, not to be carried off without awareness into the memories of the past, or into anxiety about the future."

....

— Jon Kabat-Zinn

Dr. Bernie Siegel, in his best-selling book *Love, Medicine and Miracles* (Harper & Row, 1986) states that "scientific research and my own day-to-day clinical experience have convinced me that the state of the mind changes the state of the body by working through the central nervous system, the endocrine system and the immune system. Peace of mind sends the body a "live" message, while depression, fear and unresolved conflict give it a "die" message." He continues: "Exceptional patients manifest the will to live in its most potent form. They take charge of their lives even if they were unable to so before, and they work hard to achieve health and piece of mind. They do not rely on doctors to take the initiative but rather use them as members of a team, demanding the utmost in technique, resourcefulness, concern, and open-mindedness. If they're not satisfied, they change doctors."

I have had a similar experience in working with many of my patients. That is, I have found that exceptional HIV(+) patients are aggressive, confident, open-minded, and willing to work hard to heal on all levels. This commitment and dedication usually translates, on a biochemical level, into healthy immune-system functioning and a prolonged period of good health and stability.

Other helpful tips for creating a healthful emotional environment include:

1) Maintain good reasons for living. The more good reasons you have for being here and remaining alive, the greater the chance you will continue to do so.

2) Set goals to achieve and remind yourself of them often. Celia, a 12-year-old girl with cancer, wrote down so many goals she wanted to achieve that she eventually realized there wasn't any time to die. Now she is 17, in remission, and picking out a dress for her high school prom.

3) Find a purpose for living your life. Maybe it's to gain insight into yourself, to do volunteer work, to be a good parent, or to help others. As long as it feels right to you, it's fine. Be creative!

4) Allow yourself to have some form of work or daily activity that is both stimulating and fulfilling. Find a job that provides you with more than just a paycheck at the end of the week. Full-time employment is particularly draining to someone with a life-challenging condition unless their work gives them something beyond monetary reward.

5) Work on improving your relationships with friends, family, and loved ones. Do not allow resentments to go on for a long time without expression or resolution.

These suggestions can help lessen the inertia many of us feel in these particular areas of our lives. Remember, it's just as important to heal and strengthen your emotional self as it is to heal and strengthen your physical body. They are integrally related.

Tanya

In 1991, a charming and attractive young woman came into my office for her initial consultation. Her name was Tanya and she had been exposed to HIV in 1988 through a heterosexual relationship. Tanya was European, worked as a flight attendant, and was asymptomatic. She had started a combination of AZT/DDI a few months before coming to see me and was tolerating her medications well. However, her CD4 count was continuing to fall and was now 110 cells/mm3.

After a thorough evaluation, I recommended that Tanya significantly increase her protein intake, start acupuncture, take immune-enhancing herbs, and begin prophylaxis medication with Septra DS 3x/week to prevent Pneumocystis pneumonia. Her comprehensive stool analysis revealed intestinal parasites, and we treated these successfully with the Parasite Elimination program (see Chapter 8). I also advised her to change her antiviral medications with the hope of better suppressing her viral infection.

During the next couple of years, Tanya was able to maintain her CD4 count in the 100 to 200 range with a variety of antiviral combinations. In addition to her antiviral and prophylaxis program, Tanya also continued to eat a healthy diet, get regular exercise, maintain a positive attitude, and get frequent acupuncture treatments. During this time Tanya felt extremely well, continued to work full-time, and began studying to be an acupressurist.

At the beginning of 1996, Tanya's CD4 count again fell to 97 cells/mm3 with a viral load of 80,000 copies/ml Because her prior antiviral program had clearly lost its effectiveness, we needed to make a complete change to her regimen. I therefore recommended that Tanya begin protease-inhibitor therapy with a triple combination of D4T/3TC/ritonavir (the most effective protease inhibitor available at the time).

During the next 12 months, Tanya's viral load became undetectable and her CD4 count rose to 350 cells/mm3. She also became involved in a very nurturing relationship and got married.

Tanya and I are extremely pleased with her progress. While one might argue that the majority of her improvement was due to the inclusion of a protease inhibitor, I would like to highlight her positive attitude and fighting spirit. She never gave up hope. She never gave into her illness. She maintained her smile, balanced outlook, and charm, without letting HIV prevent her from achieving her goals. She fell in love and got married, improved her living situation, and changed her career. She is presently healthy, happy, and planning to stay alive for a very long time. She is a shining example of healing HIV in action.

Your Healing Hour

This exercise is extremely beneficial for increasing your CD4 cells and treating fatigue; it is very potent when practiced regularly. The benefit comes from the fact that the probability of accomplishing any goal is heightened when time is spent concentrating on its accomplishment.

Consider what you are reading as a guide to facilitating the learning of this technique. After several practice runs, you will be able to do this technique by heart.

Take 1 hour a day to devote to your healing. Focus on what you are doing without any distractions such as television, loud music, or reading the newspaper. You may want to begin by lighting a candle and invoking this prayer: "May the time I now take bring true love and healing to my body, mind, and spirit."

During your healing hour, it is very important to make sure that you minimize any disturbances. Disconnect the phone or make sure that your answering machine is turned down so that you cannot screen your calls. If those you live with ask what you are doing, just tell them that you are taking some time for healing once a day. Then get back to your healing. Do not worry about what they may think; you are doing what's right for you.

Now lie down and allow your body to get comfortable. Don't just read this exercise; you need to practice it. Take a few deep breaths. Allow everything to quiet and to settle. Allow your thoughts to begin to have a lot of space between them. When you are ready, place your hands on any part of your body that needs healing. If you are attempting to heal the immune system or an emotional imbalance, place your hands first on your heart and then on any other part of your body that needs your healing touch. Love yourself…Be with yourself…Heal yourself…

✳

Feel your body. Notice any areas of tension, hurt, or pain. Gently…Just begin to notice them. Make no judgments. Acknowledge the pain's presence. And then, slowly, allow your awareness to move a little closer to this area, the area where you feel the pain. As you go, breathe deeply, expanding your abdomen completely, and then your back, and then the front of your chest. Deep breathing is very important. Allow your awareness to come as close to your pain as you feel comfortable and, then, just be with it. Just experience the place that exists between pain and no pain, between tension and no tension. Just sit there, on the boundary of your pain, and be with it for a little while. As it softens, take 1 small step closer. Just be with it. Be with it for a while longer and continue to breathe deeply. Nowhere to go, nothing to do, just to be with yourself and your pain. Give it the attention that it's pleading for. Give yourself 1 hour each day to focus on complete healing. Aren't you worth 1 hour each day? Isn't your healing worth 1 hour each day? You can create the most potent healing environment possible for yourself during this hour.

✳

You are definitely worth it. You *can* create for yourself an environment during this time that is better than any other place you could be to heal. As you develop experience at being with pain in 1 area of your body, allow your awareness to go to any other part of your body that needs your lovingkindness and attention. If it has taken you 10 or 15 minutes to get this far, you are doing just fine. You are doing what is necessary to regain balance, vitality, health, and strength. Take a nice, long, deep breath, and relax further.

*

Many people do not take time just to be with themselves or to ask these questions: What needs to surface? What needs to come up? What do I need to become aware of to heal? A good deal of illness manifests as a means for your body to get your attention so that its needs can be met. Pain and fatigue are early signs. Physical illness often comes if those go unheeded. Let whatever you need to learn from this experience rise to the surface. Listen to yourself closely.

The environment that you create during this hour can be anything that you want. You can be watching the ocean or listening to a creek in a forest. It can be day or night. Consider practicing your healing hour in a setting that helps you remain comfortable and relaxed. A room in your house or a place in your garden without distractions can suffice. Spend the hour keeping yourself comfortable and nurtured. Spend the hour not "doing" anything. Notice how your mind will constantly think of things for you "to do" during this time. Just notice it, try to calm and reassure it, and allow your body to continue relaxing. Work on your healing, 1 hour each day, every day, and you will continue to make progress.

*

As your healing hour progresses, allow your body to find its own natural positions. As healing occurs, repressed emotional energy that has been stored in your body will begin to surface and release. This may occur as a series of deep, cleansing sighs. These are significant when they occur. They help to lighten your overall state. They may be looked at as individual steps on your path toward healing.

Remember, you are creating the environment for yourself that is the most nurturing possible during this hour. Allow yourself to feel safe, comfortable, and protected. Allow your healing process to unfold. Allow your natural needs and rhythms to express themselves. Get in touch with your heart and with your body.

If you feel uncomfortable during this time, do not be afraid. There is a part of you that is hurt, crying, and in pain. A part of you that needs your love and attention. You can provide this to yourself.

During this time, allow the space for any repressed emotional energy to come up and move out of your body. Tell the part of you that is hurting that you love it, care for it, and will do everything in your power to support it. As this process continues, be aware of any areas of your body that are in pain or that need your attention and just be with them, send love to them.

Continue to take deep breaths. Continue to let everything become quiet and settled. Let go of whatever you don't need. Continue to make healing progress toward balance. Allow yourself at least a full hour for this important work every day.

At this point it would be helpful to stop reading and allow 15 minutes of silence to pass so your state of relaxation can deepen.

Isn't it amazing what thoughts you begin to have? Isn't it amazing what you can feel in the parts of your body that have been in pain? It may feel like you have been wound up like a spring and are now just beginning to unwind. Just notice these things. You have already moved closer toward balance. Now, have the courage to do this every day. Its effect on your healing can be remarkable.

❋

Remember, your hands have healing touch. The only thing that you need to do to tap into your own inner healing potential is to slow down, become relaxed, love yourself, and breathe deeply. You know this is healthful for you to do. You know this is necessary. Place your hands wherever your healing needs to occur. Then just get out of the way and allow your healing to unfold. Let the process begin and gain momentum on a daily basis. You deserve it!

Follow Your Heart!

"Just listen to your heart," I advised Robert. "Just listen to whatever your heart wants you to do and follow it."

"I can't understand how that's going to help me," he said. "I just can't understand how not listening to my mind and just following my heart is going to be of any benefit at all."

Whenever you listen to your heart, you listen to the part of you *that is most interested in your well-being.* Your heart's concern is that you experience joy, love, and happiness. It has no other agenda. It is very important to tune into your heart's needs and desires when you are trying to heal. You may also imagine this technique as tuning into a part of you that is commonly called your intuition.

"Let's try a simple experiment," I said to Robert. "Any decision that you need to make, try to follow your heart's desire. I'll write a helpful aid down on this card."

Robert looked down at the card:

My head says to…
My heart says to…

He turned the card over. It said:

Follow my heart!

"Let's see how it works," I said. "Tell me something that you need to make a decision about today."

Robert began, "Well, I'm off from work today. I need to decide whether to drive back across the Bay Bridge to my home in Oakland for lunch, or to stay here in San Francisco and eat . My head tells me to drive back home to Oakland because it's more practical and less expensive to eat there. But my heart tells me to enjoy myself in San Francisco and spend some time in the city and have lunch here."

"Don't you see how your heart just wants you to experience joy?" I said. "Can you see how your enjoyment of life is its foremost concern? Your heart wants you to enjoy your time in the city rather than get in your car and drive back home. Your heart's interest is that you get the most joy out of every decision you make."

When you follow your heart's desires, as opposed to what your head tells you to do, you will undoubtedly follow the path that is right for you. Your heart wants you to experience the positive emotions of joy, happiness, and love. Your heart wants you to have experiences that are invigorating and life-affirming. These are emotions that you need to experience for healing to occur.

Your head, on the other hand, has values and beliefs that were instilled in it by other people. These "old tapes" were usually inserted by parents, peers, teachers, and other authority figures in the past. They may not have had your enjoyment of life as their primary concern. Their agenda and programming messages can be misleading and less helpful to you now.

If you can quiet your mind and follow your heart, no matter how small the decision, you will begin to learn how to follow the path that is right for you. This is your path toward healing.

Following your heart allows you to do the things that are most nurturing for you. It's time to surrender and stop trying to control things with your mind. Just allow your heart to lead you through life. There is no need to be afraid. It is the path that you were meant to follow.

Write down the following saying on a card as a reminder:

Side 1 :   My head says to…
               My heart says to…

Side 2 :   *Follow my heart!*

It's important to have confidence in this technique for it to work. Refer to it whenever you have a decision to make. Practice this technique to help you tune into your heart's desires. Begin with small decisions. For example, what shall I do this afternoon? Shall I stay home and watch TV, or shall I go for a walk in the park? If your heart wants to go for a walk in the park, go for a walk in the park. Test it out. See if you are happy that you followed your heart's advice.

Another example: Shall I go to the movies with my friends, or shall I stay home tonight and rest? Your heart knows what's best for you and for your body. If your heart wants you to stay home and rest, then it's clear that you do not have the surplus energy necessary to go out to the movies with your friends. Therefore, you need to stay home and rest.

Often it will be helpful to say these sentences aloud to enable you to "tune in" to the desires of first your head and then your heart. *Your head's* desire can be perceived as coming from your thoughts. *Your heart's* desire is most often a *feeling* coming from within. Follow your heart!

If you need to heal, the decisions that best meet the needs of your body are the best decisions to make. They will help keep you in balance and keep you on the path toward joy, love, and healing. Listen to your heart. It knows what is best for you when it comes to any decision. The more you practice this technique for making small decisions, the more confidence you will have in it when it comes to the big ones.

Robert's comment at the end of our session was: "That's radical!"

Support Groups

I have facilitated a support group for HIV(+) patients since 1989. This group provides a time and place where members can relax their defenses and honestly express their feelings. The members of my support group share not only the negative aspects of their situation but the creative approach to living they each practice as well.

A positive group experience is enhanced when all of the group's members are following a similar healing approach. It helps when they are also being cared for by a physician or physicians who share this philosophy. This provides everyone in the group with a strong sense of community, and we rarely lose time arguing about whose approach is better. When everyone's treatment approach is basically the same, time can best be spent on expressing feelings and pursuing emotional and spiritual growth.

This kind of support group experience is different from some HIV support groups where participants often come to "dump" their problems. If this is occurring, it can be very stressful to the other members and does not have a healing effect. Support groups benefit from a finely tuned, complementary blend of individuals who share friendship and mutual support.

The results of an interesting study performed at Stanford University were released in 1989. At the beginning of the study, 86 middle-aged women with metastatic breast cancer were divided into 2 treatment groups. For the study, 1 group received medical treatment alone, while the other group received similar medical treatment plus weekly group therapy for 1 year. The therapy group focused on expressing emotions such as fear, anger, anxiety, and depression. They also practiced relaxation techniques. By the end of the year, those attending the support group reported fewer mood swings and a higher sense of "vigor." The group therapy sessions were limited to only the first year of the study.

When the data was reviewed 10 years later, it revealed that the women in the support group component of the study lived almost twice as long as the women without the benefit of the support groups.

"I must say that I was quite stunned," reported Dr. David Speigal of Stanford University to the American Psychiatric Association annual meeting in May 1989. "My original goal was to design a study that would refute the very hypothesis that I ended up supporting."

Support groups provide an experience that can be strengthening to an individual faced with the hard work of healing. They can encourage the expression of deeply held feelings and emotions. This can help diminish tension, fatigue, anxiety, and depression, all of which can weaken the immune system. Consider participating in a support group to strengthen your Healing HIV program. If you can't find one that meets your needs, don't be afraid to start your own. You need only to find 2 other people who share your views on healing for the core of a beneficial support group to be created.

Positive Affirmations

• •

"Healing does not come out of little bottles;
it comes from within."

• •

— Jon Kaiser

Your subconscious beliefs play a very important role in determining how your immune system functions. If you can change your negative beliefs into positive ones, you can alter the biochemical messages that your brain sends to your immune system.

Negative beliefs are like faulty computer code buried deep within a program. They are formed by events or statements you have experienced in the past, which subsequently cause you to behave in an ineffective and unskillful manner. These beliefs were probably contributed to by your parents, teachers, relatives, or friends. Now that you are older and have a greater appreciation for your own needs, you can choose to replace these negative beliefs with positive ones that will serve you better throughout your daily life. Working with affirmations can help encourage this transformation to occur.

For the most part, many of our parents were doing the best they could as they raised us. The statements they made usually came from a place of love and a desire to provide for our well-being. But *you* can do a better job at creating a positive belief system. You know yourself, your abilities, and your desires much better than anyone else. You know what it is you want out of life and what you need to do to get it. *Eliminate the subconscious fears that are holding you back, and many of the obstacles to achieving your goals will disappear.* These deep fears are what prevent many of us from acting decisively in the pursuit of growth.

Affirmations can be used to reprogram the "chatter" of your subconscious from negative and destructive, to positive and life-affirming. The first step is to write out a list of the negative beliefs (fears) that commonly arise to block you from pursuing your goals. These may include statements such as:

- "I am not good enough to succeed in life."
- "I can't heal — it's too much work."
- "I'll never have enough money to satisfy my needs."

These negative beliefs, when played loudly over and over in the subconscious, can have a degenerating effect on the immune system. It is important to first identify these negative beliefs before trying to replace them with positive ones.

The next step is to take each negative belief and write a positive response to it that more accurately describes the belief *that you would like to have in its place*. A few examples follow below:

Old belief: "I am not good enough to succeed in life."
New belief: "I have what it takes to be happy, successful, and fulfilled in my life."

Old belief: "I can't heal — it's too much work."
New belief: "The potential to heal is inherent in every human being. As long as I have life energy, I can heal. I will make changes 1 at a time, and I will be successful with each of them."

Old belief: "I'll never have enough money to satisfy my needs."
New belief: "The universe will provide for all my needs with abundance."

Additional examples include:
Old belief: "I am afraid of becoming sick. I am afraid that my CD4 count will continue to go down."
New belief: "I am a healthy human being, and my healthy emotions and thoughts will manifest a healthy body. I am not defined by my CD4 count."

Old belief:	"I am afraid to express my sexuality. I am afraid that when I feel sexual feelings toward another person that I am being dirty."
New belief:	"It is healthy for me to express my sexuality. Experiencing my sexuality is an expression of the love that is inside of me.

Old belief:	"I am afraid to express my feelings. I fear that they are not worthy or that I will be ridiculed for expressing them."
New belief:	"It is healthy to express the way I feel when I feel it. I can always express my feelings as they arise in a gentle and loving manner. It is healthy for me to express my feelings."

As you can see, the new beliefs are positive, spiritually uplifting statements that directly address the "negativity" of the old belief. Evolving the old belief into a more positive one can help you reprogram your subconscious to feel more deserving of good health and an abundance of love in your life. Positive beliefs can help you manifest a positive reality.

The final step is repetition: repetition, repetition, repetition, and more repetition. This is the way that you learn to integrate positive affirmations. This is the way that you transform and evolve the "negative chatter" of your subconscious. After you have come up with a list of positive beliefs, repeat them over and over again until you know them by heart. Once you know them to this extent, they can begin working for you in wonderfully subtle and transforming ways.

You can practice your affirmations in many ways. You can read them several times a day. You can post them on your mirror so that you see them often. You can record them as part of an affirmations tape and listen to it daily. Be creative. The transforming effect of affirmations occurs best when utilizing all of the above techniques in combination. The more they are repeated, the faster the process of evolving your belief system can occur.

Another helpful technique is to focus on 5 affirmations at a time. Write them out every day. Say them several times to yourself. Each week replace 1 affirmation that you have learned by heart with a new one that you would like to begin integrating. Make the repetition of your affirmations a normal part of your daily routine. It may seem a little like work, but it will pay off.

Although working with affirmations can help you to spiritually transform your everyday life, utilizing them as part of your treatment program for HIV can evoke positive physical outcomes. Gay men, people of color, IV drug users, and many other individuals who make up the HIV(+) community have been told for the majority of their lives that they are not as good or deserving as everyone else; that they are "deficient" in some way. These are not life-affirming beliefs. All who are HIV(+) must strive to believe in themselves as proud, lovable, and profoundly important human beings who can have a positive effect on society.

Another reason to work with affirmations (even if you don't think you need to) is that negative beliefs can be deep-rooted and not available to your conscious awareness. Just as taking vitamins can provide a beneficial insurance policy to help protect you from a nutritional deficiency, working with affirmations can help provide a beneficial insurance policy to help protect you against deep-rooted negative beliefs. It can also assist you in eliminating chronic states of fear, depression, and anxiety.

Intensive affirmation work is most helpful for individuals who are following comprehensive healing programs for HIV and feel fine physically, but are watching a gradual decline in their CD4 cells. It is my belief that this decline can often be traced to fear, panic, and negative beliefs held deeply within the subconscious. This situation responds very well to affirmation work.

Wil Garcia, an inspirational friend and spiritual guide, said that our emotions arise when our beliefs interact with reality. If our beliefs maintain that life is hard and filled with suffering, then those beliefs will interact with reality to produce pain and resentful feelings. On the other hand, if our beliefs incorporate trust, hope, and an exploration of our experiences for knowledge and growth, then these beliefs will interact with our reality to produce feelings of positivity, hope, and joy.

＊

The following is a list of positive, spiritually uplifting statements that you may choose to incorporate within your new system of beliefs:

"I am connected to the power of the universe."

"I breathe in love and light and exhale fear and darkness."

"I am confident and powerful."

"I am at peace with myself."

"I will listen to my body's guidance throughout my healing journey."

"I listen quietly and trust my body to tell me the truth."

"I imagine myself walking in a heavenly garden where I joyfully pick flowers that brighten my soul. The flowers are my teachers, my books, and my guides. The bouquet I make is my own unique spiritual practice."

"I am willing to listen to the whispers of my life."

"I let go of all limiting beliefs and allow fate to unfold moment by moment."

"What I thought were obstacles, I now see as doorways to new possibilities and new beginnings."

"What I saw as blockages, I now see as opportunities for growth."

"I am confident and hopeful."

"I surround myself with confident, nurturing, and loving people."

"I commit to giving all my needs direct and kind attention."

"I trust that the universe will take care of me with love, mercy, and kindness."

"I radiate joy and vibrant health from the deepest core of my being."

"I will create pleasing and beneficial job situations that abundantly provide for my needs."

"I love and approve of myself exactly as I am."

"I have the time, patience, and desire to develop meaningful and joyful relationships."

"I take the time to nurture myself."

"I deserve to be loved and admired by all the people who know me."

"All experiences are provided to me so that I may learn and grow."

"Opening my heart helps to heal my body."

"I am bathing my body with warmth, positivity, and love."

"Whatever is causing me pain and discomfort I will explore fully."

"I will explore my pain with love and openness."

"Sending love toward any situation helps it to heal."

"I give thanks for today. It is complete and unfolds for me in wondrous and miraculous ways."

"I have confidence in myself and in all that I do."

"I surround myself with love, peace, and harmony."

"I trust the universe to provide for all my needs with abundance and love."

"There is a special place within me that is quiet, beautiful, and peaceful. I arrive at this place through quiet time, meditation, and prayer."

"I am comfortable, relaxed, and balanced whenever I am in this place."

"I heal to the greatest extent possible whenever I am in this place."

"I am happy to be exactly who I am."

"I give thanks to life for today."

"I see the magic, the wonder, and the enlightenment in each moment as it unfolds."

"Today is perfect for me."

"I am happiness, gratitude, spontaneity, inspiration, laughter, creativity, prosperity, faith, intuition, love, wisdom, peace, harmony, balance, forgiveness, trust, health, and joy. I am all of these things."

"I love myself fully."

"I am one with all of life. I am safe and comfortable."

"Everything is going to work out just fine."

Faith

To begin the process of true healing, each of us must make the leap of faith described by the French poet Guillaume Apollinaire, who wrote:

> *Come to the edge.*
> *No, we will fall.*
> *Come to the edge.*
> *No, we will fall.*
> *They came to the edge.*
> *He pushed them, and they flew.*

Another quote that I find inspirational in the setting of emotional and spiritual healing comes from the words of a song by Robert Hunter, lyricist for the Grateful Dead, who wrote:

> *Comes a time…*
> *when the blind man takes your hand,*
> *and says: "Don't you see?"*
> *You've got to make it somehow…on*
> *the dreams you still believe.*
> *Don't give it up…you've got an*
> *empty cup.*
> *Only love can fill. Only love can fill.*

Letters to the Virus

When my first book, *Immune Power*, was released, a section that received consistent praise from patients and reviewers alike was "Letters to the Virus." This technique encourages an individual who is struggling with a chronic illness to express emotional energy which otherwise would not find expression. Most of the time, these emotions include anger and fear.

When negative emotions are held inside (repressed), they can be very damaging. They can cause fatigue, depression, and a depressed immune system. Since physical health is clearly linked to emotional health, alleviating emotional distress can produce profound physical benefits.

Letters to HIV: Why Write Them?

Many of my patients have expressed a measure of appreciation that HIV has become a part of their lives. Its presence has helped them to make changes that they have always wanted to make. They eat better, get plenty of rest, meditate, pray, love themselves and others more fully, and express their emotions more often. In many situations, the presence of HIV has motivated them to make the positive changes necessary for healthful growth to occur.

A good diet, exercise, and a minimum of stress can help you stay balanced *physically*. But as many of my patients have discovered, physical treatments are not always enough. It is not enough just to balance and support your physical body. It is not enough just to take your vitamins and medications. It is also crucial to explore your feelings, emotions, and the needs of your heart. Whether this is accomplished through meditation, attending church or synagogue, seeing a therapist, or by practicing some of the techniques described in this section, processing your emotional energy is extremely important. We are all here to open our hearts as much as possible, and to connect with the love that is our true, basic nature. We are all here to grow and to heal.

HIV becomes a part of the DNA of your cells. That is why it is so difficult to eradicate completely. At present, finding ways to keep it completely suppressed is the most effective strategy. Feelings of calm, joy, satisfaction, forgiveness, and self-love help create a peaceful emotional environment that, through the direct action of neurotransmitters and hormones, encourages the immune system to remain strong and participate fully in the suppression of HIV activity.

Writing Your Letters to HIV

When you write a letter to HIV, you are putting down on paper the way you truly feel about your relationship to HIV. It is a conscious expression of your thoughts, feelings, and emotions about your current situation. Nobody knows what will be released until the pen hits the paper and the feelings begin to flow.

The feelings expressed in the letter that HIV writes *back to you* is a reflection of your *subconscious* beliefs about yourself and your situation. If HIV writes to you that it is going to do everything possible to kill you in a short period of time, then that is what *you believe* is going to happen. If it writes that it is providing you with an opportunity to learn, heal, and grow, and that as long as you continue to explore this path it will remain quiescent and dormant, then these are beliefs you hold deep within your subconscious. The goal of this technique is to open a continuing dialogue with your condition. Through this dialogue, a more positive belief system will begin to emerge. A cooperation between you, your body, and your spirit, in the pursuit of healing is the goal. At the very least, expressing deeply felt emotions, and developing a more positive attitude, can help alleviate the immune-depressing effects caused by fear, depression, and chronic anxiety.

Give this exercise a try. Just see what happens. First, take a piece of paper and write a letter "to" the HIV virus. Express all of the thoughts and feelings you have toward it. Stop here until you have completed this part.

Now, notice if you have sent any hate, anger, or intense fear to the virus, and therefore to yourself (since it is within you). If you notice that you have, try to explore your feelings around this. Then, after completing this first letter, write a letter from HIV back to you. How would you feel if you were in its position? If you were forced to live in an environment that was constantly hostile and threatening? Would you want to fight back, possibly to the death, or might some common ground or mutual agreement for coexistence be arranged?

Your body possesses many mechanisms for suppressing chronic viral infections. Chicken pox, Epstein-Barr virus, several strains of herpes, and multiple other viruses are kept fully suppressed for the majority of our adult years. We must do everything we can to enhance these virus-suppressing mechanisms inherent within our own immune systems. Anger and fear are inflammatory emotions that can produce inflammatory physical effects. And chronic inflammation has clearly been shown to stimulate HIV replication.

I know this exercise may sound strange to some of you (especially those who don't live in California!) but give it a try. You are working with your own subconscious beliefs. Whatever this exercise accomplishes, it may help lessen any feelings of hate, panic, and intense fear, all of which have depressing effects on the immune system.

Eventually, try to extend this technique into a dialogue with the virus. You can accomplish this in 1 of 2 ways. You can write a letter to it and then have it write a letter back on a continual basis (such as once every couple of weeks) or you can get a piece of paper and put a line down the middle. Begin a running dialogue, 1 sentence or question from you to the virus on the left and 1 answer or question from the virus back to you on the right, as if you were having a conversation.

The following letters were written by a patient of mine who is regularly practicing this technique. I hope his letters provide you with some insight into the growth-promoting capabilities this technique possesses.

Matt's Letter to the Virus

Virus,

So, I guess we've been together for quite some time. I am afraid of you in many ways. First, that someone will find out about you and hold it against me. Maybe they will hate me or look down upon me. What will they think when they find out you exist inside of me?

Second, will I get so sick I can't take care of myself? Will I look so bad that no one will want to see me? Will I be in a lot of pain?

Third, will I lose everything I own because it costs so much to keep you under control?

I really try hard not to think about you. I just wish you would stay calm and not take over my body. I don't want to share my life with you. All I want is for you to leave me alone. However, for now, I have to live with you as part of me. I ask that you to stay where you are and leave my good cells alone. Please don't knock at the door of doom. I am not sure how I will handle it. Some way I'll get through this. I just need your help to stay away.

Sometimes you make me cry, but only when I'm alone. You have made me hold all my feelings inside — maybe because I feel this way you will not get the better of me.

Sometimes I hear people talk of the good things they've learned since you came into their lives. I would be very happy if you weren't in mine. However, I guess in some ways I look at things differently. I now say what I think, and in some ways I am able to say to myself, "I don't want to look back and say I wish I had. There may not be the time." I will not give up. I just wish you would.

Matt

The Virus's Letter to Matt

Matt,

I am here and I will be for sometime. It's not you that I'm after, I just want to live too. What I do is all I know and if it kills you — that I can't help. I know you are putting up a good fight. I know that you are strong. I want you to stay that way, because I don't want to die either.

I hope we can work together so that we might both have a long life. I'll stay out of your way as long as I can. I just wish you'd stay out of my way!

Nothing personal. You're just the host.

Signed,

V

Matt's CD4 count before he wrote this set of letters was 256 cells/mm3. After he wrote them his CD4 count increased to 324 cells/mm3. There was no change in his antiviral therapy. Did this technique contribute to his improvement, or was it just a coincidence? There is no way to know for sure. It certainly did not hurt. Matt is continuing to pursue his emotional healing utilizing this and other emotional healing techniques.

The next patient has had an extremely difficult time battling HIV. He has taken an extremely aggressive approach starting with AZT monotherapy as soon as it became available in 1988.

During the past 10 years, Bruce has seen his CD4 count progressively drop to 0. Despite now taking a program which includes 7 antiviral medications, his viral load recently tested at over 400,000 copies/ml. Other than a chronic infection with CMV retinitis which is currently stable, his health has otherwise been remarkably good.

Knowing that this patient's pharmaceutical options are severely limited, and that his natural therapies program is as strong as it can be, I asked him to write a letter to his virus to help sort out some of the deep emotional issues arising from his long-term relationship with HIV.

Bruce's Letter to the Virus

Dear Virus,

Although we have been communicating for over 10 years now, this is the first time I have addressed you on paper.

And what a 10-year period we've shared! During this time, partly due to you, my life has changed greatly on so many levels. Most importantly, I am at peace with myself. I have accepted my homosexuality, grown closer to my parents and the friends around me, and become a success at my career.

Not that it has been without a struggle. Growth involves emotional and intellectual maturation and introspection, which thereby encompasses hard work. With respect to my sexuality, I have learned to exchange encounters from the dark, back rooms of the world, into the positive relationships now present in my everyday life; and to celebrate the intimacy that these interactions can offer.

Regarding my parents, both they and I have learned to respect my life in ways that I never thought possible 15 years ago. Respect, laughter, and love truly define our interactions today. And as to not feeling worthy about my career, I was circumspect as to whether I would ever succeed at anything during my twenties. Happily, I have excelled around my great strength of working with people and I am more confident of future successes. I look forward to returning to work in the future as you and I work through some important issues.

Regarding the dark side of the past 10 years, I am frustrated, angry, and tired of fighting you. When we started our mating dance, I had not even considered putting an aspirin in my mouth at the young age of 25. Since that time, I have experienced the necessity of constant pharmaceutical intervention, which only seems to have increased as the years have moved forward. Constant medical intervention including massage, herbs, medications, and surgeries have entered my experience. I am tired of your blind push to increase your numbers regardless to my condition. Remember, without me you cease to exist. I had no idea you were going to be so tenacious in your quest forward.

So, I guess that I am asking for a truce. I know that we are integrated and that we can live together, but I ask that you slow down so that we might coexist a lot longer. The lessons of diet, rest, and spiritual introspection have already increased both my quality of life and chronological moments on the planet Earth, which directly benefits both of us. Let me teach you the beauty of rest and relaxation; you need to not work so hard. Take a break, and in so doing, help me continue to live a good life and grow even more. These things will allow me to spend my energy to become an ever better host for your survival.

Looking forward to your response,

Bruce

The Virus's Letter to Bruce

Dear Bruce,

I am glad that you have taken the time to write to me and to tell me what you are thinking. I have often wondered how you felt about having me in your life. After all, we are joined at a basic molecular level.

It's funny. . . . I had never thought about the fact that, without you, I am nothing.

Virus

Bruce's letter to the virus eloquently expressed many of his thoughts and feelings about the past 10 years. He realizes that many of the experiences he has had during this time have been positive and relate to his continued growth on many levels. However, I do not think he has ever tried, or realized, that he could send a message to the entity that is presently trying to consume him. This is evident in the virus's very brief letter back to Bruce. There isn't a well-developed line of communication. This can, *and needs,* to change.

The virus's letter back in this technique reveals a person's subconscious beliefs regarding their predicament with HIV. In Bruce's case, there is very little belief there. He neither believes that HIV is a death sentence nor a positive stimulus to his growth. In fact, it's my opinion that Bruce is living out his conscious expectations of what being infected with HIV entails. This scenario includes a constant battle with an infection that requires multiple drug interventions plus aggressive alternative therapies. I think it would be very helpful for Bruce to believe that a conscious relationship between the virus and himself is possible, and this might lead to more positive results down the line.

Some 6 weeks after writing this set of letters, Bruce's CD4 count rose from 0 to 16 cells/mm3. Bruce's CD4 count had not risen above 0 for over a year. There were no changes in his medications. His viral load dropped by 66% as well. I will certainly encourage Bruce to continue working with this technique.

Cindy

The Letters to the Virus technique can easily be adapted for use by patients with other chronic medical conditions. Accessing the mind-body connection can provide a powerful tool for improving any healing program. The goal of this technique is to better understand what your mind/body/spirit needs for your healing to occur. It can also help the development of a better relationship between you and your body.

It is not unusual to frequently send anger toward your body if it is causing you difficulty or pain. It is not unusual to feel annoyed and confused. This is not helpful and often can make matters worse. Writing letters to your body can help identify these emotions and create the proper environment for working them through.

At other times, this technique can reveal specific things your body needs from you to heal. Ultimately, writing letters to your body, your condition, your lower back, your immune system, and so forth helps you to look within and find what your body needs for the process of healing to occur.

I recently visited with Cindy, a very nice woman in her mid-fifties who has been struggling with disabling chronic fatigue, migraine headaches, fibromyalgia (muscle pain), and diminished cognitive brain function, including severe memory loss, for the past 8 years. She also has a history of severe alcohol abuse, drinking up to a quart of gin a day between the ages of 17 to 35. Fortunately she has been sober and in Alcoholics Anonymous for the past 20 years.

Cindy had been working with another physician in San Francisco for the previous 10 years. Though her prior physician was caring and sympathetic, she could only prescribe medications to help her. Surgery and medications are the only modalities available to physicians who work within the current paradigm of standard medical care. Cindy's medications included Prednisone (a steroid, immune-depressant, and anti-inflammatory), Plaquenil (an immune-depressant that can cause liver damage), Zoloft (an antidepressant), Doxepin (an antidepressant she used for sleep), Vicodin (a narcotic pain medication), and Imitrex (a migraine headache treatment).

The first recommendation I made was for Cindy to start taking an antioxidant-rich nutritional supplement program that included vitamins, minerals, and immune-supporting herbs. This consisted of about 5 pills 2x/day. Cindy also received body composition testing and nutritional counseling, and was prescribed a low dose of both DHEA and testosterone. I prescribed these hormones to Cindy because her blood levels tested low. Their supplementation was designed to provide her body with the surplus of energy that it needed to begin healing. I also asked Cindy to write a set of "Letters to Her Body" once every 2 weeks.

The underlying basis for many of these treatment recommendations are rooted in the fact that Cindy's body had been through an extraordinary amount of physical and psychological abuse during the years she was drinking. Though she stopped drinking 20 years ago — itself a tremendous accomplishment — Cindy has not provided her body all that it needs to fully heal. She thought that just stopping her drinking would be enough. However, her body is clearly asking for help in a variety of other ways. *Headaches, muscle pains,* and *fatigue* are the only language in which Cindy's body can communicate that it needs additional help.

A month after embarking upon this comprehensive treatment program, Cindy returned to my office for her follow-up visit. She brought with her the following set of letters:

Cindy's Letter to Her Body

Dear Bod:

I am tired of being in pain, of being tense, and of always being hungry. I do not like having a body that feels out of my control. I do not like being able not to trust my energy or strength from one minute to the next. Here it is 1:30 in the morning and I want to be sleeping. But no!!

Why am I awake? All too often my body cannot or will not do what I want it to.

Bod, you have given me way too much worry all of my life. I'm just dragging you around, or you drag me down. Either way, it's a drag being in this body. I am even afraid to feel hopeful about these new efforts I am making. You've *always* let me down. I am going to pray for the willingness to try new ways of relating to you. I am very fearful that I will fail. I have never been able to maintain a healthy approach to you. You've let me down, I've let you down. I hope one day we will become partners in a healthy relationship. How? Through honesty, open-mindedness, and willingness.

Cindy

The Body's Letter to Cindy

Dear Cindy,

Well, this is a which-came-first situation. You don't take care of me, and I don't take care of you. Whoever started all of this doesn't matter. If you want me to be strong, you will need to take care of me, feed me well, exercise me, and listen to me. You cannot just will me into having more energy and no pain. Wishing (even praying) will not work unless you take action. I am tired of you ignoring my needs. And guess what? Even small efforts toward improving my health will produce big results. Pray for willingness. Now turn out the light and go to sleep.

Your Body

P.S. I love you even though you don't love me. I want to be here for you. Ask for help and be ready for guidance.

Cindy's Second Letter to Her Body

Dear Bod,

Well, for 2 weeks I have been in a whirlwind trying to take care of you. Everyday I ask God for willingness to keep up this new regime. Every meal I ask, "What would you want me to eat right now?" I am taking all of my pills, I stopped eating candy, refined sugar, and white flour (at least 98% of the time), and I try to eat only 3 or 4 times a day with at least 4 hours in between.

For exercise, though I am not going for walks, I am gardening, cleaning, and baby-sitting. I am trying to be awake and out of my bed 12 hours out of every 24. But, every 3 or 4 days I crash and sleep during the day. I tell myself to remember that all this is about my immune system and not about diets or morality. I am trying very hard to help you recover. And I am sorry for neglecting you for so long. Pat at the Wellness Center said I was in denial about being ill. I may have been in denial about being ill, but please believe me, I really did believe that if I stayed in bed and kept resting I would get well.

Cindy

The Body's Second Letter to Cindy

Dear Cindy,

Thanks for all of your efforts. I am really feeling more hopeful that you will take care of me. I would like you to get going with the 15-minute walks and maybe some other types of strengthening exercises. That would help me a lot. But please know how much I appreciate your efforts so far. It's a real miracle!

Love,

Your Body

During this relatively brief period of time, the frequency of Cindy's headaches dramatically declined from several per week to only 2 during the month she was writing these letters to her body. She was also able to go off many of her medications, including Prednisone, Plaquenil, and her narcotic pain medication. Furthermore, Cindy's energy level and sense of well-being were clearly on the rise. She has also lost 10 pounds, from 202 down to 192.

Most notably, Cindy no longer gets angry at her body if it feels poorly. She is cultivating a healthier, gentler relationship, one that includes an abundance of love and understanding, instead of frustration, annoyance, and anger. She now writes letters to her body on a regular basis to check in periodically, most especially when she doesn't feel well. Cindy has finally realized that by giving her body the attention, compassion, and gentle loving kindness it needs, she can now fully heal.

When working with the Letters to the Virus technique, it is important to continue your dialogue on an ongoing basis. As time goes on, you may see possible reasons for HIV's presence in your life. You may begin to notice how it can help you improve your diet and the food you put in your body. How it can help you find the courage to get out of a stressful job situation. How it can help you be more present in the moment. If there is anything that might motivate you to heal your life and grow, this can be it!

Closing Thoughts

You are not your body. You are but a being of light that is currently manifesting in physical form.

You are an aware, conscious part of Spirit, God, Jesus, Allah, and the Cosmic Buddha. You are an integral part of the whole of existence.

The universe is continuing to evolve, and you are playing an important part in its evolution.

It takes effort to evolve. It has always been a struggle. It is a struggle to be born, to grow, and to establish yourself in the world. This process moves forward whether we like it or not.

We are all here to learn, grow, give and receive as much love as possible, and contribute in a meaningful way to the dance of universal evolution. We are all part of an evolving universe.

❋

You are exactly where you need to be. You are experiencing exactly what God needs you to experience. The situation you find yourself in can provide you with an opportunity to learn, grow, evolve, and open your heart as much as possible.

Grow toward the Light. The Light is where Spirit is found. Seek it out. Spend time connected to it in prayer, meditation, dance, and joy. Jesus, Allah, Buddha, God, and Unconditional Love are all found in the same place. They exist where that light is shining forth from your heart!

Namasté.

And good luck on your healing journey!!

Appendix One

Common Abbreviations

(in alphabetical order)

AIDS - Acquired immune deficiency syndrome

CAT - Computerized axial tomography (as in CAT scan)

CDC - Centers for Disease Control and Prevention, United States

CMV - Cytomegalovirus (an opportunistic infection)

CSF - Cerebrospinal fluid

DMP-266 - A non-nucleoside reverse transcriptase inhibitor about to be released; also known as efavirenz or Sustiva

1592 - A reverse transcriptase inhibitor about to be released; also known as abacavir or Ziagen

HAART - Highly active antiretroviral therapy

HIV - Human immunodeficiency virus

HMO - Health maintenance organization,

HMO - Health minimizing organization (alternative definition)

IV - Intravenous

LP - Lumbar puncture

MAC - Mycobacterium avium complex (an opportunistic infection)

NNRTI - Non-nucleoside reverse transcriptase inhibitor

OI - Opportunistic infection

PCP - Pneumocystis carinii pneumonia (an opportunistic infection)

PI - Protease inhibitor

RTI - Reverse transcriptase inhibitor

ZI - Zinc finger inhibitor

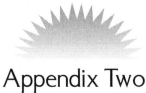

Appendix Two

Important Lab Tests

I f you have recently tested HIV(+), it is important that your initial medical work-up include several laboratory tests. These tests can help determine the current strength of your immune system and your optimal course of action. They include a CD4/CD8 lymphocyte panel, viral load assay, CBC (complete blood count), basic chemistry panel (including cholesterol, triglycerides, blood sugar, and liver function tests), hepatitis serologies, hormone levels, TB test, PAP smear (for women), and comprehensive stool analysis.

These tests can help determine the strength of your immune system, the momentum of the infection, and the presence of any concurrent infections or other complicating factors that you need to address. Several of these tests need to be repeated regularly. The interval is most often determined by the kind of test and your level of health and stability at the time. In our practice for instance, stable HIV(+) patients usually receive follow-up evaluations and routine lab testing on a quarterly basis. If instability is present, you may benefit from more frequent testing.

CD4/CD8 Lymphocyte Cell Panel

The lymphocyte cell panel measures the number of CD4 cells (T-helper cells), CD8 cells (T-suppressor cells), and the ratio of the 2 in the bloodstream. CD4 cells are the type of white blood cell that helps the body fight certain types of infections such as parasites, bacteria, and fungi. They are also the type of cell most commonly destroyed by HIV. CD8 cells help modulate immune system activity. Both of these cells play an important role in helping the body control HIV.

Information provided by the CD4/CD8 panel is analogous to taking a snapshot of the strength of your immune system. At the moment the test is performed, it tells you the current level of strength of this arm of the immune system.

Let us first look at the CD4 cells. The normal range for this lab value, depending on the laboratory, is between 400 and 1200 cells/mm3. If the level is above 300 cells/mm3, most individuals can avoid the occurrence of an opportunistic infection if they are following the recommendations of the Healing HIV program.

Because the number of CD4 cells can vary widely, any 1 test result should always be considered in the context of your previous results. I have sent *identical samples* of blood to the same lab and received test results that varied by over 50 CD4 cells. To minimize these variations, your samples should be analyzed at the same lab and drawn at about the same time of day. It is also important to get your CD4 cell test performed while you are at a stable level of health; not during an acute infection or while on antibiotics.

After looking at an individual's absolute CD4 cell number, the next important part of this panel is the CD4 cell percentage. This value has been shown to vary less from 1 test to another than the CD4 absolute number. It is therefore a more stable indicator of whether a person has improved, declined, or remained stable during any given time period.

The CD8 cell number also helps to measure the strength of your immune system. CD8 cells have been shown to produce an antiviral factor which plays an important role in suppressing HIV activity. A rising CD8 cell number is therefore beneficial but *only* if the CD4 cell percentage and/or absolute number are rising as well.

An example of a difficult-to-interpret scenario is as follows: The absolute CD4 count declines, but the CD4 cell percentage and the absolute

CD8 cell numbers both increase. If the viral load (a measure of viral activity) has not changed, my interpretation of this situation is that this patient has improved slightly or at the very least remained stable.

As you can see, interpreting these lab tests is often difficult and complex. Though I have tried to provide you with helpful guidelines, the results of these tests should always be discussed with an experienced health-care practitioner.

Viral Load Testing

The advent of viral load testing has allowed HIV treatment to move a quantum leap forward. By determining the amount of HIV replication in the blood, we can directly measure the effectiveness of specific antiviral treatments. This test has provided us with an invaluable tool for monitoring HIV disease.

The most sensitive viral load assay available can now measure between 20 and 50 HIV RNA strands (copies) per milliliter of blood. Specifically, it takes 2 HIV RNA strands to make up a single HIV viral particle. Therefore, a viral load assay reporting the detection of 1000 copies of HIV RNA is essentially detecting 500 viral particles. The ability of the viral particles to specifically infect and kill CD4 cells, referred to as the "viral fitness," is an entirely different matter. Researchers have clearly shown that a significant percentage of HIV viral particles in the blood are defective. We would all be well served if there were a test to determine the fitness, or ability to infect and kill CD4 cells, of a patient's HIV infection. Hopefully the availability of this test is not too far off.

The HIV viral load test has also been shown to be a good predictor of the disease's rate of progression. It can therefore be thought of as measuring the "momentum" of the condition. Mellors and colleagues at the University of Pittsburgh Medical School have performed numerous studies which show that the level of viral activity at any point in time has a direct impact on the progression rate to AIDS. Differences arise, however, in the interpretation of exactly what level of HIV activity demands aggressive antiviral therapy. The most important fact to consider is that the viral load test should be interpreted *in the context of a patient's CD4 cell count and level of symptoms.* When viewed as a composite, these 3 parameters allow a thorough assessment of an individual's present status and prognosis. A convenient way to think about these tests is that the CD4 count provides a measure of how strong the immune system is at any given time, whereas the viral load assay measures the potential for the disease to progress in the future.

Different Viral Load Assays

There are 2 types of viral load tests currently available. They are the PCR (polymerase chain reaction) and bDNA (branched chain DNA) tests. The PCR test is produced by Roche Molecular Systems, and the bDNA test is produced by Chiron Diagnostics. Both tests take a sample of blood and, through the wonders of modern technology, calculate the actual number of viral particles present in the sample. When comparing viral load tests in individual patients over time, it is important to compare the same type of test, performed at the same laboratory.

There are pros and cons for using each of the above-mentioned testing methods. As a general rule, the PCR is more sensitive for identifying very low levels of viral replication. The most sensitive PCR test available, known as the ultrasensitive PCR, can detect viral replication down to between 20 and 50 copies of HIV RNA. The most sensitive bDNA test currently available, known as the second-generation bDNA, can detect viral replication down to 500 copies of HIV RNA. Chiron is about to release its third generation bDNA test, which will be able to detect viral activity down to 50 copies of HIV RNA. At the present time, results from these 2 testing methods should not be directly compared to each other.

In my practice, we routinely utilize the second-generation bDNA as our mainstay viral load assay because of its lower potential for variability. We do, however, occasionally order the ultrasensitive PCR when we desire to quantify viral replication down to very low levels. As a general rule, the lower the viral load goes, the longer your current antiviral medications will work before running out of steam.

Viral Load Assays: How to Interpret Them?

It is important to understand that viral load test results must change by a factor of two- to threefold to be considered significant. For example, a viral load test which goes from 20,000 to 30,000 copies/ml does not signify a meaningful change in the level of virus in the blood. There are several reasons for this. First, the viral load level in a given patient varies from day to day. Second, the standard deviation of these lab tests is large. Therefore, changes between onefold and twofold in viral load measurements can still occur when several samples from an identical patient are run at the same lab on the same day.

HIV viral load levels that begin to rise may indicate the development of drug resistance. Remember, "A single test does not a trend make." Wait to see if you viral load is rising upward among several tests before considering a change in your therapy. One of the worst mistakes you can make is to discard an effective antiviral program based on the results of a single elevated viral load test that could have been due to lab error. Not panicking in this situation has enabled a large number of my patients to continue taking their present therapy much longer than they otherwise would have.

Additional factors which may affect a patient's viral load level include stress, malnutrition, immunizations, and the presence of other infections (i.e., sinusitis, herpes, intestinal parasites, and pneumonia). Any of these can adversely affect both the viral load and CD4 cell count. Changes in antiviral medication should never be made until at least 2 viral load levels and CD4 count measurements, taken several weeks apart, show a negative trend in their results.

Recent research has shown that the duration of response to antiviral drug therapy is predicted by the lowest viral load level reached while taking that particular therapy. It is not predicted by the starting viral load, initial CD4 count, magnitude of viral load drop, or magnitude of CD4 cell increase. Therefore, when initiating antiviral therapy, it is very important to get your viral load as low as possible so your therapeutic program will last a long time.

This is especially true if you are beginning triple-combination therapy with a protease inhibitor or NNRTI (non-nucleoside reverse transcriptase inhibitor) medication. If resistance develops to 1 of these drugs, it can possibly compromise your future use of other drugs within these classes. The protease inhibitor and NNRTI medication classes are too valuable to lose to resistance so, when initiating a new antiviral program which contains 1 of these drugs, allow approximately 3 to 6 months to see how low your viral load goes on that program. After 6 months on the same antiviral program, if your viral load has not yet become completely undetectable, it is unlikely that it will go any lower and a change in medications may be warranted to avoid the development of drug resistance.

Genotype and Phenotype Resistance Testing

Antiviral drug resistance is defined as HIV replication which takes place despite the presence of antiviral drug therapy. To develop resistance to a medication, HIV must make changes in its structure called mutations. Some mutations occur randomly and do not confer resistance. Others allow HIV to continue reproducing despite your taking antiviral therapy. These mutations are deemed successful from the virus's point of view. A successful mutant strain grows until it becomes the dominant strain of HIV in an individual. If this strain is effective at killing CD4 cells, the drugs a person is taking become completely ineffective. If the mutant strain is able to replicate, but is somehow compromised in its ability to kill CD4 cells, the drugs you are taking may still retain some value.

There are 2 lab tests which can help determine whether resistance of HIV to the antiviral medications a patient is taking has occurred. "Genotype" testing seeks to determine whether changes to a part of HIV's genetic structure are present. These changes, as mentioned above, are referred to as mutations. Mutations at specific points on the genome (viral genetic map) confer resistance to a specific antiviral drug, and several of these resistance:mutation links have been identified. In genotype testing, the laboratory maps the HIV genome and identifies any resistance-conferring mutations which may be present.

"Phenotypic" testing is a more direct, and possibly more accurate, measure of HIV resistance. Phenotypic testing examines the ability of the predominant HIV strain in the body to grow in the presence of a wide range of antiviral drugs. In its natural state, when HIV is not resistant to a particular drug, predetermined levels of various drugs completely suppress its replication. If HIV is resistant, it requires a higher level of drug to be present before its growth is suppressed. In some cases, HIV's growth is unaffected despite the presence of many drugs. These are the antiviral drugs to which the viral strain is most resistant.

Unfortunately, measuring genotypic or phenotypic resistance is laborious and expensive. Only a few laboratories perform these tests at present. Work is proceeding on increasing the availability and decreasing the cost of these technologies. At the current time, genotypic testing is being offered by Specialty Labs in Santa Monica, California, and costs about $300. Phenotypic testing at present is most easily obtained through a lab in Belgium whose test is called an "antivirogram." The antivirogram provides phenotypic resistance testing for RTIs, NNRTIs, and will soon include protease inhibitors. It costs upwards of $1000 and is currently available at only a few locations. On the West Coast of the United States, it can be obtained through the San Francisco office of Dr. Marcus Conant (415-661-2613). Since these tests are experimental, insurance companies usually do not cover their cost.

CBC (Complete Blood Count)

The CBC measures both red and white blood cell levels. It is a very inexpensive test (average cost, $12). Red blood cells provide oxygen to all of the body's cells. If the red blood cell count is low, you can feel tired and fatigued. This condition is termed *anemia* and can be caused by several factors, which can include nutrient deficiencies such as iron, vitamin B_{12}, and folic acid deficiencies. Taking a multiple-vitamin and a mineral supplement (as recommended in this program) can help prevent these deficiencies from occurring.

Anemia can also be caused by drugs such as AZT, certain antibiotics, and other medications. In addition, it can be caused by infections of the bone marrow (MAC, TB, HIV, etc.) or the "stress" a chronic disease places on this organ of the body.

The presence of anemia may need to be investigated with additional blood tests, including serum vitamin B_{12}, serum folic acid, serum iron, a reticulocyte count, serum ferritin, serum erythropoietin and TIBC (total iron-binding capacity). Your physician should be able to explain the results of these tests to you in a clear and concise manner.

If a nutritional deficiency is identified, it can be easily corrected with vitamin and/or mineral supplementation. Large doses of individual vitamins and minerals are best taken under the guidance of an experienced health-care professional. Anemia not due to a nutritional deficiency can be corrected by other measures, such as changing drugs or taking injections of erythropoietin, a naturally occurring hormone that stimulates red blood cell production. If the red blood cell count drops extremely low, a transfusion may be warranted to quickly increase the number of red blood cells in your bloodstream back to healthful levels.

The white blood cell count measures the number of free-flowing white blood cells, which constitute 1 part of the immune system. CD4 and CD8 cells are included in the white blood cell count. A normal white blood cell count is between 3000 and 10,000 cells/mm3. If your white blood cell count is significantly below 3000, the body's ability to fight off infections is diminished. Therefore, it may be necessary to take antibiotics as soon as possible if a cough or fever occurs in this setting. An *elevated* white blood cell count can signify the presence of an acute infection, usually of bacterial origin. If your white blood cell count is above normal, this warrants a full evaluation by your physician, including a physical exam and possibly additional laboratory tests. Your physician may also recommend antibiotics in this situation.

The same nutritional deficiencies that can cause low red blood cell counts may also contribute to low white blood cell counts (except iron). These include deficiencies of vitamin B_{12} and folic acid which can be identified by different blood tests.

Basic Chemistry Panel

The basic chemistry panel usually includes a collection of 12 to 24 routine blood tests to determine the concentration of specific components of the blood. These include levels of blood sugar, cholesterol, triglycerides, sodium, potassium, chloride, calcium, and a measurement of your liver and kidney functions.

The liver function tests reflect the general health of the liver. If the level of ALT, AST, or GGT enzymes are elevated above normal, the liver is in an inflamed condition. This is termed hepatitis. Hepatitis can be caused by hepatitis viruses (A, B, or C), or by other infections including CMV, MAC, and others. In addition, it can be the result of exposure of the liver to too many toxins such as alcohol, drugs, and excessive doses of natural substances such as vitamins and herbs. If your liver function tests are elevated, drinking alcohol should be completely avoided.

The kidney function tests included in the basic chemistry panel are serum creatinine and BUN. The levels of these 2 substances in the blood are kept constant by the kidneys and rise if the kidneys become weak. This is not a frequent occurrence in HIV disease but may occur due to toxicity from certain drugs (e.g., foscarnet, cidofovir, and adefovir). If this occurs, some medications which are primarily excreted from the body by the kidneys, are best given at lower dosages or at longer dosing intervals. You may want to review the list of medications you are taking with your physician if your kidney function tests begin to rise.

Other Screening Tests

The following tests are also extremely important in the management of HIV disease:

Toxoplasmosis titer

This test detects antibodies which indicate a previous exposure to toxoplasmosis, a parasite found in soil and cat excretions that can cause neurologic impairment in individuals whose immune systems have become extremely weakened (less than 100 CD4 cells). If the test is negative, you have most likely never been exposed to this parasite. If the test comes back positive, you have been exposed, but as long as you are asymptomatic, your immune system is able to suppress the parasite and there is no need for treatment. In rare cases, patients who have tested negative have been found to have the toxoplasmosis parasite when a biopsy was performed. This means that the test may not be 100% accurate in HIV-infected individuals.

Some of the same medications used to prophylax against Pneumocystis carinii pneumonia can also prevent toxoplasmosis. These include trimethoprim-sulfamethoxazole and possibly dapsone.

Regardless of this test result, HIV(+) individuals should avoid changing cat litter or, if necessary, make sure to wear plastic gloves and consider wearing a paper mask to limit your exposure to its airborne particles.

Cryptococcal antigen

This test detects the presence of a fungal infection that can affect the lymphatic and nervous systems and cause an infection known as cryptococcal meningitis. Acute infection usually produces fever, neck stiffness, and headaches. If you test positive for this fungal organism, it indicates an active infection is present. Cryptococcal infections require aggressive antifungal treatment with fluconazole, itraconazole, or amphotericin B.

TB skin test

A TB skin test can allow an individual to determine if they have been exposed to, and are therefore a carrier of, this infection. If this is the case and the immune system becomes weakened, an active case of tuberculosis may emerge. Being HIV(+) increases this risk. Carriers of this infection should therefore receive prophylactic treatment with an oral antibiotic called isoniazid (INH). This medication is usually taken for 9 to 12 months to completely eradicate the infection. Individuals manifesting active tuberculosis, as evidenced by the presence of symptoms and/or chest x-ray abnormalities, require multidrug treatment for a similar period of time.

PAP smears

HIV(+) women should have a PAP smear performed every 6 months. A PAP smear is obtained by twirling a cotton swab or stick to remove cell samples from the cervix. The risk of cervical cell abnormalities (dysplasia) is increased in women with HIV infection. Since dysplastic cells can develop into cancer of the cervix, treatment at an early stage can help prevent its progression.

Routine chest x-ray

A routine chest x-ray should be obtained by anyone who has tested HIV(+). If the chest x-ray is normal, it will establish a baseline film to which future chest x-rays can be compared in the event that respiratory symptoms develop. There are also several lung infections (i.e., tuberculosis, histoplasmosis, coccidiomycosis, etc.) that can exist in a latent phase without producing symptoms, but can be detected on a routine chest x-ray.

Hepatitis serologies

These blood tests can identify if an individual has been exposed to Hepatitis A, B, and/or C. They are best performed early in your care, and you and your current physician should know the results.

Hepatitis A: This virus produces an acute infection that is self-limited. After the initial infection resolves, antibodies provide the affected individual with lifelong immunity. If hepatitis A serologies are negative, there is a vaccine that can provide you with immunity to this disease.

Hepatitis B: This virus can produce subclinical, acute, and/or chronic infections. With additional testing, your physician can determine whether or not a previous hepatitis B infection was limited to the acute setting or has developed into chronic hepatitis. If you have never been exposed to hepatitis B, an immunization exists for it as well.

Hepatitis C: When present, this virus virtually always persists as a chronic, lifelong infection. Its symptoms may include elevated liver function tests, chronic fatigue, gastrointestinal discomfort, discolored urine, and greatly enhanced sensitivity to the toxicity of many drugs. Individuals who are infected with hepatitis C need to be especially nurturing and supportive to their livers. This includes trying to avoid taking large numbers of medications, completely abstaining from alcohol, and having their liver function tests reviewed often. You may also want to review my "Liver Support Program" printed in Appendix 9. There is currently no immunization available to prevent hepatitis C infection.

Comprehensive stool analysis

Maintaining optimal gastrointestinal health is extremely important for an HIV(+) individual to live a long and healthy life. Its level of health also directly impacts your quality of life.

In addition, the ability to tolerate many medications is often dependent on the healthfulness of the GI tract. Many patients I have treated who were previously unable to tolerate certain medication, were later able to take them after the health of their GI tract was strengthened. The most efficient way to identify the healthfulness of your GI tract is by obtaining a comprehensive stool analysis. This test is highly sensitive at identifying intestinal parasites, fungal overgrowth, and bacterial infections. Most private and hospital-based labs are unable to perform this test with the sensitivity and specificity needed to ensure accurate results. These tests must usually be obtained through the mail from a laboratory that specializes in stool analysis testing. Several of these labs are listed in the Resources section. A detailed explanation of how to interpret a comprehensive stool analysis is presented in Chapter 7.

Hormone Levels

Hormones are extremely powerful substances. Though released into the bloodstream in minute quantities, they strongly influence the mood, appetite, sex drive, muscle mass, and energy level of every individual. Though the levels of some hormones need only be checked if symptoms are occurring (e.g., checking thyroid levels if severe fatigue or depression is present), other hormone levels are best monitored routinely in all HIV(+) individuals.

The most important hormone levels to monitor routinely during the treatment of HIV infection are testosterone and DHEA (dehydro-epiandrosterone). These represent the 2 most common hormone deficiencies seen in HIV(+) individuals. Specific ways to monitor and supplement both of these hormones is discussed in Chapter 11.

Appendix Three

Exciting New Treatments

M any HIV(+) individuals have developed some level of resistance to all the currently available antiviral medications. These patients are anxiously awaiting the release of several new classes of antiviral drugs that their viral strain has never been exposed to before. In addition, some novel HIV treatment strategies hold the promise of being more effective, as well as less toxic, than currently available treatments. The purpose of this appendix is to highlight new drugs coming down the research pipeline. Efavirenz (Sustiva), abacavir (Ziagen), and adefovir (Preveon) have already arrived and will most likely be approved for use shortly after the initial publication of this book. They are covered in detail in Chapter 5.

By following the recommendations contained in this book, it is my hope that everyone who is currently HIV(+) can remain healthy and stable until these beneficial new treatments become available, and their benefits can be completely realized.

The Newest Protease Inhibitor

Amprenavir

This is the newest member of the PI class and the closest to being approved by the FDA. Also known as Glaxo-Wellcome 141W94, this drug demonstrates potent antiviral activity against HIV. Preliminary data has been published from 2 studies utilizing a combination of amprenavir and abacavir (Ziagen) 2x/day in the treatment of antiviral-naive patients. In 1 study, this combination was found to reduce plasma HIV viral activity to undetectable levels in 7 out of 7 patients at 16 weeks. The median CD4 cell count increased by 134 cells/mm3 as well. Another study found that the viral load of individuals on this combination was reduced by 99% after 4 weeks of therapy.

A study looking at dual protease combination therapy with amprenavir and either saquinavir, indinavir, or nelfinavir was performed in 14 patients completely naive to protease inhibitors. Preliminary data, after 4 weeks of treatment, found that the median decrease in viral load from baseline ranged from 2.53 to 3.18 log copies/ml (a decrease of approximately 99.9%).

Triple-combination therapy with a twice-daily regimen of AZT/3TC/amprenavir was compared with amprenavir monotherapy in antiviral naive patients. The ethics of designing research studies using monotherapy treatment in HIV patients was hotly debated when this study was presented at the 5th International Conference on Retroviruses in Chicago (1998). As expected, virologic failure occurred much more frequently in the monotherapy arm. There was detectable viral activity in 13 of 46 patients receiving monotherapy compared to 1 of 46 patients receiving the triple combination.

Amprenavir, like other protease inhibitors, is an inhibitor of the cytochrome P450 isoenzyme system (CYP3A4). Comparative studies with other protease inhibitors found that the rank order of inhibition of the P450 CYP3A4 isoenzyme was ritonovir > indinavir = nelfinavir = amprenavir > saquinavir. Inhibition of this enzyme system is probably responsible for the majority of side effects attributed to the protease inhibitor class as a whole.

In vitro data has shown that cross-resistance between amprenavir and other protease inhibitors is variable. Mutations associated with increased resistance to amprenavir resulted in decreased resistance to saquinavir and indinavir. HIV viral strains with 2 mutations to amprenavir showed decreased resistance to nelfinavir while those with triple-point mutations (46, 47, and 50) showed increased resistance to nelfinavir. All amprenavir mutant variants were less sensitive to ritonovir. The clinical significance of this data has yet to be established.

Side effects: Side effects reported in association with amprenavir administration during early investigational studies include headache, fatigue, nausea, vomiting, diarrhea, oral numbness, and rash. Laboratory abnormalities include transient mild-to-moderate increases in triglyceride levels and other metabolic parameters. Skin rashes were reported in 18% of the patients receiving amprenavir at all doses during investigational studies. They usually presented as a mild rash that appeared within 7 to 12 days after beginning therapy. Serious cutaneous adverse events were reported in 3% of patients. From preliminary safety reports, no recurrence of rash has been observed in patients rechallenged with amprenavir.

Comments: Amprenavir appears to be an additional member of the first generation of protease inhibitor antiviral medications. Its ability be taken 2x/day with or without food greatly enhances its convenience. Though it appears to be a potent antiviral at present, it has not been compared head-to-head with any other protease inhibitor for efficacy at this time. Its long-term tolerability when taken by large numbers of patients also remains to be established.

With that said, the emergence of any potent new antiviral medication should give patients with multidrug-resistant HIV another useful drug to try. To obtain a maximal effect, this medication should be taken simultaneously with 1 or 2 additional new antiviral drugs.

Second-Generation Protease Inhibitors
ABT-378
- Second-generation protease inhibitor.
- Potent against ritonavir-resistant isolates.
- More potent than ritonavir against wild-type HIV strains.
- Administered with low-dose ritonavir to enable 2x/day dosing.
- Currently entering phase lll clinical trials.

PN 140690E (tipranavir)

- Substantial activity has been shown against HIV strains resistant to the other PIs.
- Given 3x/day at present.
- Entering phase ll clinical trials.

BMS 232632

- Potent in vitro activity against HIV.
- Substantial activity has been shown against HIV strains resistant to the other PIs.
- Presently in phase l clinical trials.

DMP-450

- A new class of protease inhibitor known as a cyclic urea compound.
- Excellent oral bioavailability.
- Bypasses the cytochrome P450 pathway for metabolism.
- May therefore help avoid many commonly seen drug interactions and side effects.

New NNRTI Medications

Carboxanilide analogues

- NNRTI with a very long half-life.
- Currently requires intravenous administration.

Calanolide A analogues

- Currently in early phase I clinical trials.

PNU 242721

- Thiopyrimidine compound.
- Once-daily dosing.
- Low protein-binding characteristics.

New RTIs

FTC

- Similar to 3TC, but flourinated, thereby providing greater potency.
- Phase l and ll trials showing good results.
- Moving into phase lll clinical trials soon.

F-DDA

- Similar to DDI but with better penetration into cells and a longer half-life.
- More potent than AZT in animal studies.
- Currently in phase I clinical trials.

BCH-10652

- In vitro activity has been shown against HIV strains resistant to other RTIs.
- Good CNS penetration; resistance is slow to develop.
- Excellent preliminary safety data in animal and phase l studies.

PMPA

- Once-daily dosing; similar in mechanism of action to adefovir (Preveon).
- Favorable resistance profile, substantial anti-HIV activity.
- May possess kidney toxicity similar to adefovir.

New Classes of Antiviral Drugs

Cytokine inhibitors

- Inhibit HIV's entry into cells by blocking the interaction of the viral envelope protein gp120 with host cell membrane proteins CCR5 and CXCR4.
- These host membrane proteins probably have other important functions, so blocking them with a drug may produce significant toxicity.
- None of these agents has entered clinical trials to date.

Fusion inhibitors

- Show greater promise than cytokine inhibitors.
- Bind with HIV envelope protein gp41.
- The gp41 "fusion domain" is essential for binding of the virus to the host cell.
- A small preliminary study with the compound T-20 (pentafuside) showed encouraging results in patients with HIV.
- At present this compound needs to be delivered intravenously.
- Other fusion inhibitors entering phase 1 clinical trials include FP-21399 (Fuji ImmunoPharmaceuticals) and ISIS 5320 (ISIS Pharmaceuticals).

Integrase inhibitors

- Inhibit viral replication by blocking the integration of viral DNA into host DNA.
- Most promising compound currently being studied is AR-177.
- Presently in phase 1/11 clinical trials.
- Presently needs to be given intravenously.

Zinc finger inhibitors

- Captures viral genetic material and prevents it from producing new viral particles.
- Most promising compounds currently being studied are C-1012 and ADA.
- Currently in phase 1 clinical trials.

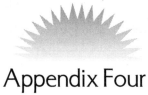

Appendix Four

Prophylaxis Recommendations

Opportunistic infections are the major cause of morbidity and mortality due to HIV. By regularly monitoring your CD4 count, you can determine when it is most appropriate to begin taking prophylactic medications which can help prevent these infections. By constructing an intelligent prophylaxis program, you can continue to remain healthy and free from these infections despite low CD4 counts.

The ideal prophylaxis program prevents opportunistic infections and is well tolerated over an extended period of time. Ideally, it is also acceptable to the patient, cost-effective, and, when possible, utilizes drugs that have activity against more than one kind of infection.

The best prophylaxis protocol is also linked to a strong antiviral strategy directed at suppressing the primary HIV infection. A strategy based solely on preventing opportunistic infections is ultimately doomed to fail, as the success of every prophylaxis regimen depends to a great extent on the overall strength of the immune system.

Recommendations for Opportunistic Infection Prophylaxis

CD4 Count	Infection	Prophylaxis
Any CD4 count	Prior genital herpes *or* shingles infection	Acyclovir 400 mg 2x/day Valacyclovir 500 mg 1x/day
Less than 200	PCP	TMP-SMX* 1 double-strength tab 3x/week *or* Dapsone 100 mg 1x/day
Less than 50	PCP	TMP-SMX 1 double-strength tab 1x/day *or* Dapsone 100 mg 1x/day.

(If using Dapsone with less than 50 CD4 cells, I recommend adding an aerosol pentamadine treatment once a month to make up for its weaker PCP protection)

Less than 50	Toxoplasmosis	TMP-SMX 1 double-strength tab 1x/day *or* Dapsone 100 mg 1x/day
	MAC	Azithromycin 1200 mg 1x/week *or* Clarithromycin 500 mg 3x/week
	Fungal	Fluconazole 100 mg 3x/week
	CMV	No prophylaxis recommended at the present time

* TMP-SMX stands for trimethoprim-sulfamethoxazole (a.k.a. Bactrim or Septra).

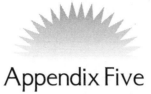

Appendix Five

Immunization Recommendations

The important decision of whether to immunize an HIV(+) individual is best treated on an individual basis. If you are HIV(+) with a CD4 count above 300 cells/mm3 and have viral activity that is suppressed to an undetectable level by antiviral medications, most immunizations are safe and effective.

If you are not on highly active antiviral therapy (HAART), immunizations may transiently increase viral activity on the order of threefold to fourfold. Although this effect is often short-lived, it can potentially lead to a drop in your CD4 cell count which may last for several months.

I list here the immunizations which are recommended to HIV(+) patients by the United States Public Health Service Working Group followed by my own comments.

Pneumococcal Vaccine

Although the efficacy of this vaccine is not well established in HIV(+) patients, the pneumococcal vaccine has been routinely administered for over a decade. The reason for this recommendation is correlated with the higher incidence of pneumococcal pneumonia seen in HIV(+)

individuals when compared to the general population.

My experience has been dramatically different. In the past 10 years of treating upwards of a thousand HIV(+) individuals, I have only had 1 patient develop a pneumococcal infection despite not routinely giving my patients the vaccine. I attribute this to the enhanced immune function of the individuals who follow my program. I believe the benefits associated with vitamin supplementation, acupuncture, stress reduction, regular exercise, and a healthy lifestyle to be responsible for my vastly different experience. My recommendations for individuals *not* following my program would be to get the vaccine. The vaccine is given as a single dose (0.5 cc IM), and revaccination should be considered every 6 years.

Influenza (Flu) Vaccine

An annual influenza vaccine is recommended for HIV(+) individuals by most physicians. It is given as a single dose, usually in October or November. This vaccine is administered to prevent influenza and its potential complications, and to prevent syndromes that may mimic opportunistic infections. Although research data are conflicting, there is evidence that influenza vaccination may lead to a temporary rise in viral load. Thus, the potential risk of increased viral replication may outweigh the benefits of the vaccine, especially in patients who are not on highly active antiretroviral therapy (HAART) or who are experiencing viral activity secondary to multidrug resistance. In addition, the immunologic response to this vaccine is low in individuals with CD4 counts less than 200 cells/mm3.

Since the first study showing the potential for increased viral activity was performed by Follansbee and colleagues at the San Francisco Consortium, I have recommended that HIV(+) patients consider not receiving the influenza vaccine. I support this recommendation based on the fact that the Healing HIV program is designed to enhance the body's ability to fight viral infections, including influenza. I prefer to place my confidence in the immune-enhancing benefits of this program rather than to risk iatrogenically (physician-caused) increased viral loads and the negative effects they may produce.

In contrast, patients with high CD4 counts on effective antiviral therapy may benefit from vaccination due to the low risk of stimulating rises in viral load when your viral load is fully suppressed by medication. The decision with regard to this vaccination is best made on an individual basis in collaboration with your primary care provider.

Hepatitis Vaccines

Although the administration of any vaccination has the potential of causing a transient rise in HIV viral activity, the benefits associated with each specific vaccination need to be weighed against the risks from the illness you are vaccinating against. While a short bout of influenza does not pose a tremendous risk to most people, HIV(+) individuals who become infected with hepatitis B are more likely to develop chronic hepatitis B infection. Chronic hepatitis B infection places a significant burden on the liver, an organ that may already be overworked due to medication side effects and infection with HIV itself.

Individuals without prior exposure to hepatitis B may benefit from the hepatitis B vaccine if they are at continued risk of infection. Hepatitis B is usually contracted through sexual transmission or exposure to bodily fluids. Hepatitis B vaccine is recommended to health-care workers, HIV(+) injection drug users, sexually active gay men, prostitutes, sexually active heterosexual men and women with a sexually transmitted disease history (including HIV), and household or sexual contacts of hepatitis B infection carriers. Recipients should first be screened for prior infection with a blood test. The vaccine is given in a series of 3 injections at 0, 1, and 6 months. The hepatitis B vaccine is a genetically engineered, inactive virus vaccine.

Hepatitis A is transmitted by fecal-oral transmission. This means that infectious particles can be passed from person to person in food, water, or from oral-anal contact. Hepatitis A causes similar initial symptoms as hepatitis B, however it almost never progresses to a chronic infection. Those at risk include individuals traveling to endemically infected areas, sexually active gay men, injection drug users, or those exposed to a community outbreak. These individuals should consider becoming vaccinated. The hepatitis A vaccine is given in a series of 2 injections at 0 and 6 months.

Hepatitis C is most often acquired through IV drug use, sexual contact, or through blood transfusions. It frequently persists in the body to become a chronic, lifelong infection. Coinfection with HIV and Hepatitis C requires special attention to nurture and support your liver. At present, there is no effective vaccine for hepatitis C.

Tetanus-Diphtheria Vaccine

Recommendations for the tetanus-diphtheria (dT) vaccine in HIV(+) individuals are the same as those for immunocompetent adults. A single booster is given every 10 years for adults who have completed the primary series. HIV(+) individuals should continue this vaccination schedule.

Vaccinations for International Travel

The inactivated typhoid vaccine can be used in place of the live oral vaccine when traveling to an endemically infected area. Hepatitis A vaccine is recommended when traveling to developing countries. Japanese B encephalitis vaccine, inactivated polio vaccine, and hepatitis B vaccine can also be given safely when indicated. Cholera vaccine has poor efficacy and is no longer recommended for travel to any country. Yellow fever vaccine is never indicated for individuals with HIV.

Important: Attenuated live virus or live bacteria vaccines, with the exception of the measles-mumps-rubella (MMR), should not be given to HIV-infected individuals. Although it is a live-virus vaccine, the measles-mumps-rubella (MMR) is considered safe for HIV-infected patients and the indications for administering it are the same as in immunocompetent adults. All other live vaccines are contraindicated, including BCG, oral polio vaccine, oral typhoid vaccine, varicella-zoster vaccine (chicken pox), and yellow fever vaccine. If polio vaccination is indicated for HIV(+) individuals or their household contacts, the enhanced potency, inactivated vaccine (eIPV) should be used.

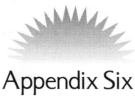

Appendix Six

Overview on Women and HIV

No book on the comprehensive treatment of HIV would be complete without mentioning the differences between men and women. For the most part, the Healing HIV program treats the needs of men and women similarly. That is, the goal of the treatment program is to support an HIV(+) individual's immune system so it is able to suppress HIV activity with as little need as possible for drugs. However, if medications are necessary, they will be more effective, work longer, and have less adverse side effects, if the body is well supported in many natural ways. That said, there are still a few very important differences to mention.

Men and women are not the same: In general, women are more sensitive than men. This is sometimes true emotionally, and it is usually true physically. Women's bodies often don't tolerate strong medications as well as, or for as long as, men's bodies. Hence, when possible, many medications are best given in somewhat gentler dosages to women than to men. These include drugs such as antibiotics, antidepressants, and occasionally antivirals. Always check with your physician before making any changes in the dosages of your current treatment program.

Another important fact is that most women weigh less than men. Giving a standard dosage of medication to a 110-pound women will produce a higher blood level than to a 180-pound man. This can increase the risk of side effects in women as well.

A woman's anatomy is different than a man's: Women who are HIV(+) should see their gynecologist twice a year. The vagina, cervix, and uterus can all develop abnormalities due to an impaired immune system. Possibilities include the occurrence of vaginal candidiasis (yeast infections), pelvic inflammatory disease (PID), sexually transmitted diseases (herpes, syphilis, chlamydia), condylomata (genital warts), and cervical cancer. Because the detection of these conditions can be difficult, 2 semiannual visits with your gynecologist, which include a Pap smear, are essential to the optimal treatment of an HIV(+) woman.

Women need to be especially nurturing to their bodies: Due to their lower testosterone levels and other biologic differences, such as less muscle mass, women are not usually as physically strong as their male counterparts. A healthy diet, adequate rest, regular exercise, massage, meditation, prayer, and stress reduction are extremely important for a woman's body to healthfully coexist with HIV for a long and healthy lifetime.

If you are an HIV(+) woman, honor your womanhood and femininity. Make sure to keep your stress as low as possible. Work to find a nurturing job, relationship, and support system. Consider joining (or starting) an HIV(+) women's support group. Strive to create a safe harbor for yourself and your life. Give your heart, your body, and your soul the opportunity to grow and flourish in a supportive and nurturing environment, and you will be happy and thrive. Putting these suggestions into practice can enable you to maintain the long-term balance and stability that is essential for excellent and long-lived good health.

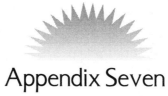

Appendix Seven

Antiviral Drug History Form

Drug Combination	Dates	Side Effects	Level of Resistance*

* None, Low, Moderate, or High

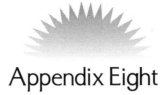

Appendix Eight

Intestinal Health Score

1) How's my appetite?

_____ Good [1]　　　_____ Medium [2]　　_____ Poor [3]

2) What is my weight compared to one year ago?

_____ Higher [1]　　　_____ Same [2]　　　_____ Lower [3]

3) How many bowel movements do I have a day (on average)

_____ Greater than 5 [3]　_____ 3 – 5 [2]　　　_____ Less than 3 [1]

4) What is their most common appearance?

_____ Watery diarrhea [4]　　_____ Loose and unformed [3]

_____ Soft and pasty [2]　　　_____ Well formed [1]

5) Are any of the following symptoms present most of the time?

_____ Heartburn [2]　_____ Gas/gurgling [2]　_____ Nausea [2]

_____ Bloating [2]　　_____ Smelly gas [2]　　_____ None [0]

6) What is my "TP" index (how many pieces of toilet paper do I usually have to tear off before I am completely clean)?

_____ Greater than 5 [3]　　　_____ 3 – 5 [2]　_____ Less than 3 [1]

To find out the general health of your gastrointestinal system, add up the small numbers next to your answers and refer to the scoring key below:

5-10 = Excellent health

10-15 = Intermediate health

Greater than 15 = Unhealthy

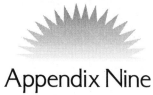

Appendix Nine

Integrative Medicine Protocols

A) Chronic Viral Infection: Nutritional Supplement Recommendations
B) Liver Support Program
C) Dr. Kaiser's Intestinal Parasite Elimination Program
D) Prevention and Natural Treatment of Sinus Infections

A) Chronic Viral Infection Nutritional Supplement Recommedations

AM: High-potency multiple vitamin . . . . . . 1 tab   (with breakfast)
High-potency multiple mineral . . . . . . 1 tab   "
Vitamin C 1000 mg . . . . 2 caps   "
Vitamin E 400 iu . . . . 1 cap   "
Vitamin B₆ 100 mg . . . . 1 cap   "
Coenzyme Q-10 30 mg . . . . 1 cap   "
N-acetyl cysteine 500 mg . . . . 1 cap   "
Acidophilus . . . . 1 cap   "

PM: High-potency multiple vitamin . . . . . . 1 tab   (with dinner)
High-potency multiple mineral . . . . . . 1 tab
Vitamin C 1000 mg . . . . 2 caps   "
Vitamin E 400 iu . . . . 1 cap   "
Vitamin B₆ 100 mg . . . . 1 cap   "
Coenzyme Q-10 30 mg . . . . 1 cap   "
N-acetyl cysteine 500 mg . . . . 1 cap   "
Acidophilus . . . . 1 cap   "

B) Liver Support Program

1) **Absolutely no alcohol!**
2) Flush your system with **8 glasses of water a day.**
3) Daily fresh-squeezed **vegetable juices and steamed vegetables.**
4) **Lipotropic complex** (Tyler Encapsulations, 800-869-9705): 3 caps, 2-3x/day between meals.
5) **Ganoderma and Reishi mushroom capsules** (check your local health food store): 3 caps, 2-3x/day between meals.
6) **Daily fiber supplement** (psyllium seed husks, oat bran, etc., available in health food stores): 2 tablespoons in juice 2x/day.
7) **Castor oil packs:** Spread a thin layer of castor oil on a piece of clean white cotton flannel or tee shirt, place it on the abdomen over the liver and gallbladder area, cover with either a hot water bottle or heating pad, and lie flat for 30 minutes. Do this at least once a day. Very effective for decreasing liver inflammation, improving jaundice, decreasing pain, and drawing toxins out of the abdominal organs.

C) Dr. Kaiser's Intestinal Parasite Elimination Program

Extremely effective against Blastocystis hominis, Endolimax nana, Iodamoeba butschlii, Entamoeba histolytica and Entamoeba coli.

	Frequency	Duration
1) **Paromomycin (Humatin)***		
2 capsules	3x/day	10 – 14 days
250 mg capsules *and/or*		
Iodoquinol (Yodoxin)*		
1 capsule	3x/day	10 – 20 days
650 mg capsules		
2) **Psyllium seed husks**		
2 teaspoons	3x/day	10 – 14 days
Add to water or juice		
3) **Black walnut tincture**		
2 droppersful	3x/day	10 – 14 days
Add to water or juice		

*Paromomycin and iodoquinol are prescription medications that are very effective and better tolerated than the more commonly prescribed metronidazole (Flagyl). If 2 or more parasites are present, which is frequently the case, I usually recommend taking both paromomycin and iodoquinol concurrently for at least 10 days, then continuing iodoquinol alone for an additional 10 days.

Add #2 & #3 to water or juice, and take together with #1 on an empty stomach (one-half hour before or 2 hours after meals). All of the above must be taken together for maximum efficacy. It is essential that this program only be taken under medical supervision.

D) Prevention and Natural Treatment of Sinus Infections

1) **Physical-therapy hot packs:** Neck muscle tension blocks the natural flow of energy and drainage of lymph fluid from the head to the rest of the body, causing sinus congestion and headaches. Massage, hot towels, and physical-therapy hot packs applied to the neck 3 times per week can provide therapeutic benefit.

2) **Immuplex lozenges** (Tyler Encapsulations , 800-869-9705): This is an impressive lozenge formulation containing astragalus root, zinc, echinacea, vitamin C, slippery elm, and licorice. Dissolve 1 in mouth 4 to 8 times a day.

3) **Zand herbal mist** (McZand Herbs, Santa Monica, CA): Another impressive herbal formulation. Contains echinacea, goldenseal, licorice, isatis root, and hyssop. Strengthens the upper respiratory mucosal barrier against viral, bacterial, and fungal infections. Use 3 sprays, 3–5x/day as needed.

4) **Tea tree oil:** Add five drops of tea tree oil to one-third glass water. Gargle, *spit out,* and then swallow the residue 2 to 3 times per day. Tea tree oil is a natural antibiotic, antifungal, and antiviral.

5) **Garlic:** Garlic is a very potent natural antibiotic, antiviral, and antifungal substance. Spread a minced clove of fresh garlic on buttered toast 1–2x/day or take 2 capsules, 2–3x/day.

6) **Licorice root tincture:** Take 2–3 droppersful of tincture dissolved in 1 oz of water 4x/day. Excellent for increasing energy and supporting adrenal gland function, which in turn helps boost immune function.

A combination of the above treatments may be utilized to treat chronic sinusitis, chronic bronchitis, and sore throats. They can be used in a preventive fashion as well.

Appendix Ten

Meditation on Taking Medicine Within

(To be read slowly to a friend or silently to oneself)

Sitting comfortably in a chair, or lying easily in bed, pick up the medicine container or bottle and just feel it in your hand. Feel its shape, its denseness, its texture, its quality of coldness or warmth.

Let your hand make contact; feel the sensations generated there.

Let your fingers open the container with awareness. Notice any strain or urgency and soften all about it.

Feel the pills, as they drop into the palm of your hand. Take a deep breath.

Take a moment to look at the pills.

Take a moment to notice if you regard the pills wholeheartedly as a medium for healing, or if there is a measure of shame or failure that accompanies taking them. Focusing on the healing quality inherent within the medication, look on the medicine for its healing potential.

Let the body open to receive the healing within.

Sense the treatment's potential to enter fully into any areas of discomfort, its power to bring equanimity and balance to your situation.

See the pills there in your hand. Feel their weight against the sensitive nerve endings in your palm.

Listen to the medicine. Does it have something to say? What is its tone of voice? Is there any sense of helplessness in your relationship to the medicine? Just notice it.

Meet with mercy and awareness any resistance you may have previously ingested along with your treatments. Look on these treatments with loving kindness and gratitude.

Thank the pills for whatever healing they may have to offer and place them gently in your mouth.

Feel them on your tongue, feel the liquid taken to swallow them entering across the lips. Feel the tongue moving the pills into position to be swallowed. Feel the swallowing. Let the pills be drawn past the heart and into the stomach.

Sense the movement of the pills down your esophagus, gently received by the body. Feel the medications settling into your stomach, radiating like soft golden light. Feel the medication conveyed into the place of greatest need.

With loving kindness, direct its healing quality to the area of greatest need. Feel the area absorb the healing.

Let it in.

Receive the medication as a blessing.

Find an image which opens you to the healing in your medication. See it as a gift from a great teacher, as a sacred communion between the outer and inner worlds, as a balancing force, or as a smile of unbearable compassion.

Let the healing in without resistance. Absorb it.

Allow loving kindness to combine with the treatment and direct it into the area which calls for healing.

Allow the medication to be drawn in, mercy and awareness binding to each molecule sent wholeheartedly into the cause of suffering.

Feel the medication dissolving the resistance of a lifetime, dispelling the tension and difficulty felt around the illness.

Feel it enter directly. Feel it melting the injury and illness away.

Let the medication help heal and make you whole again.

✳

The above meditation was written by Stephen Levine, a noted healer and meditation teacher. It can be found in his excellent book *Healing Into Life and Death* (Anchor Doubleday Books, 1987). Used by permission.

✳

It is extremely important not to be angry if you need to take medication. It is wiser to cultivate gratitude that the medication exists for your benefit. It is also wise to learn that the need to take medication does not represent a failure to heal in other ways. The best healing program makes use of all that is available, without judgment on the merits of what is bringing forth that healing.

Does it feel strange to utter a meditation each time you take medicine? Why? It is important to utilize everything your mind can offer in your attempt to heal. After the first few times, you may only need to say a few significant words of gratitude to remind yourself that the mind can play an ongoing role in your healing process.

In Eastern cultures, it is very common for words of prayer or chanting to be uttered with each dose of medication. This process helps tap into the mind-body connection, using awareness to enhance the body's healing potential. In Tibet, medication is often placed *upon the temple altar for up to 2 years* before it is administered to patients with serious illness. It would be helpful to appreciate the healing potential this practice holds. Visualizing the medicine working within your body can help facilitate its healing effects and eliminate any unconscious resistance that you may hold toward it.

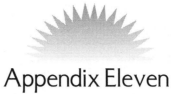

Appendix Eleven

Resources Section

Comprehensive Stool Analysis Laboratories

Great Smokies Diagnostic Laboratory 800-522-4762

Diagnost-Techs 800-87-TESTS

Institute of Parasitic Diseases 602-955-4211

Please refer to Chapter 7 for specific information on what tests may be useful in treating HIV. My advice is to call each lab and find the one that best meets your needs for cost, availability, and access.

Cookbooks

Positive Cooking: Cooking for People Living with HIV – by Lisa Mcmillan, Jill Jarvie, and Janet Brauer – 1997, Avery Publishing Group, Garden City Park, NY (ISBN 0-89529-734-5)

Cooking For Life: A Guide to Nutrition and Food Safety for the HIV(+) Community – by Robert Lehmann – 1997, Dell Publishing, New York (ISBN 0-44050-759-7)

Positive Nutrition for HIV and AIDS – by Stacy Bell and R. Armour Forse 1996, Chronimed Publishing, Minneapolis, MN (ISBN 1-56561-089-X)

Eating Positive: A Nutritional Guide and Recipe Book for People With HIV/AIDS – by Jeffrey Huber and Kris Riddlesperger – 1998, Harrington Park Press, Binghamton, NY (ISBN 1-56023-893-3)

Legal Advice

HIV Law (Three Rivers Press, 1997) is a book by Paul Hampton Crocket, an attorney and a person living with HIV. *HIV Law* presents practical solutions to the most important challenges posed by a complicated legal system and government bureaucracies. Mr. Crocket practices law in Miami Beach, Florida, and specializes in HIV-related issues. His book provides a valuable resource for those dealing with the legal issues that living with HIV can produce.

Hotlines

AIDS Clinical Trials Information 800-TRIALS-A
CDC National AIDS Hotline 800-342-AIDS
CDC National AIDS Hotline, Spanish 800-344-SIDA
CDC National AIDS Information Clearing House 800-458-5231
National Native American AIDS Hotline 800-283-AIDS
National Teens AIDS Hotline 800-234-TEEN
Project Inform's Hotline. 800-822-7422

Regional Buyers Clubs

New York: DAAIR, Direct AIDS Alternative Information Resources,
31 East 30th Street, Suite 2A, New York, NY 10016
Phone (toll free outside of NY): 888-951-5433
Phone (inside NY): 212-689-6471
E-mail: info@daair.org
Website: www.immunet.org/daair

California: Healing Alternatives Buyers Club
1748 Market Street, #204, San Francisco, CA 94102
Phone: 800-219-2233/415-626-4053

Embrace Life Nutritional Supplements
2070C Wharf Rd.
Capitola, CA 95010
Phone: 800-448-1170

Internet Websites

To find out more about Dr. Jon Kaiser's events and projects (lecture schedule, Wellness Center address, phone consults, etc.): www.jonkaiser.com

Legal

HIV InfoWeb legal information & resources: www.jri.org/infoweb/legal/
AIDS Law Updates: www.thebody.com/hanssens/updates.html

Health Options

HIV InSite: hivinsite.ucsf.edu
   Provides comprehensive, accurate and current information on HIV disease from one of the country's leading health science institutions.
Project Inform On Line: www.projinf.org
   Information clearinghouse on state of the art treatments for HIV/AIDS.
San Francisco AIDS Foundation: www.sfaf.org/beta.html
   Monthly bulletin of experimental treatments for AIDS (BETA).

Miscellaneous Health-Related

www.medscape.com
www.healthcg.com
www.actis.org/aidsabs
www.retroconference.org
www.aegis.com/areas
www.ncbi.nlm.nih.gov/pubmed/
(PubMed is now the predominant means of accessing Medline.)
Office of Alternative Medicine, National Institutes of Health – altmed.od.nih.gov
Alternative Medicine Digest – www.alternativemedicine.com
Ask Dr. Weil – www.hotwire.com/drweil
Natural Health Village – www.naturalhealthvillage.com
   One of the most popular advice sites for integrative medicine.
HealthWorld On-line – www.healthy.net/index.html

Alternative Medicine Connection – arxc.com/arxchome.htm
Websites offering information on clinics, practitioners, and referrals.
Alternative Health Search Resource – www.althealthsearch.com

Advocacy Groups
Gay Men's Health Crisis (GMHC) – www.gmhc.org
National Association of People with AIDS – www.thecure.org/
National Native American AIDS Prevention Center – www.nnaapc.org/

Pharmaceutical Companies
www.merck.com
www.crixivan.com
www.agouron.com
www.roche.com
www.fortovase.com
www.abbott.com/health/hivinfection,htm
www.ext.amgen.com/cgi-bin/genobject
www.bms.com/indexpage.htm
www.chiron.com
www.dupontmerck.com
www.gilead.com
www.glaxowellcome.co.uk/home.html
www.nexstar.com
www.pharmacia.se.home.html
www.roche.com
hiv.roxane.com
www.tripharm.com
www.vpharm.com

Miscellaneous
POZ Magazine – www.poz.com
CDC National AIDS Clearinghouse Web Server – www.cdcnac.org
FDA HIV/AIDS Page – www.fda.gov/oashi/aids/hiv.html
Index of AIDS Links – www.critpath.org/aric/pwarg/links.htm

Association of Nurses in AIDS Care – www.podi.com/aids/
International AIDS Vaccine Initiative – www.iavi.org
Safer Sex Page – www.safersex.org
Travel Health On-line – www.tripprep.com/index.html

Clinical Trials

AIDS Clinical Trials Information Service – www.actis.org
AIDS Clinical Trials Research Database – www.actis.org/database.html
Australia National Center for HIV Research – www.hiv.edu.au
Canadian HIV Trials Network – www.hivnet.ubc.ca/ctn.html
CenterWatch Clinical Trials Listing Service – www.centerwatch.com
Community Programs for Clinical Research on AIDS – www.cpcra.org
Trials Database at U.C. San Francisco – sfghaids,ucsf,edu/ucsfresearch.html

Conference Reports

Geneva World AIDS Conferencs – www.aids98.ch
Hamberg Conference October 1997 – www.euro-aids97.com
NATAP Conference Reports – www.natap.org
Oxidative Stress and Redox Regulation – www.immunet.org/redoxabs/

International

AVERT AIDS Education and Research Trust (England) – www.avert.org
British Columbia Persons with AIDS society (Canada) –
     www.bcpwa.org/bcpwa.htm
British Medical Association Foundation for AIDS (England) –
     www.bmaids.demon.co.uk/
United Nations program on HIV/AIDS (Switzerland) – www.us.unaids
Un Rincon de Esperanza (Argentina) – www.fundamind.org.arc/sida/
Toronto People with AIDS Foundation Newsletter –
     www.connection.com/martyg/surfsup.htm

Social Contact

HIV Connection-—Personal Ads – www.mm.com/user/kennyg/hiv/
HIV Positive Heterosexual Dating Service –
    www.users.cts.com/king/l/lclark/hivweb/hivdates.html
Intropoz Magazine – www.intropoz.com/
The Lifeboat – www.thegrid.net/popeye/
Aids, Medicine, and Miracles – www.csd.net/amm/

Women and Children

Pediatric AIDS Foundation – www.pedaids.org/
Positively Kids – www.aidsinfonyc.org/posikids/index.html
Project Inform Women and HIV/AIDS – www.projinf.org/fs/women/html
Women and Children with HIV –
    www.hivpositive.com/f-women/wochildmenu.html
Women Alive – www.thebody.com/wa/waphee.html

Alternative Therapies

Alternative Medicine in AIDS – www.aids-info.com/medical/Alt.html
Alternative Medicine Digest –
    www.alternativemedicine.com/alternativemedicine/
Bastyr University – www.bastyr.edu/
DHEA Homepage – //gator.naples.net/ nfn03605/
Immune Enhancement Project – www.creative.net/ iep/index.html
Institute for Traditional Medicine – www.europa.com/itm/hiv.htm
Keep Hope Alive – www.execpc.com/keephope/keephope.html

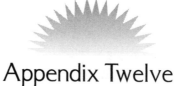

Appendix Twelve

References

This section lists reference materials used in compiling the following chapters. The sequence matches the flow of information in the text.

Chapter 4: Private Practice Data

Carpenter CCJ, et al. Antiretroviral therapy therapy for HIV infection 1997: Recommendations of an international panel. *JAMA* 1997; 277: 1962–69.

Feinberg M. Hidden dangers of incompletely suppressive antiretroviral therapy. *Lancet* 1997; 349: 1408–9.

Chapter 5: Antiviral Medications

Hammer SM, et. al. The AIDS Clinical Trials group study 175 study team. A trial comparing nucleoside monotherapy with combination therapy in HIV(+) adults with CD4 counts from 200–500 cells/mm3. *NEJM* 1996; 335: 1081–1090.

Cooley TP, et al. Once daily administration of DDI in patients with the Acquired Immunodeficiency Syndrome or AIDS-Related Complex. *NEJM* 1990; 322: 1340–45.

Faletto MB, et al. Unique intracellular activation of the potent anti-HIV virus agent 1592U89 *Antimicrobe Agents Chemother.* 1997; 41: 1099–1107.

Staszewski S, et al. Preliminary long term open label data from patients using abacavir (1592) containing antiviral treatment regiments. In: Abstracts of the 5th Conference on Retroviruses and Opportunistic Infections. Chicago, IL, Feb 1–5, 1998, Abstract no. 658, p. 203.

Montaner J, et al. A randomized, double blind trial comparing combinations of nevirapine, didanosine, and zidovudine for HIV-infected patients. *JAMA*: 1998; 279.

Hammer SM, et al. A placebo-controlled trial of indinavir in combination with two nucleoside analogs in HIV-infected persons with CD4 counts < 200 cells/mm3. In: Programs and Abstracts of the 8th Congress of Clinical Microbiology and Infectious Diseases; May 25–28, 1997; Lausanne, Switzerland. Abstract 90A.

Isaacs R, et al. 16 week follow-up of indinavir administered Q 8 hours vs. Q 12 hours in combination with efavirenz (MSD protocol 067). 12th World AIDS Conference; Jun 28, 1998; Geneva, Switzerland.

Fessel W, et al. A phase 3 double-blind placebo-controlled multicenter study to determine the effectiveness and tolerability of a combination of efavirenz and indinavir vs. indinavir in HIV-1 infected patients receiving nucleoside analog therapy at 24 weeks. 12th World AIDS Conference; Jun 28, 1998; Geneva, Switzerland.

Tashima KT, et al. Cerebrospinal fluid HIV-1 RNA levels and HIV-1 RNA levels and efavirenz concentrations in patients enrolled in clinical trials. 12th World AIDS Conference; Jun 28, 1998; Geneva, Switzerland.

Mayers D, et al. A double-blind placebo-controlled study to assess the safety tolerability and antiretroviral activity of efavirenz in combination with open label zidovudine (ZDV) and lamivudine (3TC) in HIV-1 infected patients. 12th World AIDS Conference; Jun 28, 1998; Geneva, Switzerland.

Kotler DP. *Clinical Care Options for HIV.* Healthcare Communications Group, 1998.

Yound CW, et al. Inhibition of DNA synthesis by hydroxyurea: structure-activity relationships. *Cancer Res* 1967; 27: 535–40.

Lori F, et al. Hydroxyurea as an inhibitor of human immunodeficiency virus-type 1 replication. *Science* 1994; 266: 801–5.

Lori F, et al. Long term suppression of HIV-1 by hydroxyurea and didanosine. *JAMA* 1997; 277(18): 1437–38.

Rutschmann OT, et al. A placebo-controlled trial of didanosine plus stavudine, with and without hydroxyurea for HIV infection. *AIDS* 1998; 12(8): 71–77.

Chapter 6: Clinical Treatment Scenarios

Carpenter CCJ, et al. Antiretroviral therapy therapy for HIV infection 1997: Recommendations of an International Panel. *JAMA* 1997; 277: 1962–69.

Feinberg M. Hidden dangers of incompletely suppressive antiretroviral therapy. *Lancet* 1997; 349: 1408–9.

Schacker TW, et al. HSV suppression is associated with a significant decrease in plasma levels of HIV RNA. 5th International Conference of Retroviruses and Opportunistic Infections, 1998. Abstract no. 260.

Chapter 7: Optimizing Intestinal Health

Haenel JH, et al. Progress in Food and Nutrition *Science* 1975; 1(1): 21–64.

Gorbach SL. *Review of Infectious Diseases* 1984; 6(1): 85–90.

Chung KT, et al. *J Nat Cancer Instit* 1975; 54(5): 1073–78.

Goldin BR. *Dietary Fat in Cancer* 1986: 655–85.

Hill MJ. *Microbial Metabolism in the Digestive Tract.* CRC Press, Inc.

Thorne GM. *Infect Dis Clin North Am* 1988; 2(3): 747–51.

Johnston TS. *Drug Intell Clin Pharm* 1981; 15(2): 103–10.

Chapter 8: Intestinal Parasites

Markell EK, et al. *Medical Parasitology* 1986. 6th ed.: 6–9.

Lee MG, et al. *Ann Rheum Dis* 1990; 49(3): 192–93.

Veraldi S, et al. *Int J Derm* 1991; 30: 376.

Corcoran GD, et al. *Lancet* 1991; 338: 254.

O'Gorman MA, et al. *Am J Gastroenterol* 1989; 84: 1192.

Radvin JL. *J Infect Dis* 1989; 159: 420–29.

The Medical Letter. Drugs for Parasitic Infections. Dec 1993; 35(911): 111.

Chapter 9: Body Cell Mass and the Immune System

Perelson A et al. HV-1 dynamics in vivo: Virion clearance rate, infected cell life span, and viral generation time. *Science* 271: 1582–85. Mar 15, 1996.

Chlebowski RT, et al. Nutritional status, gastrointestinal dysfunction, and survival in patients with AIDS. *Am J Gastroenterol* 1989; 84(10): 1288–93.

Kotler DP, et al. Magnitude of body cell mass depletion and the timing of death from wasting in AIDS. *Am J Clin Nutr* 1989; 50: 444–47.

Grunfeld C, et al. Metabolic disturbances and wasting in the Acquired Immunodeficiecy Syndrome. *NEJM* 1992; 327(5): 329–37.

Kotler DP, et al. Body composition studies in patients with the Acquired Immunodeficiency Syndrome. *Am J Clin Nutr* 1985; 42: 1255–65.

Grunfeld C. What causes wasting in AIDS? *NEJM* 1995 Jul 13; 333: 124–24.

Hellerstein M. Metabolic alterations in HIV infection: Clinical significance for the wasting syndrome. In: Miller T, Gorbach S, eds. *Nutritional Aspects of HIV Infection* (in press). Chapman and Hall, 1998.

Mooney M. Gorilla steroid anadrol returns to USA. *Metabolics: The Program for Wellness Restoration Newsletter* vol. 2, no. 2, Nov 1997.

Ishak K, et al. Hepatotoxic effects of the anabolic/androgenic steroids. *Seminars in Liver Disease* Thieme Medical Publishers, Inc., vol. 7 no. 3, 1987.

Fisher AE, et al. The effects of oxandrolone on body weight and composition in patients with HIV-associated weight loss (abstract). 12th World AIDS Conference, Geneva, Switzerland. Jun 1998. Abstract no. 42351.

Hengge U, et al. Oxymetholone promotes weight gain in patients with advanced human immunodeficiency virus infection. *Br J of Nutr* 1996; 75, 129–38.

Chapter 11: Hormonal Therapy

Schwartz FL, Miller RJ. Androgens and anabolic steroids. *Modern Pharmacology*, 2nd ed. Little, Brown & Company; 1982: 905–24.

Fox M, et al. Oxandrolone: A potent anabolic steroid. *J Clin Endocrin Metabol* 1962: 22: 921–24.

Pappo R, Jung CJ. 2-Oxasteroids: A new class of biologically active compounds. *Tetrahedron Letters*. 1962: 9: 65–371.

Schambelan M, et al. Recombinant humane growth hormone in patients with HIV-associated wasting: A randomized, placebo-controlled trial. *Ann Intern Med* 1996 Dec 1; 125: 873–82.

Berger DS, et al. A Phase III study of recombinant human growth hormone in patients with AIDS wasting (abstract). 11th International Conference on AIDS. 1996 Jul 7–12; 1: 26.

Berger JR, et al. Oxandrolone and AIDS-wasting myopathy. *AIDS*. 1996. 10: 1657–62.

Oxandrolone as a treatment for AIDS-related weight loss and wasting. IDSA Conference. 1996.

Yang JY, et al. Inhibition of 3' Azido-3'deoxythymidine-resistant HIV-1 infection by dehydroepiandrosterone in vitro. *Biochemical and Biophysical Research Communications* 201: 3. Jun 30, 1994.

Hasheeve D, et al. DHEA: A potential treatment for HIV disease. Houston Immunology Institute. International Conference on AIDS 1994, Aug 7–12; 10(1): 223 (Abstract number PB0322).

Dyner TS. An open label escalation trial of oral dehydroepiandrosterone tolerance and pharmacokinetics in patients with HIV disease. *Journal of Acquired Immune Deficiency Syndromes*, 1993 May; 6(5): 459–65.

Wisniewski TL, et al. The relationship of serum DHEA-S and cortisol levels to measures of immune function in human immunodeficiency-related illness. *American Journal of Medical Science*, Feb; 305(2): 79–83.

Henderson E, et al. Dehydroepiandrosterone(DHEA) and synthetic DHEA analogues are modest inhibitors of HIV-1 replication. *AIDS Res Hum Retroviruses*,1992 May; 8 (5): 625–31.

Mulder JW. Dehydroepiandrosterone as predictor for progression to AIDS in asymptomatic human immunodeficiency virus-infected men. *Journal of Infectious Diseases* 1992 Mar; 165(3): 413–18.

Jacobson MA, et al. Decreased serum dehydroepiandrosterone is associated with an increased progression of human immunodeficiency virus infection in men with CD4 cell counts of 200–499. *J of Infect Disease* 1991 Nov; 164(5): 864–68.

Chapter 12: Preventing and Treating Fatigue

Súllivan PS, et al. Epidemiology of Anemia in Human Immunodeficiency Virus-Infected Persons: Results From the Multistate Adult and Adolescent Spectrum of HIV Disease Surveillance Project. *Blood*, vol. 91, no. 1: 301–8, 1998.

Beck EJ, et al., *Int J STD AIDS*, May–Jun 1992.

Saah AJ, et al. *Am J Epidemiol*, May 1992.

Saah AJ, et al, Factors Influencing Survival After AIDS: Report from the Multicenter AUDS Cohort Study (MACS) *J AIDS*, 1994; 7: 287–95.

Swanson CE, et al. Factors Influencing Outcome of Treatment with Zidovidine in Patients with AIDS in Australia. *AIDS*, 1990; 4: 749–57.

Glascon P, et al. Immunologic Abnormalities in Patients Receiving Multiple Blood Transfusions. *Ann Intern Med*, 1984; 100: 173–77.

Chapter 14: Preventing and Treating Kaposi's Sarcoma

Rutherford GW, et al. The epidemiology of AIDS-related Kaposi's sarcoma in San Francisco. *J AIDS*; S4–S7, 1990.

Beral V, et al. Risk of Kaposi's sarcoma and sexual practices associated with faecal contact in homosexual and bisexual men with AIDS. *Lancet* 339: 632–39, 1992.

Chang Y, et al. Identification of herpesvirus-like DNA sequences in AIDS-associated Kaposi's sarcoma. *Science* 266: 1865–69, 1994.

Moore PS, et al. Detection of herpesvirus-like DNA sequences in Kaposi's Sarcoma in patients with and without HIV infection. *NEJM* 332: 1181–85, 1995.

Beral V, et al. Kaposi's Sarcoma among persons with AIDS: A sexually transmitted infection? *Lancet* 335: 123–28, 1990.

Peters BS, et al. Changing disease patterns in patients with AIDS in a referral center in the United Kingdom: The changing face of AIDS. *Br Med Journal* 302: 203–6, 1991.

Samaniego F, et al. Inflammatory cytokines increased in HIV-1-infected individuals stimulate AIDS-Kaposi's sarcoma (AIDS-KS) cell growth and this effect is blocked by antisense oligonucleotides against basic fibroblast growth factor (bFGF). Poster at the 1993 Annual Meeting of the Laboratory of Tumor Cell Biology, Bethesda, 1993.

Barillari G, et al. Effect of cytokines from activated immune cells on vascular call growth and HIV-1 gene expression. *J of Immunology* 149: 3727–34, 1992.

Borden EC, et al. Comparative antiproliferative activity in vitro of natural interferons alpha and betafor diploid and human cells. *Cancer Res* 42: 4948–53, 1982.

Ross M, Presentation at the Oncology Drug Advisory Committee Meeting to the Food and Drug Administration. Jun 8, 1995.

Northfelt DW, et al. Randomized comparative trial of Doxil vs. adriamycin, bleomycin and vincristine (ABV) in the treatment of severe AIDS-related Kaposi's sarcoma. American Society for Hematology, 1995.

Saville MW, et al. Treatment of HIV-associated Kaposi's sarcoma with paclitaxel. *Lancet* 346: 26–28, 1995.

Li CJ, et al. Inhibitors of HIV-1 transcription. *Trends Microbiol.* 2: 164, 1994.

D'Amato RJ, et al. Thalidomide is an inhibitor of angiogenesis. *PNAS* 91: 4082–85, 1994.

Pluda JM, et al. A phase I trial of an angiogenesis inhibitor, TNP-470 (AGM-1470) administered to patients with HIV-associated Kaposi's sarcoma (abstract). *Proc Am Soc Clin Oncol* 13: 51, 1994.

TeVelde AA, et al. Interleukin-4 (IL-4) inhibits secretion of IL-1b, tumor necrosis factor a and IL-6 by human monocytes. *Blood* 76: 1392–97, 1990.

Krown SE, et al. Kaposi's sarcoma: Medical management of AIDS patients. *Med Clin North Am* 76: 235–57, 1992.

Taperro JW, et al. Caution in the use of local therapies for Kaposi's sarcoma. (Letter). *Arch Dermatology* 129: 42, 1993.

Supapannachart N, et al. Isolation of human immunodeficiency virus type 1 in cutaneous blister fluid. *Arch Dermatology* 127: 1998–2000, 1991.

Taperro JW, et al. Kaposi's sarcoma: Epidemiology pathogenesis, histology, clinical spectrum, staging criteria and therapy. *J Am Acad Dermatol* 28: 371–95, 1993.

Lucatorto FM, et al. Treatment of oral Kaposi's sarcoma with a sclerosing agent in AIDS patients. A preliminary study. *Oral Surg Oral Med Oral Path* 75: 192–98, 1993.

Kahn JO, et al. Intralesional recombinant tumor necrosis factor alpha for AIDS-associated Kaposi's sarcoma: A randomized double-blind trial. *J AIDS*; 2: 217–23, 1989.

Taperro JW, et al. Pulsed-dye laser therapy for cutaneous Kaposi's sarcoma associated with acquired immunodeficiency syndrome. *J Am Acad Dermatol* 18: 297–300, 1992.

Nisce LZ, et al. Radiation therapy for Kaposi's sarcoma. *Infect Med* 10(3): 54–58, 1993.

Staddon, et al. A randomized dose finding study of recombinant platelet factor 4 (rPF4) in cutaneous AIDS-related Kaposi's sarcoma (KS). *Proc Am Soc Clin Onco* 13: 50, 1994.

Gill PS, et al. The effects of preparations of human chorionic gonadotropin on AIDS-related Kaposi's sarcoma. *NEJM* 335: 1261–69, 1996.

Chapter 15: Aggressive Natural Therapies

Lemp GF, et al. Survival trends for patients with AIDS. *JAMA* 263: 402–6, 1990.

National Research Council, Recommended Dietary Allowances, Washington, DC: National Academy of Sciences, 1974: 34.

Sanchez A, et al. Role of sugars in human neutrophilic phagocytosis. *Am J Clin Nutr* 26: 180, 1973.

Bernstein J, et al. Depression of lymphocyte transformation following oral glucose ingestion. *Am Clin Nutr* 30: 613, 1977.

Jacobsen BK and Hansen V. Caffeine and health (letter). *Brit Med J* 296: 291, 1988.

Riddick H. U.S. Dept. of Agriculture, personal conversation, May 1991.

National Food Consumption Survey, U.S. Department of Agriculture, Nutrition Monitoring Division, 1986.

Halsted CH, and Rucker RB. *Nutrition and the Origins of Disease.* Academic Press, 1989.

Werbach M. *Nutritional Influences on Illness,* Third Line Press, 1988.

Levy JA. *Nutrition and the Immune System, Basic and Clinical Immunology,* 4th ed. Lange Medical Publications, 1982, pp. 297–305.

Alexander M, et al. Oral beta carotene can increase the OKT4+ cells in human blood. *Immunol. Lett* 9: 221–24, 1985.

Watson RR (ed.). *Nutrition, Disease Resistance and Immune Function.* Marcel Dekker, 1984, pp. 345–54.

Cohen B, et al. Reversal of postoperative immunosuppression in man by Vitamin A. *Surg Gynecol Obstet* 149: 658–63, 1979.

Chandra RK. Nutrition and immunity: basic considerations, Part 1. *Contemp Nutr* 11: 1986.

Nuwayri-Salti N, Murad T. Immunologic and anti-immunosuppressive effects of Vitamin A. *Pharmacol* 30: 181–87, 1985.

Castleman M. *Cold Cures.* Fawcett, 1987.

Harakeh S, Jariwalla R, Pauling L. Suppression of human immunodeficiency virus replication by ascorbate in chronically and acutely infected cells. *Proc Natl Acad Sci* USA, 87: 7245–49, 1990.

Meydani S, et al. Vitamin E supplementation enhances cell-mediated immunity in healthy elderly subjects. *Am J Clin Nutr* 52: 557–63, 1990.

Prasad JS. Effect of Vitamin E supplementation of leukocyte function. *Am J Clin Nutr* 33: 606–8, 1980.

Beisel WR, et al. Single nutrient effects on immunologic functions. *JAMA* 245: 53–58, 1981.

Lim TS, et al. Effect of Vitamin E on cell-mediated immune responses and serum corticosteroids in young and maturing mice. *Immunol* 44: 289, 1981.

The effect of vitamin E on immune responses, *Nutr Rev* 45: 27–29, 1987.

Beisel WR. Single nutrients and immunity. *Am J Clin Nutr* 1982; 35: 417–68.

Chandra RK. *Nutrition, Immunity and Infection: Mechanisms of Interactions.* Plenum Publishing, 1977.

Baum MK, et al. Association of vitamin B6 status with parameters of immune function in early HIV-1 infections. *J AIDS* 1991; 4: 1122–32.

Baum MK, et al. Toxic levels of dietary supplementation in HIV-1 infected patients. *Arch AIDS Res* 1990; 4: 149–57.

Cheslock KE, et al. Response of human beings to a low vitamin B6 diet. *J Nutr* 1960; 70: 507–13.

Folkers K, et al. Evidence for deficiency of coenzyme Q10 in human heart disease. *Int J Vit Nut Research* 40: 380–90, 1970.

Hashiba K, et al. *Shinzo* 4: 12: 1579–89, 1972.

Iwabuchi T, et al. *Rinsho To Kenkyu* 49: 9: 2604–8, 1972.

Langsjoen PH, et al. Effective treatment with coenzyme Q10 of patients with chronic myocardial disease. *Drug Exp Clin Res* 8: 577, 1985.

Bliznakov E, et al. Coenzymes Q: Stimulants of the phagocytic activity in rats and immune response in mice. *Experentia* 26: 953–54, 1970.

Bliznakov E. Restoration of impaired immune functions in aged mice by coenzyme Q. Proceedings of the 4th International Congress of Immunology, Paris, France, Jul 21–26, 1980.

Herzenberg, LA, et al. Glutathione deficiency as associated with impaired survival in HIV disease. *Proc Nato Acad Sci USA* vol. 94, pp. 1967–72, Mar 1997.

Buhl R, et al. Systemic glutathione deficieny in symptom-free HIV seropositive individuals. *Lancet,* 1294–98, Dec 1989.

Baruchel S, et al. The role of oxidative stress and disease progression in individuals infected by the human immunodeficiency virus. *Journal of Leukocyte Biology* vol. 52, pp 111–14, Jul 1992.

Witschi A, et al. The systemic availability of oral glutathione *Eur Jour Clin Pharm* vol. 43; 667–69, 1992.

Mowrey DB. *The Scientific Validation of Herbal Medicine.* Cormorant Books, 1986.

Tierra M. *The Way of Herbs.* Washington Square Press, 1983.

Green J. *The Male Herbal.* Crossing Press, 1991.

Tragni E, et al. Evidence from two classic irritation tests for an anti-inflammatory action of a natural extract, Echinacina B. *Food Chem Toxicol* 23: 317–19, 1985.

Wacker A, Hilbig A. Virus inhibition by Echinacea purpurea. *Planta Medica* 33: 89–102, 1978.

Kulkarni SK, et al. Pharmacological investigations of berberine sulphate. *Jap J Pharmacol* 22: 11–16, 1972.

Dutta NK, Panse MV. Usefulness of berberine in the treatment of cholera. *Ind J Med Res* 50: 732–36, 1962.

Lahiri SC, Dutta NK. Berberine and chloramphenicol in the treatment of cholera and severe diarrhea. *J Ind Med Assn* 48: 1–11, 1967.

Waller CW, Gisvold O. A phytochemical investigation of *Larrea Divaricata* (American Chaparral). *J Am Pharmacol Assn* 34: 78–81, 1945.

Hunan Medical College. Garlic in crypotococcal meningitis. A preliminary report of 21 cases. *Chinese Med. J* 93: 123–26, 1980.

Dharmananda S. Chinese herbal therapies for the treatment of immunodeficiency syndromes. *Oriental Healing Arts Intl Bull* 12: 24–38, 1987.

Young M. Chinese herbal therapies and HIV infection: A clinical report. Reprints available from the Institute for Traditional Medicine. Portland, OR (503-233–4907).

Chu D, Wong W, Mavligit G. Immunotherapy with Chinese medicinal herbs. Immune restoration of local xenogenic graft-versus-host reaction in cancer patients by fractionated astragalus membraneceus in vitro. *J Clin Lab Immunol* 25: 119–23, 1988.

Chu D, Wong W, Mavligit G. Immunotherapy with Chinese medicinal herbs. Reversal of cyclophosphamide-induced immune suppression by administration of fractionated astragalus membranaceus in vivo. *J Clin Lab Immunol* 25: 125–29, 1988.

Chu D, Wong, W, LaPushin R, Mavligit G. Fractionated extract of astragalus membranaceus, a Chinese medicinal herb, potentiates LAK cell cytotoxicity generated by a low dose of recombinant interleukin-2. *J Clin Lab Immunol* 26: 183–87, 1988.

Zhao KS, et al. Enhancement of the immune response in mice by astragalus membranaceus extracts. *Immunopharmacol* 20: 225–34, 1990.

LaPerriere AR, et al. Exercise intervention attenuates emotional distress and natural killer cell decrements following notification of positive serologic status for HIV-1. *Biofeedback Self Regulation* 15: 229–42, 1990.

Kusnecov AV, et al. Decreased herpes simplex viral immunity and enhanced pathogenesis following stressor administration in mice. *J Neuroimmunol* 38: 129–37, 1992.

Glaser R, et al. Stress induced modulation of the immune response to recombinant hepatitis B vaccine. *Psychosom Med* 54: 22–29, 1992.

Bonneau R, et al. Stress-induced suppression of herpes simplex virus (HSV)-specific cytotoxic T lymphocyte and natural killer cell activity and enhancement of acute pathogenesis following local HSV infection. *Brain, Behavior and Immunity* 5: 170–92, 1991.

Appendix References

Todd J, et al. Quantitation of Human Immunodefiency Virus plasma RNA by branched-DNA and reverse transcription coupled polymerase chain reaction assay methods: A critical evaluation of accuracy and reproducibility. *Serodiagn Immunother Infect Dias* 1994; 6: 233–39.

Volberding PA. Treatment Dilemmas in HIV Infection. *Hosp Pract* 1994; 29: 49–60.

Mellors JW, et al. Quantitation of HIV-1 RNA in plasma predicts outcome after seroconversion. *Ann Intern Med* 1995; 122: 573–79.

Cao Y, et al. Clinical evaluation of branch DNA signal amplification for quantifying HIV type 1 in human plasma. *AIDS Research and Human Retroviruses* 1995; 1: 353–61.

Dewar RL, et al. Application of branch DNA signal amplification to monitor human immunodeficiency virus type 1 burden in human plasma. *J Infect Dis* 1994; 170: 1172–79.

Mellors J, et al. Antiretroviral effects of therapy combining abacavir (1592) with HIV protease inhibitors. In: Abstracts of the 5th Conference on Retroviruses and Opportunistic Infections. Chicago, IL, Feb 1–5, 1998, Abstract no. 4, p 79.

Bart PA,et al. Combination 1592/141W94 therapy in HIV-1-infected antiretroviral naive subjects with CD4 counts greater than 400 cells/mm3 and viral loads greater than 5000 copies/ml. In: Abstracts of the 5th Conference on Retroviruses and Opportunistic Infections. Chicago, IL, Feb 1–5, 1998, Abstract no. 365, p 147.

Eron J, et al. Preliminary assessment of 141W94 in combination with other protease inhibitors. In: Abstracts of the 5th Conference on Retroviruses and Opportunistic Infections. Chicago, IL, Feb 1–5, 1998, Abstract no. 6, p. 80.

Index

Figures and charts are listed in bold.